Preventing Medical Emergencies

Use of the Medical History in Dental Practice

Preventing Medical Emergencies

Use of the Medical History in Dental Practice

THIRD EDITION

Frieda Atherton Pickett, RDH, MS
Adjunct Associate Professor, Graduate Division
Department of Dental Hygiene
Idaho State University
Pocatello, Idaho

JoAnn R. Gurenlian, RDH, PhD
Professor and Graduate Program Director
Division of Health Sciences
Department of Dental Hygiene
Idaho State University
Pocatello, Idaho

Wolters Kluwer

Philadelphia • Baltimore • New York • London
Buenos Aires • Hong Kong • Sydney • Tokyo

Acquisitions Editor: Jonathan Joyce
Product Development Editor: Paula Williams
Marketing Manager: Shauna Kelley
Production Project Manager: Alicia Jackson
Manufacturing Coordinator: Margie Orzech-Zeranko
Design Coordinator: Teresa Mallon
Compositor: Integra Software Services Pvt. Ltd.

351 West Camden Street
Baltimore, MD 21201

Two Commerce Square
2001 Market Street
Philadelphia, PA 19103

Printed in China

Library of Congress Cataloging-in-Publication Data

Pickett, Frieda Atherton, author.
Preventing medical emergencies: use of the medical history / Frieda Atherton Pickett, JoAnn R. Gurenlian. — Third edition.
p. ; cm.
Includes bibliographical references and index.
ISBN 978-1-4511-9418-0
I. Gurenlian, JoAnn R., author. II. Title.
[DNLM: 1. Dental Offices—Examination Questions. 2. Emergencies—Examination Questions. 3. Iatrogenic Disease—prevention & control—Examination Questions. 4. Medical History Taking—Examination Questions. WU 18.2]
RK308.3
617.6'0751—dc23

2014012813

To purchase additional copies of this book, call our customer service department at (800) 638-3030 or fax orders to (301) 824-7390. International customers should call (301) 714-2324.

Visit Lippincott Williams & Wilkins on the Internet: http://www.LWW.com. Lippincott Williams & Wilkins customer service representatives are available from 8:30 am to 6:00 pm, EST.

10 9 8 7 6 5 4

CCS1018

Preface

Taking and reviewing the medical history is considered to be the most effective strategy to prevent a medical emergency in dental practice settings. The oral healthcare practitioner determines modifications for treatment and potential risks during treatment as each response is considered on the health history. As the health history is used by all professionals in dental practice settings, it should be the focus of instructional materials for identifying potential risks during treatment. ***Preventing Medical Emergencies: Use of the Medical History in Dental Practice, Third Edition,* is the only textbook to discuss each component on a comprehensive health history that identifies clinical implications and risks for an emergency situation**. It is written as a reflection of the critical thinking process that occurs when gathering health history information and is designed to be used as a reference during the health history review. Significant features of the text include the following:

- Listing of relevant follow-up questions to gain necessary historical information for those situations that require additional information.
- Discussion of each medical condition in terms of the pathophysiology, the clinical implications for the treatment plan, and potential medical emergencies. The third edition includes a detailed discussion of clinical management for the patient with special needs.
- Strategies for preventing potential emergency situations, followed by management procedures to follow should an emergency occur.

Because prevention of medical emergencies is strongly related to taking and analyzing a comprehensive medical or health history, a Health History Form is used as a guideline. The Health History Form is comprehensive; it contains questions related to the most significant medical information needed before providing oral health care or dental treatment, and it reflects information necessary to identify potential emergency situations.

The text is written to accommodate a 15-week self-study format. It can be used as a supplement to clinical instruction textbooks during preclinical education, and it can also be used as a stand-alone textbook for courses dealing with dental office medical emergencies. Information provided in clinical texts will not be repeated unless required to explain points made in the text. As most semesters are 15 weeks long, this text is designed to be assigned to students for weekly study during the preclinical education period. At the end of the preclinical semester, the text will have been completed. As students begin providing clinical treatment during the following semester, the text can be used as a reference during the medical history review. Some discussion of information in the text may be included as a weekly supplement to the preclinical technique laboratory course. If used in this manner, assignment of the reading could be made as a didactic preparation for the preclinical laboratory course. The self-study format will assist the course instructor in reducing the class time necessary to explain significant information contained in the text.

The text is written to follow a logical section on a Health History Form and identifies clinical implications for potential emergencies related to specific items on the form. The text follows the same critical thinking process that occurs when a practitioner analyzes questions on the health history. For example, stress-related medical emergencies are among the most frequent emergency situations to occur during oral healthcare procedures and are most likely to occur in the client who has experienced them in the past. For this reason, they are discussed with the question on the Health History Form that deals with experiencing problems during past dental treatment. Another common emergency during oral healthcare procedures is postural hypotension. Because it most commonly occurs as a result of a side effect from various medications, it is discussed in the section on medications being taken by the client. Emergency situations that might be experienced in the client with diabetes are discussed in the medical section dealing with diabetes; potential emergencies during oral healthcare procedures for the pregnant client are discussed as part of the questions related to pregnancy. Appropriate follow-up questions for relevant conditions are included along with brief explanations of the relevance to clinical modifications and risks for a possible medical emergency during oral healthcare procedures.

The latter part of the Health History Form includes a variety of medical conditions and symptoms related to medical conditions.

NEW TO THIS EDITION: A new section added in the third edition is management of patients with special needs. In addition, several national guidelines were updated between 2011 and 2014. New guidelines for antibiotic prophylaxis for the client with a prosthetic joint were released, updated guidelines for the prevention of mucositis in cancer therapy became available and JNC8 guidelines for blood pressure evaluation, including changes in blood pressure levels in diabetes were released. Video presentations of management procedures for the most common medical emergencies will be placed on The Point site. Information contained in the POINT site is expanded, and Web site information has been moved to this site to accommodate for URL changes that occur. The authors have attempted to organize the medical conditions according to system relationships for the individual chapters in the text. For example, all of the conditions listed in the medical condition section that deals with being immunocompromised are discussed together. Each medical condition includes a discussion of pathophysiology, appropriate follow-up questions related to treatment risks, clinical implications, potential emergencies, and prevention and management of the emergency.

Each chapter includes self-study questions that review significant information. These questions are designed to parallel item types that appear in the National Dental Hygiene Board Examination (NDHBE). Readers should attempt to answer each item as they proceed through the chapter. Correct responses are found at the end of each chapter with the appropriate page noted to provide a resource for the correct response. At the end of each chapter, the reader will find case studies and a group of related case-based questions. Completing these questions will reinforce key points and strengthen the understanding of the application of information presented in the text and reflect case-based questions on the NDHBE. When using *Preventing Medical Emergencies: Use of the Medical History in Dental Practice, 3rd Edition*, if issues arise that are not discussed in the text, the course instructor should notify the publisher so subsequent editions can include appropriate information.

It is hoped that this focused format will assist students and practitioners in effective use of the health history interview to identify potential risks in treatment as part of a thorough health history review. In addition, the text can be used as a tool to calibrate clinical faculty to assure that faculty members are guiding students to gain the same information during the health history review.

Additional Resources

Preventing Medical Emergencies: Use of the Medical History in Dental Practice, 3rd edition, includes additional resources for both instructors and students that are available on the book's companion Web site at http://thePoint.lww.com.

Instructor Resources

Approved adopting instructors will be given access to the following additional resources:

- PowerPoint Presentations
- Image Bank

Student Resources

Students who have purchased *Preventing Medical Emergencies: Use of the Medical History in Dental Practice, 3rd edition*, have access to the following additional resources:

- Summary Case Studies
- Interactive Quiz Bank
- Videos
- Image Bank

Purchasers of the text can access the resources online at the *Preventing Medical Emergencies: Use of the Medical History in Dental Practice, 3rd edition*, Web site at HYPERLINK "http://thePoint.lww.com/Engelkirk10e" http://thePoint.lww.com. See the inside front cover of this text for more details, including the passcode you will need to gain access to the Web site.

Acknowledgments

I would like to acknowledge those who participated in the generation of the concept for this book and those who reviewed materials and made important recommendations to ensure *Preventing Medical Emergencies: Use of the Medical History in Dental Practice, 3rd Edition* would meet the needs of oral healthcare practitioners.

To Linda Meeuwenberg, RDH, MA, MA, former Professor of Dental Hygiene, Ferris State University, goes my gratitude for encouraging JoAnn and me to prepare a reference text that reviews the health history.

To Ruth Tornwall, RDH, MS, Instructor IV of the Lamar Institute of Technology Dental Hygiene Program and Kathleen B. Muzzin, RDH, MS, Clinical Associate Professor at Caruth School of Dental Hygiene, Baylor College of Dentistry, Texas A&M University Health Science Center, thank you for the in-depth review of chapter information accuracy and clinical relevance.

To Cynthia A. Stegeman, RDH, M ED, RD, CDA, Associate Professor, Dental Hygiene Program, University of Cincinnati, for reviewing the sections on diabetes and eating disorders and providing recommendations.

Finally, sincere thanks to my coauthor, JoAnn Gurenlian, RDH, PhD, without whose constant encouragement and support, this project would not have gone forward.

Frieda A. Pickett, RDH, MS

Like Frieda, I would like to acknowledge key colleagues for their support during the preparation of this self-study textbook.

To Linda Meeuwenberg, RDH, MA, MA, for bringing Frieda and me together at a continuing education program and suggesting that we collaborate on this endeavor. Your words of encouragement turned into a reality, and we are now on this third edition.

To my family, Tom, Laura and Adam, and T.J., who encouraged me to keep writing. Thank you for understanding what this project meant to me.

Especially, to Frieda Pickett, RDH, MS, my coauthor, for keeping an open mind about making this a self-study text and for being the driving force throughout this publication. Frieda deserves the credit for the content herein.

JoAnn R. Gurenlian, RDH, PhD

Contents

Chapter One

Using the Medical History to Prevent Emergencies: Risk Assessment

Objectives

After completing the self-study chapter the reader will be able to:

- Describe strategies for gaining complete medical history information.
- Use medical history information and functional capacity level to identify risks for medical emergencies during oral health treatment.
- Identify normal limits of vital sign measurements and their relevance in assessing potential medical risks during dental treatment.
- Apply the American Dental Association's policy on screening for hypertension in the dental office to planning oral health care.

Key Terms

Atrial tachycardia: rapid heart rate ≥150 beats per minute (bpm)

Bradycardia: a heart rate less than 60 bpm, with normal electrocardiogram (ECG)

Bronchodilator: an inhaler device that delivers medication to dilate bronchioles and allows increased airflow to lungs; commonly prescribed for asthma

Client: the person seeking oral healthcare treatment

Clinician: the dental professional providing oral healthcare treatment

Continuing care: appropriately timed maintenance care

Diastolic blood pressure: the pressure in arteries when the heart rests, or between beats

Electrocardiogram (ECG): primary test used to identify and diagnose arrhythmia

Functional capacity: the ability to complete various physical activities, a measure used in cardiac risk assessment

Hypertension: blood pressure measurements of 140/90 mm Hg or higher

Metabolic equivalents (METs): a measurement of the ability to perform common daily tasks

Positive Responses: response on the medical history for which the client indicates "yes"

Reappointment: appointments after initial oral healthcare treatment in which treatment could not be completed in one appointment

Systolic blood pressure: the pressure in arteries during ventricular contraction, or when the heart beats

Tachyarrhythmia: a fast, irregular heart rate, usually over 150 bpm

Tachycardia: a heart rate in excess of 100 bpm with normal ECG

MEDICAL CONDITION

INTRODUCTION

This chapter will discuss the role of the medical history information (also called health history) and the analysis and interpretation of **functional capacity** and vital signs in identifying the **client** at risk for experiencing a medical emergency during oral procedures. Risk management includes measures to detect, evaluate, prevent, and control untoward situations. It often involves strategies to reduce financial loss due to claims of negligence associated with malpractice lawsuits. When a dental hygienist or any healthcare professional fails to provide reasonable care and that failure results in injury to the client, a malpractice claim may be the result. Essentially, risk management in oral health care is the practice of collecting and interpreting available information for the safety and success of providing oral care. Managing risk can be as simple as maintaining proper patient records and documentation, communication of risks to the client, and following procedures that the reasonable practitioner would complete, related to providing safe treatment.

ROLE OF THE MEDICAL HISTORY IN PREVENTION OF EMERGENCIES

The taking and reviewing of an adequate medical history is the best strategy to follow for preventing medical emergencies in dental practice settings.

Unanticipated emergencies (such as choking, emergencies related to fear of treatment, or unknown disease conditions) can occur; however, many emergencies in clinical practice settings can be predicted if adequate information is gathered from the client on the medical history and properly followed up in the subsequent review. For this reason, *it is essential that all questions be answered on the history form.*

Clients may leave a question unanswered because of misunderstanding the question. Other reasons for unanswered items may involve a feeling that the question is an invasion of privacy, or result from inadvertently skipping a question. Follow-up questioning can often resolve these issues. The medical history should be dated and signed to document the client's verification of accurate information. For minors, the parent or guardian would provide medical information and date/sign to document participation and give permission to treat the minor.

Methods to gain medical history information include the interview method and the questionnaire method. Clinical textbooks contain a variety of advantages and disadvantages for whatever method is selected to gain medical history information. This text will focus on specific questions needed to gain essential historical information, no matter what method is used.

RISK ASSESSMENT

The key to successful management of the client who presents for oral care is a thorough evaluation and assessment of potential risks to determine whether a patient can safely tolerate planned procedures. This includes a thorough investigation of the nature and severity of the client's medical status, determination of the physical tolerance for procedures (also referred to as functional capacity), the emotional status of the client, and the type and duration of the procedure planned.

Four general guidelines pertain to acquiring information with the medical history (Box 1-1). These include:

1. Making sure all questions have been answered.
2. Following up all positive responses with further questioning, and recording a concise summary of the additional information on the history form.
3. Observing the client for signs of stress and coordinate signs with vital sign values.
4. Updating the medical information to ensure current, accurate status of health.

Whether the medical history is completed by the client or by the **clinician** during the interview, the clinician must focus on those responses that

Table 1.1	Energy Requirements for Activities and Metabolic Equivalents (METs)
1 MET	Eat, dress oneself, use toilet Walk indoors around house Walk a block on level ground at 2–3 mph
4–9 METs	Light housework, dusting, washing dishes Climb a flight of stairs carrying groceries Walk at 4 mph on treadmill Run a short distance Heavy housework, scrub floors, move furniture Participate in moderate activities like golf, bowling, dancing, doubles tennis
10 METs	Participate in strenuous activities, singles tennis, football, skiing, etc.

(Adapted from Fleisher et al. ACC/AHA 2007 Perioperative Guidelines. Circulation 2007.)[2]

Box 1-1

Criteria for Reviewing the Medical History

- Ensure that all questions have been answered
- All positive responses should be followed up with questions related to history and control of disease, and a concise summary of responses should be recorded
- Observe client for signs of stress and coordinate with vital sign values
- Update health information to reflect the current medical status

indicate a loss of health has occurred. Generally, those are questions answered with a "yes" response. Questions worded in the format "Are you in good health?" would be exceptions to this rule. As each disease is discussed in later chapters, questioning related to anticipating potential emergencies will be identified. Fear and anxiety frequently precipitate medical emergencies in the dental office. These are often referred to as stress-related emergencies. Because stress-related emergencies are common in dental treatment, the clinician must be very observant for signs of stress in the client. Chapter 2 will discuss the most common stress-related emergencies and their relationship to fear of dentally related treatment. It is essential to have accurate information regarding the client's health status and medical condition in order to make proper judgments on how to proceed with care. This requires a regular update of information at each appointment for oral care.

FUNCTIONAL CAPACITY

Following the gathering of complete medical history information, additional clinical data (vital signs, level of functional capacity, extraoral examination) are needed to determine whether the client can safely withstand oral procedures. A method for the determination of cardiac risk has been described by the American College of Cardiology and the American Heart Association (ACC/AHA).[1] It is based on the client's ability to perform basic daily activities and is described as "functional capacity." Adequate functional capacity is defined as being able to perform activities that meet a 4 metabolic level of endurance or 4 METs. Table 1.1 includes activities for various MET levels. A MET is a unit of oxygen consumption needed for physical activity. This unit of measurement must be added to the vocabulary of healthcare providers. Identifying the level of physical activity (as expressed in METs) provides a means of quantifying the client's general physical status. The ACC/AHA has proposed that the risk for occurrence of a serious cardiac event (myocardial infarction [MI], heart failure) is increased when the client is unable to meet a 4 MET demand during normal daily activity. Questioning should include "Can you walk on the treadmill at 4 mph? Can you climb a flight of stairs carrying groceries? Can you run a short distance?" If the answers are "yes", one can conclude that the client meets the minimum 4 MET level of endurance and has a low risk for a cardiac emergency. On the other hand, the client who cannot walk up a flight of stairs without shortness of breath, fatigue, chest tightness, or pain is at increased risk for cardiac problems during oral procedures.

American Society of Anesthesiologists Risk Categories

The American Society of Anesthesiologists (ASA) developed a risk classification system to estimate the medical risks in treatment associated with anesthesia for a surgical procedure. Since the initial development, the classification system has been used to estimate risks in treatment even when anesthesia is not planned. The classification system is described as ASA I through ASA V and is detailed below.[2]

ASA I: Healthy client without systemic disease
ASA II: Client with mild systemic disease that does not interfere with daily activity; or a healthy client with significant risk factors
ASA III: Client with moderate to severe systemic disease that limits activity but is not incapacitating
ASA IV: Client with an incapacitating systemic disease that is a constant threat to life
ASA V: Client not expected to survive 24 hours with or without an operation
ASA E: Emergency operation of any variety, with E preceding the number to indicate the client's physical status (e.g., ASA E-III)

Clients requesting oral health care would be placed in classifications I through IV. The practical use of this system is limited as it does not include specific information about treatment modifications.[3] General treatment decisions for oral health care are as follows:

ASA I

Clients should be able to tolerate oral healthcare procedures with no added risk of serious complications. They should have adequate functional capacity or physical endurance and be able to walk up a flight of stairs without distress, shortness of breath, undue fatigue, or chest pain. Treatment modification is usually not required for these clients.

ASA II

This classification includes the client with mild disease that does not interfere with daily physical activities, or one who is healthy, but has significant risk factors (e.g., smoking, obesity, substance abuse), or one who is very fearful or anxious about receiving oral healthcare treatment. These clients are less able to tolerate stressful situations; however, they represent minimal risks during treatment. Routine treatment is allowed with consideration given to the influence of the specific problem on oral procedures. For example, anti-anxiety drugs may be given to the anxious client, epinephrine doses in local anesthesia may be limited when cardiovascular disease exists, and appointments may be of short duration. The ASA II classification means to proceed with caution.

ASA III

This classification is applied to the client with severe systemic disease that limits activity but is not incapacitating. When rested, the ASA III client shows no signs of distress, but when physiologic or psychological stressful situations occur the client may tolerate them poorly. Elective oral procedures are not contraindicated, but the clinician should proceed with great caution because the risk during treatment is increased. An example of this category may include the client who has suffered a recent heart attack and has regained adequate functional capacity. Although this client may be able to respond to the increased cardiac demands during oral procedures and the risk for a cardiovascular emergency is low, the client may need short appointments, a stress reduction protocol, low concentrations of epinephrine, and adequate pain control procedures to prevent excessive cardiac stress.

ASA IV

Clients in this category have a medical condition that incapacitates them and is a threat to their lives. Whenever possible, elective treatment should be postponed until the condition has improved and the client has moved into the ASA III category. These clients have low functional capacity and cannot meet a 4 MET level of endurance, cannot walk up one flight of stairs, and cannot run a short distance or walk two city blocks without stopping. They feel stress even when rested. They exhibit signs and symptoms of their medical condition when at rest. When a dental emergency occurs, the dentist should consider providing oral care at an acute care facility (such as a hospital) where emergency response equipment is available. For some conditions, there is a high risk for serious consequences or death during the time following the event. For example, the ACC National Database Library defines recent MI as more than 7 days but less than or equal to 1 month.[1] This is a dangerous time for reinfarction. An example of a client in this category is one who has had a heart attack within the past 4 weeks or a stroke within the past 6 months.[1,3]

The ASA classification system is helpful in determining the treatment risks with various medical conditions. It relies on the ability of the practitioner to assess the relevant medical situation accurately. ASA I, II, and III conditions can receive both elective and emergency treatments if the practitioner makes plans to reduce the risks associated with the specific medical condition.

FOLLOW-UP QUESTIONS: WHAT, WHEN, WHY?

When a question such as "Do your gums bleed when you brush?" is answered "yes," it signals the clinician to pursue further information. Following the format "When, what, why, how resolved" is a good plan for most positive responses. Questions should be worded in an "open-ended" style, requiring the client to answer with an explanation rather than simply "yes" or "no." An example is "Why do you think your gums bleed?" This provides the clinician with more information related to the specific issue being investigated, the client's understanding of causative factors, and helps to direct the oral care plan.

As the reader continues this self-study, examples of appropriate follow-up questions will be provided. A discussion of the reasons for asking the follow-up question will be included, and required actions based on the client's answers will be identified. In some cases, the questions in the first section of the American Dental Association (ADA) health history are specific and require no follow-up questioning. These medical history items will have a concise discussion of clinical implications for a positive response. This text is not intended to replace a clinical textbook, and *the reader should refer to clinical textbooks for rationale and technique issues.* However, it seems logical to include the clinical implications when the medical history question requires consideration of any treatment plan modification. In the last section of the self-study (Chapters 9–14) that specifies diseases experienced by the client, the discussion will include:

1. The pathophysiology of the disease.
2. The potential risks for a medical emergency as a result of the disease.
3. The clinical management for the client with the disease.
4. Strategies for resolving the potential medical risks and preventing an emergency situation. For conditions which result in a medical emergency during oral healthcare treatment, a protocol for managing the specific emergency will be included.

THE AMERICAN DENTAL ASSOCIATION HEALTH HISTORY FORM

The 2007 ADA Health History Form is illustrated in this chapter as Figure 1.1. This two-page form includes most conditions of concern before oral treatment. As dental practice settings become more automated, it is anticipated that this medical history form will be entered into the office computer system. In that way, the form can be tailored to meet the needs of the client population of the practice. For example, the current ADA Health History Form does not include a section for recording vital sign values. Adding this physical assessment information would make a more reliable document to assess and document client's health.

SIGNIFICANCE OF VITAL SIGNS IN DETERMINING THE RISK FOR AN EMERGENCY

Generally, in dental practice settings, vital signs that need to be measured include a combination of one or more of the following: blood pressure (BP), pulse, respiration, temperature, height, and weight.

Measurement of Blood Pressure

BP can be simply described as the pressure in the arteries exerted by the circulating volume of blood. It is affected by the volume of blood, the size and elasticity of the arteries, and the force of the cardiac contraction. The measurement is illustrated as 120/80 mm Hg (millimeters of mercury). BP is more accurate if taken when the client has rested, and has not smoked or had caffeine within the past 30 minutes.[4] The area of the arm used should be at the level of the heart. The appropriate cuff size should be used. The client is seated with legs uncrossed, feet on the floor. An upright position promotes this arrangement. Either arm can be used, but measurements will vary from one arm to another. For this reason, the client's position and the arm used are usually noted when the values are recorded so that the same arm is used for subsequent measurements. This is illustrated in question 6 of the self-study questions. The BP is a significant piece of information in assessing the client's physical health. For example, elevated BP is associated with potential cardiovascular

Health History Form

ADA®
American Dental Association
www.ada.org

E-mail: Today's Date:

As required by law, our office adheres to written policies and procedures to protect the privacy of information about you that we create, receive or maintain. Your answers are for our records only and will be kept confidential subject to applicable laws. Please note that you will be asked some questions about your responses to this questionnaire and there may be additional questions concerning your health. This information is vital to allow us to provide appropriate care for you. This office does not use this information to discriminate.

Name: (Last / First / Middle) Home Phone: *Include area code* ( ) Business/Cell Phone: *Include area code* ( )

Address: (Mailing address) City: State: Zip:

Occupation: Height: Weight: Date of birth: Sex: M F

SS# or Patient ID: Emergency Contact: Relationship: Home Phone: ( ) Cell Phone: ( ) *Include area codes*

If you are completing this form for another person, what is your relationship to that person?

Your Name Relationship

Do you have any of the following diseases or problems: *(Check DK if you Don't Know the answer to the question)*	Yes	No	DK
Active Tuberculosis	☐	☐	☐
Persistent cough greater than a 3 week duration	☐	☐	☐
Cough that produces blood	☐	☐	☐
Been exposed to anyone with tuberculosis	☐	☐	☐

If you answer yes to any of the 4 items above, please stop and return this form to the receptionist.

Dental Information *For the following questions, please mark (X) your responses to the following questions.*

	Yes	No	DK
Do your gums bleed when you brush or floss?	☐	☐	☐
Are your teeth sensitive to cold, hot, sweets or pressure?	☐	☐	☐
Does food or floss catch between your teeth?	☐	☐	☐
Is your mouth dry?	☐	☐	☐
Have you had any periodontal (gum) treatments?	☐	☐	☐
Have you ever had orthodontic (braces) treatment?	☐	☐	☐
Have you had any problems associated with previous dental treatment?	☐	☐	☐
Is your home water supply fluoridated?	☐	☐	☐
Do you drink bottled or filtered water?	☐	☐	☐
If yes, how often? Circle one: DAILY / WEEKLY / OCCASIONALLY			
Are you currently experiencing dental pain or discomfort?	☐	☐	☐

What is the reason for your dental visit today?

How do you feel about your smile?

	Yes	No	DK
Do you have earaches or neck pains?	☐	☐	☐
Do you have any clicking, popping or discomfort in the jaw?	☐	☐	☐
Do you brux or grind your teeth?	☐	☐	☐
Do you have sores or ulcers in your mouth?	☐	☐	☐
Do you wear dentures or partials?	☐	☐	☐
Do you participate in active recreational activities?	☐	☐	☐
Have you ever had a serious injury to your head or mouth?	☐	☐	☐

Date of your last dental exam:

What was done at that time?

Date of last dental x-rays:

Medical Information *Please mark (X) your response to indicate if you have or have not had any of the following diseases or problems.*

	Yes	No	DK
Are you now under the care of a physician?	☐	☐	☐

Physician Name: Phone: *Include area code* ( )

Address/City/State/Zip:

	Yes	No	DK
Are you in good health?	☐	☐	☐
Has there been any change in your general health within the past year?	☐	☐	☐

If yes, what condition is being treated?

Date of last physical exam:

	Yes	No	DK
Have you had a serious illness, operation or been hospitalized in the past 5 years?	☐	☐	☐

If yes, what was the illness or problem?

	Yes	No	DK
Are you taking or have you recently taken any prescription or over the counter medicine(s)?	☐	☐	☐

If so, please list all, including vitamins, natural or herbal preparations and/or diet supplements:

Figure 1.1 ■ American Dental Association Health History Form.

Medical Information ***Please mark (X) your response to indicate if you have or have not had any of the following diseases or problems.***

(Check DK if you Don't Know the answer to the question) **Yes No DK**

Do you wear contact lenses? ☐ ☐ ☐

Joint Replacement. Have you had an orthopedic total joint (hip, knee, elbow, finger) replacement? ☐ ☐ ☐
Date: ____________ If yes, have you had any complications?____________

Are you taking or scheduled to begin taking either of the medications, alendronate (Fosamax®) or risedronate (Actonel®) for osteoporosis or Paget's disease? ☐ ☐ ☐

Since 2001, were you treated or are you presently scheduled to begin treatment with the intravenous bisphosphonates (Aredia® or Zometa®) for bone pain, hypercalcemia or skeletal complications resulting from Paget's disease, multiple myeloma or metastatic cancer? ☐ ☐ ☐
Date Treatment began: ____________

Yes No DK

Do you use controlled substances (drugs)? ☐ ☐ ☐

Do you use tobacco (smoking, snuff, chew, bidis)? ☐ ☐ ☐
If so, how interested are you in stopping?
(Circle one) VERY / SOMEWHAT / NOT INTERESTED

Do you drink alcoholic beverages? ☐ ☐ ☐
If yes, how much alcohol did you drink in the last 24 hours? ____________
If yes, how much do you typically drink In a week? ____________

WOMEN ONLY Are you:
Pregnant? ☐ ☐ ☐
Number of weeks: ____________
Taking birth control pills or hormonal replacement? ☐ ☐ ☐
Nursing? ☐ ☐ ☐

Allergies - Are you allergic to or have you had a reaction to: **Yes No DK**
To all **yes** responses, specify type of reaction.

Local anesthetics ____________ ☐ ☐ ☐
Aspirin ____________ ☐ ☐ ☐
Penicillin or other antibiotics ____________ ☐ ☐ ☐
Barbiturates, sedatives, or sleeping pills ____________ ☐ ☐ ☐
Sulfa drugs ____________ ☐ ☐ ☐
Codeine or other narcotics ____________ ☐ ☐ ☐

Yes No DK

Metals ____________ ☐ ☐ ☐
Latex (rubber) ____________ ☐ ☐ ☐
Iodine ____________ ☐ ☐ ☐
Hay fever/seasonal ____________ ☐ ☐ ☐
Animals ____________ ☐ ☐ ☐
Food ____________ ☐ ☐ ☐
Other ____________ ☐ ☐ ☐

Please mark (X) your response to indicate if you have or have not had any of the following diseases or problems.

Yes No DK

Artificial (prosthetic) heart valve ☐ ☐ ☐
Previous infective endocarditis ☐ ☐ ☐
Damaged valves in transplanted heart ☐ ☐ ☐
Congenital heart disease (CHD)
  Unrepaired, cyanotic CHD ☐ ☐ ☐
  Repaired (completely) in last 6 months ☐ ☐ ☐
  Repaired CHD with residual defects ☐ ☐ ☐

Except for the conditions listed above, antibiotic prophylaxis is no longer recommended for any other form of CHD.

Yes No DK

Cardiovascular disease ☐ ☐ ☐
Angina ☐ ☐ ☐
Arteriosclerosis ☐ ☐ ☐
Congestive heart failure ☐ ☐ ☐
Damaged heart valves ☐ ☐ ☐
Heart attack ☐ ☐ ☐
Heart murmur ☐ ☐ ☐
Low blood pressure ☐ ☐ ☐
High blood pressure ☐ ☐ ☐
Other congenital heart defects ☐ ☐ ☐

Yes No DK

Mitral valve prolapse ☐ ☐ ☐
Pacemaker ☐ ☐ ☐
Rheumatic fever ☐ ☐ ☐
Rheumatic heart disease ☐ ☐ ☐
Abnormal bleeding ☐ ☐ ☐
Anemia ☐ ☐ ☐
Blood transfusion ☐ ☐ ☐
  If yes, date: ____________
Hemophilia ☐ ☐ ☐
AIDS or HIV infection ☐ ☐ ☐
Arthritis ☐ ☐ ☐

Yes No DK

Autoimmune disease ☐ ☐ ☐
Rheumatoid arthritis ☐ ☐ ☐
Systemic lupus erythematosus ☐ ☐ ☐
Asthma ☐ ☐ ☐
Bronchitis ☐ ☐ ☐
Emphysema ☐ ☐ ☐
Sinus trouble ☐ ☐ ☐
Tuberculosis ☐ ☐ ☐
Cancer/Chemotherapy/ Radiation Treatment ☐ ☐ ☐
Chest pain upon exertion ☐ ☐ ☐
Chronic pain ☐ ☐ ☐
Diabetes Type I or II ☐ ☐ ☐
Eating disorder ☐ ☐ ☐
Malnutrition ☐ ☐ ☐
Gastrointestinal disease ☐ ☐ ☐
G.E. Reflux/persistent heartburn ☐ ☐ ☐
Ulcers ☐ ☐ ☐
Thyroid problems ☐ ☐ ☐
Stroke ☐ ☐ ☐
Glaucoma ☐ ☐ ☐

Yes No DK

Hepatitis, jaundice or liver disease ☐ ☐ ☐
Epilepsy ☐ ☐ ☐
Fainting spells or seizures ☐ ☐ ☐
Neurological disorders ☐ ☐ ☐
  If yes, specify: ____________
Sleep disorder ☐ ☐ ☐
Mental health disorders ☐ ☐ ☐
  Specify: ____________
Recurrent Infections ☐ ☐ ☐
  Type of infection: ____________
Kidney problems ☐ ☐ ☐
Night sweats ☐ ☐ ☐
Osteoporosis ☐ ☐ ☐
Persistent swollen glands in neck ☐ ☐ ☐
Severe headaches/ migraines ☐ ☐ ☐
Severe or rapid weight loss ☐ ☐ ☐
Sexually transmitted disease ☐ ☐ ☐
Excessive urination ☐ ☐ ☐

Has a physician or previous dentist recommended that you take antibiotics prior to your dental treatment? ☐ ☐ ☐

Name of physician or dentist making recommendation: Phone:

Do you have any disease, condition, or problem not listed above that you think I should know about? ☐ ☐ ☐
Please explain:

NOTE: Both Doctor and patient are encouraged to discuss any and all relevant patient health issues prior to treatment.
I certify that I have read and understand the above and that the information given on this form is accurate. I understand the importance of a truthful health history and that my dentist and his/her staff will rely on this information for treating me. I acknowledge that my questions, if any, about inquiries set forth above have been answered to my satisfaction. I will not hold my dentist, or any other member of his/her staff, responsible for any action they take or do not take because of errors or omissions that I may have made in the completion of this form.

Signature of Patient/Legal Guardian: Date:

FOR COMPLETION BY DENTIST

Comments: ____________

____

____

____

Figure 1.1 ■ continued

Self-Study Review

1. The best strategy for preventing medical emergencies in dental practice settings is keeping a medical emergency kit readily available because quick action is needed to save a life.
   a. Both the statement and reason are correct and related.
   b. Both the statement and reason are correct, but NOT related.
   c. The statement is correct, but the reason is NOT.
   d. The statement is NOT correct, but the reason is correct.
   e. NEITHER the statement NOR the reason is correct.
2. One of the best ways to anticipate a potential emergency when reviewing the medical history is to:
   a. complete follow-up questions for all "yes" responses.
   b. obtain a medical clearance for each client.
   c. ask the client if he or she thinks an emergency is possible at the appointment.
   d. verify information with the supervising dentist.
3. Clients may fail to provide complete medical history information as a result of all of the following reasons EXCEPT ONE. Which is the EXCEPTION?
   a. Client does not understand question.
   b. Feelings of invasion of privacy.
   c. Client had assistance completing the form.
   d. Client may skip questions.
4. Determining cardiac risk based on the client's ability to perform daily activity describes:
   a. cardiac equivalents.
   b. functional capacity.
   c. ASA risk classification.
   d. vital signs.
5. A client presents with a medical history of obesity, smoking, diabetes, and hypertension. He is currently participating in weight loss and walking programs. What ASA classification does this client represent?
   a. I
   b. II
   c. III
   d. IV

emergencies. The BP should be monitored for all clients who present for oral care.

The **systolic BP** reflects arterial pressure when the heart muscle contracts and forces blood into the circulation. It is influenced by a variety of conditions, such as:

- the elasticity of arteries (arteries hardened by atherosclerosis will not dilate to accommodate changes in BP as well as healthy arteries)
- the degree of hydrostatic pressure in the body (such as water retention)
- the degree of anxiety related to anticipation of treatment and subsequent physiologic stimulation of major organ systems through the autonomic nervous system
- influences on blood vessel muscle response (e.g., exercise promotes vasodilation, smoking promotes vasoconstriction)

The **diastolic BP** reflects the arterial pressure between heartbeats when the heart muscle rests.

Hypertension in adults is defined as a systolic BP of 140 mm Hg or higher, a diastolic BP of 90 mm Hg or higher, or taking medication to reduce BP.[4] The ranges of normal, prehypertension, and stages of hypertension as defined by the Seventh Report of the Joint National Committee on Prevention, Detection, Evaluation, and Treatment of High Blood Pressure (JNC7) published in May 2003 are provided in Table 1.2. These guidelines are in the process of being updated and are expected in 2014. New guidelines for treatment of hypertension (JNC8)[4] released in early 2014 did not change diagnosis of hypertension from JNC7 values, so JNC7 values will be used. JNC8 did recommend treatment for individuals with diabetes and chronic kidney disease (CKD) to bring them below 140/90 mm Hg, higher than treatment values in JNC7 [formerly ≤130/80 mm Hg)]. The pathophysiology of hypertension will be discussed in Chapter 10. This chapter will discuss the issue of how often BP should be measured as part of the physical evaluation process. For adults with no history of hypertension or hypertension-related diseases (e.g., diabetes, kidney disease) and having BP within normal limits, the current recommendations of the Joint National Committee advise remeasurement for every 2 years.[4] A new category was included in the 2003 guidelines called prehypertension and includes values that were formerly considered to be BP within normal limits (a systolic measurement of 120 to 139 mm Hg and a diastolic measurement of 80 to 89 mm Hg). Clients with prehypertension are at increased risk for progression to hypertension and are advised to undertake

Table 1.2 Classification of BP for Adults Age 18 and Older[a]

Category	Systolic BP (mm Hg)		Diastolic BP (mm Hg)
Normal	<120	and	<80
Prehypertension	120–139	and	80–89
Hypertension[b]			
Stage 1	140–159	or	90–99
Stage 2	≥160	or	≥100

[a]Not taking antihypertensive drugs and not acutely ill. When systolic and diastolic BPs fall into different categories, the higher category should be selected to classify the individual's BP status. For example, 160/92 mm Hg should be classified as stage 2 hypertension. In addition, to classifying stages of hypertension on the basis of average BP levels, clinicians should specify the presence or absence of target organ disease and additional risk factors.

[b]Based on the average of two or more properly measured, seated readings taken at each of two or more office visits.

(Adapted from Chobanian AV, et al. The Seventh Report of the Joint National Committee on Prevention, Detection, Evaluation, and Treatment of High Blood Pressure. National Heart, Lung, and Blood Institute. JAMA 2003;289:2560–2578.)

lifestyle modifications to get measurements into the normal range. They should have BP monitored annually. Lifestyle modifications include weight reduction and consuming a diet high in fruits and vegetables and food low in fat and sodium. Dental personnel are encouraged to reinforce hypertension-related lifestyle modifications recommended by physicians to improve client lifestyles and BP control. If the BP is at or above 140/90 mm Hg, the pressure should be measured more often as a part of medical treatment to return levels to normal limits. Target BP goals in clients with diabetes or chronic kidney disease are <140/90 mm Hg in the 2014 guidelines. More recently the AHA established ≤130/80 targets for men and women with established coronary artery disease (CAD) or who are at a high risk for developing CAD (e.g., carotid blockage, peripheral artery disease, abdominal aortic aneurysm, or a 10-year Framingham risk score of ≥10%)[5]. The AHA further stated that in individuals with heart failure, the target BP rate should be <120/80 mm Hg.[5] The guidelines state that 30% of the US population who have hypertension are unaware of having the disorder and, of those being treated for hypertension, only 34% are controlled. For this reason, the ADA advises that BP be taken at continuing-care dental visits as a screening mechanism for undiagnosed or uncontrolled hypertension.[6] Proper technique and appropriate cuff size for the diameter of the arm are essential to get accurate measurements. A cuff that is too small yields falsely elevated levels, whereas a cuff that is too large yields falsely low values. The auscultation method of BP measurement (sphygmomanometer and stethoscope) is universally accepted and is advocated by the AHA.[3] It is recommended that BP be measured at least twice during the appointment, separated by several minutes, and the average taken as the final measurement.[3,4]

Pediatric Blood Pressure

Diagnosing hypertension in children follows a different set of guidelines compared to diagnosing high BP in adults. In adults, the BP values are compared to a set of standard numbers and clients are categorized based on where their values fall. In children and adolescents, high BP is diagnosed using a statistical scale that adjusts the measured BP for factors such as height, sex, and age and compares the adjusted number to a set of averages. Research has shown that not only is obesity on the rise in children, but also comorbidities such as hypertension, dyslipidemia, and early-onset type 2 diabetes mellitus (metabolic syndrome) are increasing. In 2004, the Fourth Report on the Diagnosis, Evaluation, and Treatment of High Blood Pressure in Children and Adolescents was published.[7] The new guidelines recommend that all children over 3 years of age have BP measured when presenting at any healthcare facility and that a cuff is used which accommodates the size of the child's upper arm.

The 2004 guidelines depend on BP measurements over time, not on isolated measurements. The role of the oral health professional is to monitor BP in patients over the age of 3 years, according to the current pediatric BP guidelines, and refer children/adolescents for medical evaluation when values are

Table 1.3 Pediatric BP Values Needing Further Evaluation. Values Represent the Lower Limit for Abnormal BP by Age and Gender

	Females		Males	
Age (years)	Systolic BP (mm Hg)	Diastolic BP (mm Hg)	Systolic BP (mm Hg)	Diastolic BP (mm Hg)
3	100	59	100	59
4	101	64	102	62
5	103	66	104	65
6	104	68	105	68
7	106	69	106	70
8	108	71	107	71
9	110	72	109	72
10	112	73	111	73
11	114	74	113	74
12	116	75	115	74
13	117	76	117	75
14	119	77	120	75
15	120	78	120	76
16	120	78	120	78
17	120	78	120	80
18	120	80	120	80

(Adapted from *The Fourth Report on the Diagnosis, Evaluation, and Treatment of High Blood Pressure in Children and Adolescents* [2004] and *The Seventh Report of the Joint National Committee on Prevention, Detection, Evaluation, and Treatment of High Blood Pressure: The JNC7 Report* [2003].) These values represent the lower limit for abnormal BP by age and gender. Any BP readings at or higher than these values represent BP s in the prehypertension, stage 1 hypertension, or stage 2 hypertension range and therefore should be further evaluated by a physician.

above normal limits, rather than identify whether the child is in the prehypertension or hypertension levels. For the child with prehypertension, rechecking BP in 6 months is recommended. For stage 1 hypertension, clients should be referred for medical evaluation (time unspecified), however for stage 2 hypertension values referral within 1 week is indicated (see Table 1.3 for values).[7]

Relevance of Dental Appointment Measurements of Blood Pressure

Elevation of BP above normal limits is an important consideration as hypertension is a major risk factor for stroke, myocardial infarction (heart attack), heart failure, and kidney dysfunction. Clients with hypertension pose a risk for medical emergencies during oral healthcare treatment involving stress. The inability to respond to stress experienced during oral healthcare treatment is a major factor leading to several emergency situations. These will be identified in the medical section (Chapters 9–14) that deals with potential emergencies associated with specific disease conditions. Clients reporting a history of medical conditions related to increased BP (e.g., hypertension, cardiovascular disease, hyperthyroidism, kidney disease, or diabetes) should have BP measured and evaluated at every oral healthcare appointment (Box 1-2). Should an emergency occur during the appointment, these baseline values are used for comparison with postemergency values. When drugs that can alter BP values (e.g., anesthetics or local anesthetics with vasoconstrictor)

Box 1-2

Disease Conditions Associated with Hypertension

- Stroke
- Myocardial infarction
- Heart failure or congestive heart failure
- Kidney dysfunction
- Hyperthyroidism
- Diabetes

are planned for the appointment, a baseline BP should be available. For situations where treatment is not completed in one appointment and the client is rescheduled, the BP should be remeasured on subsequent appointments only in clients whose medical condition or drug treatment suggests there is a risk for having abnormal values leading to a potential emergency situation. For example, a client with elevated BP values at the initial appointment should have BP remeasured at subsequent appointments. Clients taking antihypertensive medication should have BP measured at each appointment. As well, if local anesthesia with a vasoconstrictor is to be used during the appointment, the BP should be measured. The client with BP values within normal limits at the initial appointment and who has a medical history with no medical conditions associated with elevated BP does not need to have BP remeasured at **reappointments** (unless a drug is planned to be used that requires it). These are suggestions to assist the clinician in using critical thinking to determine when BP should be taken before oral health care. It is helpful to use a national standard recommended by a credible authoritative body. The JNC7 recommendations illustrated in Table 1.2 are for the general public. BP values for children are included in Table 1.3.[7] The determination of BP for children and adolescents was changed in 2004 to include prehypertension and stage 1 and stage 2 hypertension.[7] Table 1.3 provides values according to age and sex that represent the levels at which the child/adolescent should be referred for medical evaluation. BP values for the specific age and sex ideally should be lower than the values in the table, unless the child is in the higher height categories. Since it is difficult to determine the height category used for determining BP and since there is a range of error when taking BP measurement, the table should still be used to identify the child needing referral for medical evaluation. There is evidence that childhood hypertension is rising and the main reason is thought to be childhood obesity. The report states that children older than 3 years (and some medically complicated children at age 3) who are seen in a medical setting should routinely have the BP measured using a child sized cuff. Adolescents (aged 10 to 17 years) with BP values of 120/80 mm Hg or higher should be considered prehypertensive and referred for medical evaluation. Pediatric hypertension is defined as having systolic BP or diastolic BP at or above the 95th percentile for sex, age, and height on three separate occasions.[7] The ADA's policy for screening of BP in the dental office is discussed below.

AMERICAN DENTAL ASSOCIATION POLICY ON SCREENING FOR BLOOD PRESSURE

The ADA suggests BP be measured at the initial appointment for all new dental clients, including children, as a screening tool to identify undiagnosed hypertension.[6] Recent communication with ADA officials verifies this policy is still in force. The association policy also recommends that BP be measured at annual or 6-month continuing-care appointments. Some texts consider routine measurement of BP prior to providing oral health care to be the standard of care in dentistry.[8] Table 1.4 illustrates recommendations by the authors of this self-study for the client with elevated BP values needing oral treatment. The recommendations use BP values specified in the JNC7 report identified above and in clinical texts.[3,9]

Blood Pressure Readings above Normal Limits

The appropriate follow-up question for elevated BP with a negative history of hypertension is *"Have you ever been told you have high BP?"* For the client reporting hypertension, the follow-up questions are *"When was the last time your physician evaluated your BP? What changes were made in your therapy?"* When elevated values are identified, the clinician should determine whether the client is aware of the elevated pressures. The client should be informed of the values found at each appointment and referred to the physician if values are consistently above normal ranges. Hypertension is never diagnosed on an isolated reading. The general rule is that two or more consecutive high readings on separate occasions must occur before a diagnosis of hypertension is made. For more than two-thirds of those taking antihypertensive medication, their failure to adhere to antihypertensive therapy and lifestyle changes are the largest contributing factors to insufficient BP control.[4]

Clinical Management

For the client with elevated BP, short appointments and use of effective pain control methods are recommended (refer to Table 1.4). Painful treatment will cause the stress response to be activated, increasing the heart rate and need for more oxygenated blood by the heart muscle. Narrowed arteries from atherosclerosis reduce the amount of blood to the muscle. This sets the stage for a

Table 1.4 Dental Considerations for the Hypertensive Client Age 18 and Older

Blood Pressure (mm Hg)	Dental Treatment Considerations
≤140/90	1. Routine dental treatment can be provided. 2. Remeasure BP at continuing-care appointment as a screening strategy for hypertension.
140–159/90–99	1. Remeasure BP after 5 minutes when client has rested. 2. Measure prior to any appointment; if client has measurements above normal range on two separate appointments, and has not been diagnosed as hypertensive, refer for medical evaluation. 3. Inform client of BP measurement. 4. Routine treatment can be provided.
160–179/100–109	1. Remeasure BP after 5 minutes when client has rested. 2. If still elevated, inform client of readings. 3. Refer for medical evaluation within 1 month; delay treatment if client is unable to handle stress or if dental procedure is lengthy. Use local anesthesia with 1:100,000 vasoconstrictor if required, limit to two cartridges. 4. Routine treatment can be provided. Consider using a stress reduction protocol that includes anti-anxiety medication during dental treatment and keep appointment short.
≥180/110	1. Remeasure BP after 5 minutes when client has rested. 2. Delay elective dental treatment until BP is controlled, require a medical consultation form approving oral healthcare treatment to be completed and signed by client's physician. 3. If emergency dental care is needed, it should be done in a setting in which emergency life support equipment is available.

BP, blood pressure.

cardiovascular (CV) emergency. In general, older clients should be appointed in the late morning or early afternoon when BP is naturally lower.[3] Nitrous oxide can be used to reduce BP if anxiety is the cause of the elevated readings. Limit the use of epinephrine in local anesthesia to no more than two cartridges of 1:100,000 epinephrine and check BP after injection of local anesthetics.[3] BP values ≥180/110 mm Hg contraindicate dental treatment (ASA IV) and should be referred for immediate medical evaluation.[3,9]

Measuring the Pulse Rate

The pulse rate can be defined as the heart rate or a reflection of the heartbeat. The pulse rate is usually taken by palpating the radial artery for 1 minute, mentally noting the force of the pulse and the regularity (described as the quality). **Atrial tachycardia** is a fast, irregular pulse rate that indicates cardiovascular instability and is associated with symptoms leading to cardiac arrest. In fact, arrhythmia (more correctly called **tachyarrhythmia**) is identified as the most common sign preceding cardiac arrest.[10] **Tachycardia** is the term used to describe a pulse rate above the limits of normal, and **bradycardia** describes the pulse rate below the normal range. These can occur with a normal rhythmic quality and are measured by an ECG.

Self-Study Review

6. BP is most accurate if taken when the client is:
   a. seated in a supine position.
   b. seated in an upright position.
   c. rested.
   d. standing.

7. The ADA Council on Scientific Affairs recommends that BP be measured at the initial appointment. If the BP reading is within the normal limits, the client does not have hypertension.
   a. Both statements are true.
   b. Both statements are false.
   c. The first statement is true, and the second statement is false.
   d. The first statement is false, and the second statement is true.

8. A 12-year-old boy presents with a BP of 118/84 mm Hg, right arm, representing stage 2 hypertension. Treatment should be delayed until the BP is better controlled.
   a. Both statements are true.
   b. Both statements are false.
   c. The first statement is true, and the second statement is false.
   d. The first statement is false, and the second statement is true.

9. Your client presents with a BP of 148/86 mm Hg, right arm, sitting. Treatment considerations for this client include (circle all that apply):
   a. performing routine dental or dental hygiene procedures.
   b. delaying treatment until the BP is better controlled.
   c. referring the client to a physician for a medical evaluation.
   d. using a stress-reduction protocol during dental and dental hygiene procedures.

10. Your client presents with a BP of 165/100 mm Hg, right arm, sitting. Treatment considerations for this client include all of the following EXCEPT one. Which is the EXCEPTION?
   a. Performing routine dental or dental hygiene procedures.
   b. Delaying treatment until the BP is better controlled.
   c. Referring the client to a physician for a medical evaluation.
   d. Using a stress-reduction protocol during dental and dental hygiene procedures.

For adults, a rate of 60 to 80 bpm is considered normal. Some texts list pulse rates up to 100 bpm as being within normal limits.[3,11] Children may have upper limits of 120 bpm. A client with a pulse rate less than 60 bpm may not pose a risk for an emergency situation. People in excellent physical condition often have low pulse rates. However, pulse rates above 120 bpm (whether regular or irregular) may indicate cardiovascular disease. Increased pulse rate can be a side effect of some medications (such as decongestants), so the clinician should investigate the cause. An increased pulse rate (or severely decreased rate) for no apparent reason is the basis for referral for medical evaluation. Clients should be required to have a medical consultation form completed by their physician specifying the degree of cardiovascular health with recommendations regarding oral treatment. When an irregular pulse rate above 120 bpm occurs, and the cause is unknown, a potential emergency exists and elective oral health care would best be delayed until a normal quality is restored. The normal pulse rate is determined using the radial artery; however, during an emergency situation, the carotid pulse is more reliable than the radial pulse. The carotid pulse is found in the middle of the neck along the sternocleidomastoid muscle. Refer to a clinical practice textbook for more information on the technique of measuring the pulse.

Measurement of Respiration

Respiration is defined as the inhalation and exhalation of air. The respiration rate includes the number of times the chest rises (inhalation) in 1 minute. The quality (noiseless? deep or shallow?) of respiration should also be assessed. The normal respiration rate for adults is 14 to 20 breaths per minute.[11] For children younger than 5 years of age, it can be as high as 22 breaths per minute. Respiration rates over 28 indicate an abnormal condition, and rates over 60 represent a medical emergency.[11] Before assessing respiration rate and qualities, the clinician should tell the client that the pulse is being retaken to verify the rate, so that the client does not realize breathing qualities are being observed and unconsciously alter breathing patterns.

Self-Study Review

11. All of the following are true for a fast, irregular pulse EXCEPT one. Which one is the EXCEPTION?
   a. The client is in excellent physical condition.
   b. A potential medical emergency can occur.
   c. A sign of cardiovascular instability.
   d. High risk for cardiac arrest.

12. A client who presents with a pulse rate over 100 bpm and an irregular rhythm should be referred to a physician for medical evaluation because he may have bradycardia.
   a. Both the statement and reason are correct and related.
   b. Both the statement and reason are correct, but NOT related.
   c. The statement is correct, but the reason is NOT.
   d. The statement is NOT correct, but the reason is correct.
   e. NEITHER the statement NOR the reason is correct.

13. During an emergency, the pulse should be taken from which artery?
 a. Brachial
 b. Carotid
 c. Femoral
 d. Radial

When noting respiration rates, the clinician should watch for depth of respiration and listen for sounds during respiration. Normal respiration can be shallow or deep but should be noiseless. Sounds heard during respiration indicate airway obstruction. The clinician must determine what is causing the sounds. Anxious clients may have fast respiration rates that may lead to hyperventilation. Increased respiration should be followed up by observing whether the client is displaying signs of anxiety, such as clutching the arms of the chair (called white knuckle syndrome) or having facial perspiration. If these behaviors are observed, stress reduction procedures may be necessary before oral procedures begin.

Stress Reduction Protocol

Stress reduction procedures can include a variety of strategies to relieve anxiety, such as developing rapport with the client and gaining his or her trust, leading the client to focus on pleasant experiences rather than oral procedures, prescribing an anti-anxiety medication or using nitrous oxide conscious analgesia, ensuring good pain control, and appointing the client for short periods at a time of day when he or she is relaxed (usually early morning; Box 1-3). Hyperventilation is a stress-related medical emergency characterized by fast, irregular respiration. It will be discussed in the next chapter within the section that deals with questions on the medical history that identify clients who are anxious about having oral healthcare treatment.

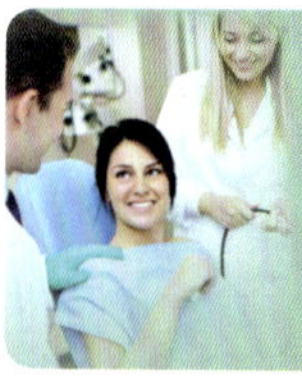

Follow-up Questions

"Are you aware of noises when you breathe? Do you know what is causing this sound?"

Normal respiration is noiseless. Sounds indicate respiratory obstruction. The condition causing the airway obstruction must be evaluated in terms of its impact during the oral procedure. In the asthmatic client, the clinician should ensure that the client has brought a **bronchodilator** inhaler to the appointment for use in case of bronchoconstriction during treatment. Respiration noise in the nonasthmatic patient implies other possibilities, such as an infectious respiratory disease or congestive heart failure. Dental considerations include determining whether the client is contagious and, if not, upright positioning to prevent airway blockage during treatment. If use of a rubber dam is planned and the client has respiratory difficulty, the procedure may have to be rescheduled. The same is true when use of an ultrasonic scaler with associated water lavage is planned. This instrument will cause aerosols that could compromise respiration. To protect the oral healthcare practitioner, any patient with a contagious respiratory disease must be rescheduled until the condition is resolved.

Box 1-3

Stress Reduction Strategies

- Talk to client to gain trust, develop rapport
- Influence client to focus on pleasant experiences
- Consider prescribing an anti-anxiety drug
- Use nitrous oxide gas for conscious sedation
- Ensure good pain control
- Make short appointments, early in day

Self-Study Review

14. Normal respiration rate for adults is:
 a. 10–18 breaths per minute.
 b. 14–20 breaths per minute.
 c. 16–22 breaths per minute.
 d. 18–24 breaths per minute.

15. When evaluating respiration, the clinician should observe:
 a. rate of respiration.
 b. depth of respiration.
 c. presence of sounds.
 d. all of the above.

16. An ultrasonic device to debride teeth can safely be used in a client with compromised respiration. Suction devices will eliminate aerosols and reduce the potential for contamination.

a. Both statements are true.
b. Both statements are false.
c. The first statement is true, and the second statement is false.
d. The first statement is false, and the second statement is true.

Measurement of Temperature

The range of normal body temperature is 96.8°F to 99.58°F.[10] The significance of including temperature in the vital sign assessment relates to the risk for disease transmission to the healthcare worker from the presence of contagious diseases. For this reason, the temperature should be measured at every appointment for oral services. The client with a normal temperature at the initial appointment can develop a contagious infection within a few days. Masks, which usually would provide protection, are not usually worn during the medical history review. Disease passed by droplet infection in an active state may be discovered by noting an elevated body temperature. This is particularly true with children, who may have contagious childhood diseases. Postponing treatment and referral for medical care is recommended for clients with elevated temperature readings as a result of suspected illness or infection. The clinician should rule out temporary causes of elevated oral temperature (recent ingestion of hot beverages, cigarette smoking).

Risk of Disease Transmission

There is a risk of disease transmission when treatment is provided to a person with an elevated temperature of unknown origin. One exception to this is when a client reports for emergency oral care and it is determined that the temperature elevation relates to a dental infection. In this case, there is no risk of disease transmission to the oral healthcare provider. However, the client experiencing elevated temperature is less able to tolerate stress, and treatment should be limited to resolving the oral infection and associated discomfort.

Self-Study Review

17. Normal body temperature ranges from:

a. 95.8°F to 98.58°F.
b. 95.8°F to 99.58°F.
c. 96.8°F to 99.58°F.
d. 97.8°F to 100.58°F.

18. Treatment considerations for a 10-year-old boy who presents with a body temperature of 100.5°F include all of the following EXCEPT one. Which one is the EXCEPTION?

a. Postponing treatment
b. Referral to a physician to identify the type of infection or illness
c. Asking the client to rinse with mouthwash before providing treatment
d. Identifying any temporary causes of elevated temperature

CHAPTER SUMMARY

This chapter provided an introduction to taking and reviewing the medical history. Follow-up questions and the relevance of determining functional capacity and vital signs to evaluate clients for potential emergency situations were addressed. Guidelines for identifying hypertension and for providing dental treatment to clients with hypertension were presented. The recommendations of the ADA related to measurement of BP in the dental office were identified. The next chapter will continue to discuss questions on the medical history form, as well as address stress-related emergency situations.

Review

1. Define the following terms: BP, systolic pressure, diastolic pressure, pulse, respiration, functional capacity, and METs.
2. Why should all questions on the medical history form be answered?
3. What guidelines should be used when considering oral treatment for a client who presents with a BP of 180/100 mm Hg, right arm?
4. The majority of individuals taking antihypertensive medication continue to have insufficient BP control. What is the clinical relevance of this finding?
5. According to the latest guidelines on screening for hypertension, at what age should the BP be measured in a dental office?
6. Describe the technique for taking the pulse during an emergency.
7. What information related to "quality" is needed before determining a client's respiration status?
8. What is the risk of treating a client with an elevated body temperature?

Case Study

Case A

Mr. Farnsworth, a 48-year-old man, presents for a dental examination and restorative appointment. Before performing the examination, vital signs are measured. His pulse is 72 bpm, respiration is 16 breaths per minute, and BP measures 126/86 mm Hg, right arm. His height is 5′8″ and weight is 200 lbs.

1. What category of BP does Mr. Farnsworth's reading rate?
2. What health recommendations should be made on the basis of Mr. Farnsworth's vital signs?
3. What dental considerations should be made when considering oral treatment for this client with his BP values?

Mr. Farnsworth returns for a dental hygiene appointment 1 year later. Upon updating the medical history, the clinician learns that this client had a myocardial infarction approximately 4 months ago. He is currently taking aspirin 81 mg and Norvasc daily, but he left his medication at home and cannot recall the dosage. Vital signs at this appointment are pulse 80 bpm, respiration 18 breaths per minute, temperature 97.8°F, and BP 145/88 mm Hg, right arm. When questioned about functional capacity, Mr. Farnsworth reports that he has difficulty climbing stairs, cannot dance or play tennis without shortness of breath, and has difficulty walking the dog more than a few blocks.

4. What category of BP does Mr. Farnsworth's reading rate now?
5. Which ASA classification does this client represent?
6. Based on the client's vital signs and METs, what treatment considerations should be made?

Chapter Two

The American Dental Association Health History Form

Objectives

After completing the self-study chapter the reader will be able to:

- Describe the dental management for a client who reports a history of tuberculosis (TB) disease or who demonstrates signs of TB disease.
- Differentiate between TB infection and TB disease.
- Describe the criteria used for determining a noninfectious status in clients with a history of active TB.

Key Terms

Contagious: a disease that may be transmitted to another person by direct or indirect contact

Induration: hardness of a tissue, such as a positive skin test for tuberculosis

Infectious: capable of causing an infection

Mantoux TB skin test: a skin test that screens for tuberculosis infection

Tuberculosis (TB): an infectious, inflammatory disease caused by *Mycobacterium tuberculosis* that primarily affects the pulmonary system

MEDICAL CONDITION

INTRODUCTION

The 2007 American Dental Association (ADA) Health History Form includes a section for e-mail contact information and the date of the initial completion of the health history at the top of the first page. A statement that the office policy adheres to federally required privacy of information and assurance of confidentiality and nondiscrimination follows. The health history documentation begins by asking for personal data (information related to telephone contact information, address, occupation, height, weight, sex, and so forth), whom to contact should an emergency occur, and family information. Next, screening questions related to identifying an individual with active **tuberculosis** (TB) or one having signs and symptoms of active TB are included. This section of four questions ends with a request for the individual to return the form to the receptionist if "yes" is the answer to any of the screening questions for TB. The relevance of this request is discussed in the next sections. The Health History portion begins with questions related to dental information and experiences, followed by a comprehensive section for medical information.

PERSONAL DATA

This section deals with client data related to setting up the file for business purposes. Client information including height, weight, age, and sex can be important when determining treatment considerations. A person under the age of 18 would need parent or guardian approval for treatment and verification for the accuracy of health history information. The parent or legal guardian must be available when the history is reviewed and must sign the form verifying accuracy. Some clients will not provide their social security numbers because of fear of identity theft or misuse. This information may not be essential to establish the client record and can be replaced with a patient ID number. A nondiscrimination statement to the client explaining how the health history information is used and confidentiality assurances to comply with Health Insurance Portability and Accountability Act of 1996 (HIPAA) regulations begins this section. HIPAA laws will be discussed in Chapter 15.

SCREENING QUESTIONS FOR ACTIVE TUBERCULOSIS

"Do you have any of the following diseases or problems: Active TB? Persistent cough for greater than 3-week duration? Cough that produces blood? Have you been exposed to anyone with TB?

If your answer is 'yes' to any of the four items above, please stop and return this form to the receptionist."

One-third of the world's population is infected with TB, which is also a leading cause of death in HIV-infected persons. Current statistics revealed that a total of 10,528 TB cases were reported in the United States in 2011. Fortunately, the number of TB cases reported has continued to decrease over the past decade.[1] This number represents a 6% decline compared to 2010 figures and was the lowest recorded number of cases since reporting began in 1953. This can be attributed to the increased funds to establish TB control programs in the United States. In 2011, 62% of TB cases occurred in foreign-born individuals, approximately 11.5 times greater than the cases among US-born individuals.[1] States with more than 3.4 cases per 100,000 population include Hawaii, California, Nevada, Arizona, Texas, Louisiana, Georgia, Florida, New York, and the District of Columbia. Racial/ethnic populations at the greatest risk for TB include Asians and Native Hawaiians or Pacific Islanders.

The Centers for Disease Control and Prevention (CDC) has advised dental facilities to add screening questions for active TB to the medical history.[2] While gathering information at the initial medical history and at periodic updates, oral health professionals should routinely question clients regarding exposure to TB, if they have a history of TB disease or have symptoms of active TB. A persistent cough for more than 3 weeks and a cough that produces blood are two significant symptoms of active TB disease. Other symptoms are night sweats, unexplained fever, loss of appetite, and malaise. Individuals who have spent time with a person having active TB is also at a great risk for becoming infected with the bacterium. The instruction to the client to immediately return the history form to the receptionist if "yes" is answered to any of the four items is designed to identify **contagious** persons before being seated for oral procedures and to isolate them from others in the facility. There is one report of TB transmission in the dental setting.[3] Guidelines for infection control (IC) were published in 2003 and suggest establishing an IC team knowledgeable in **infectious** diseases in the facility.[4] The training of the IC team is based on the degree of risk for TB in the local area where the dental office or healthcare setting is located. The team would follow up the patient with health history responses that suggest active TB. Information from public health offices (where all TB case information is held) would be gained when there is a strong suspicion of TB disease.

IC guidelines discuss testing dental personnel for TB disease or infection with a skin test. All staff should have a baseline test to rule out TB disease or infection. Negative tests, especially in a community at a low risk for TB, allow healthcare workers (HCWs) to prolong time between screenings unless the risk in the local community increases. For staff who test positive, a chest X-ray should be made to rule out active TB and then annual screening examinations.

PATHOPHYSIOLOGY

Infection occurs when a susceptible person inhales droplet nuclei containing *Mycobacterium tuberculosis*, which then travel to the alveoli of the lungs. Usually within 2 to 12 weeks after initial infection, the immune response prevents further spread of the bacterium, although bacilli can remain alive in the lungs for years, a condition termed latent TB infection. Only the person with active disease (individual has symptoms) is contagious and presents a risk for transmission of TB.

The CDC advises to provide masks when the client is coughing to reduce the numbers of airborne bacilli (also referred to as droplet nuclei) or to instruct the person to cover the mouth with cupped hands.[2] Surgical masks do not prevent inhalation of TB droplet nuclei, and therefore, standard precautions are not sufficient to prevent disease transmission.[2] The main administrative goal of a TB infection-control program is early detection of a person with active TB disease and prompt isolation from susceptible persons to reduce the risk of transmission. Clients suspected of having active disease should be immediately referred for medical evaluation. The local public health department maintains records of TB diagnoses and can be contacted to determine if the patient in question has been diagnosed. Referrals can be made to the public health clinic for testing and medical evaluation. *Elective dental care is contraindicated in the client with active TB disease.*

Self-Study Review

1. Screening questions on the medical history form concerning active TB are recommended by the:
   a. Centers for Disease Prevention and Health Promotion.
   b. Centers for Disease Control and Prevention.
   c. National Institutes of Health.
   d. National Center for Health and Disease Prevention.
2. Symptoms of active TB include all of the following EXCEPT one. Which is the EXCEPTION?
   a. Persistent cough for > 3 weeks
   b. Cough that produces blood
   c. Unexplained weight gain
   d. Flu-like symptoms
3. Mr. Cheng presents with a history of coughing up blood for 3 weeks. He had seen a physician, but does not know his diagnosis. What resource would you use to determine if this client was diagnosed with TB?
   a. Centers for Disease Control and Prevention
   b. National Institutes of Health
   c. State agency for infectious diseases
   d. Local public health department

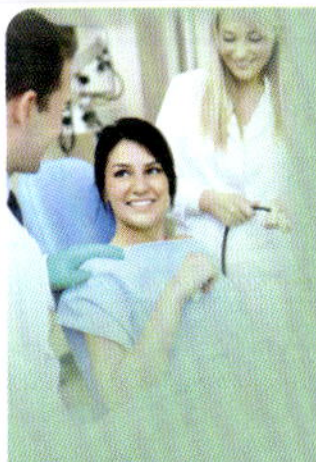

Follow-up Questions

If the client replies "yes" to any item in the questionnaire, investigation for the presence of other signs of active TB, such as night sweats and unexplained weight loss, should be pursued.

"Have you seen a physician about the persistent cough? Do you wake up during the night from sweating? Have you recently had unexplained weight loss? Do you know anyone who has had TB?"

If the client answers only that he or she knows of someone who has had TB but has not spent much time with the person, the proper follow-up question is *"Have you been tested for exposure to TB with a skin test?"* It is important to understand that there are two manifestations of TB: (1) TB *infection* and (2) TB *disease.* In 2013, the CDC updated the core curriculum on TB and reported that guidelines are in development.[5] Study questions are included throughout each chapter to provide a review of the content and help the reader apply the content to real-life situations. The reader of this text is advised to monitor the CDC Web site for new guidelines.

TUBERCULOSIS INFECTION

A person who has inhaled the TB bacillus and whose immune system has developed antibodies to the bacillus, but who has not developed symptoms of TB as described above, is considered to be infected with the bacillus but not have active disease. This person is NOT contagious to others. This client will have a positive result on the **Mantoux TB skin test** meaning only that the bacillus has stimulated the immune system to develop antibodies against the bacillus. There is no contraindication to oral healthcare procedures in this client; however, the client must be monitored for the development of active disease in the future. It is estimated that 10% of infected people will eventually develop active TB disease, and this can occur up to 20 years later. The greatest risk of TB infection developing into active disease occurs when a person becomes immunocompromised, either from disease or from immunosuppressive medications, such as prednisone.

ACTIVE TUBERCULOSIS

TB is transmitted by airborne droplet infection. It is chiefly a pulmonary disease, although less often it can affect the skin or internal organs. The oral HCW is at risk when the client has the pulmonary form. Although the generation of droplet nuclei containing *M. tuberculosis* as a result of dental procedures has not been demonstrated, oral procedures may stimulate coughing.[2] When a person with active disease coughs, the bacillus can be found within the small aerosol droplets that are expelled in the cough. In the latter stage of active disease, violent coughing causes blood vessels in the lungs to break, and blood may be found in the sputum. This possibility relates to the ADA question about "cough that produces blood" illustrated at the beginning of the discussion. The numbers of pulmonary bacilli are highest in the latter stage of the disease, and the person is considered to be highly contagious. Because it is possible that bacilli can be in saliva, working in the mouth of the person with active disease is likely to produce aerosols containing the TB bacilli. Those aerosols are considered a vector for transmission of the bacillus organism. The dental mask will not protect against inhalation of the bacillus because it gets into the room air and can be inhaled once the face mask is removed. There is one report of active TB developing in a dentist and in the dental assistant employed in a hospital dental clinic.[3] It is unknown whether the disease was transmitted between the two dental personnel or whether they contracted TB from a client. They were reported to have followed standard infection-control procedures (mask, gloves, barriers), but because TB has an airborne transmission route these barriers are ineffective for preventing TB disease transmission. The dental clinic was in a hospital setting where HIV-positive clients were treated, a group at increased risk for TB.

People who spend time with someone in the coughing stage of TB disease are at high risk of becoming infected with TB and developing active disease in the future. This generally includes family members, coworkers, clients in long-term care facilities, residents in institutional care, and individuals who work or are placed in prisons. "*Has anyone in your family or a friend or coworker been diagnosed with TB? Have you been tested for TB infection?*" would be appropriate follow-up questions for the client who responds positively to having symptoms of unexplained cough for 3 weeks or longer or a cough that produces blood. Other populations at high risk of having TB disease include foreign persons who have emigrated from countries where TB is endemic (e.g., Vietnam, Asia, Russia, Central America, and other third world countries), people with HIV disease or AIDS, children who live in high-risk environments (where people often have TB disease), and people with malignancies.[2,4,5]

From this discussion, one can understand why dental clients should be screened for symptoms of TB and why treating a person with active TB in the dental office is contraindicated. For this reason, the instruction is added to the question:

"If you answered 'yes' to any of the four items above, stop and return this form to the receptionist."

When the client returns the form to the receptionist, the dentist is notified, and appropriate questioning identifies the client needing isolation within the facility and a medical evaluation to determine the etiology of symptoms. This practice is important in areas or facilities where TB is prevalent. Each dental office should know if TB is prevalent in the area by contacting the public health department. When active TB is suspected, the client is referred for medical evaluation. The dentist should request the physician to complete a medical clearance form verifying that treatment was successful and the client poses no risk for disease transmission.

Self-Study Review

4. A positive Mantoux skin test without symptoms indicates that the client is:
   a. infected with the TB bacillus, but not contagious to others.
   b. infected with the TB bacillus and has active disease.
   c. infected with the TB bacillus and is contagious to others.
   d. infected with the TB bacillus and immunocompromised.
5. Blood in the sputum of an individual infected with TB represents aerosols have infected and damaged blood vessels in the lungs. The client should be isolated and dental hygiene treatment should be postponed.
   a. Both statements are true.
   b. Both statements are false.
   c. The first statement is true, and the second statement is false.
   d. The first statement is false, and the second statement is true.
6. All of the populations are at a high risk of contracting TB EXCEPT one. Which one is the EXCEPTION?
   a. People infected with HIV
   b. Immigrants from third world countries
   c. People with malignancies
   d. People who are immunocompromised with diabetes mellitus

MULTIDRUG-RESISTANT TB

Multidrug-resistant TB (MDR TB) is caused by an organism that is resistant to at least isoniazid and rifampin, the two most potent TB drugs. It is a serious public health concern. Both US-born and foreign-born persons had decreases in the number and percentage of cases of MDR TB, although the decline in US-born persons has been greater. As a result the percentage of all reported primary MDR TB cases associated with being foreign born increased from approximately 25% of all MDR TB cases in 1993 to 88% in 2009.[6] In 2010, there were 89 cases reported and 98 cases in 2011. The percentage of US-born patients with primary MDR TB remains low at below 1.0% of cases. Primary MDR TB is defined as having no history of TB disease and being resistant to at least isoniazid and rifampin, anti-TB drugs used as first-line treatment. The rate of case reports of primary MDR TB in foreign-born individuals was 82.7% in 2011.[1,5]

SYMPTOM-RELATED QUESTIONS FOR ACTIVE TUBERCULOSIS

"Persistent cough for greater than 3-week duration; cough that produces blood?"

When reported together these are signs of active TB. If the client answers a positive response on just one of these items, questioning should determine whether the client knows the cause of the symptom and whether the client has had a medical evaluation of the symptom. Persistent cough can relate to other reasons, some of which can include cigarette smoking, chronic bronchitis, asthma, respiratory infection, or malignancy. Determine the correct etiology of the cough condition if possible, and if the client is unsure of the etiology, refer for medical evaluation. A recent Cochrane systematic review and meta-analysis revealed a sputum test (Xpert) to be highly effective in identifying TB, including multidrug-resistant TB. Authors state that the test is easily administered and could be performed at point-of-care appointment, increasing the time to diagnosis of TB and getting those affected into treatment.[6]

A medical clearance form should be requested from the physician assuring the client is not infectious. The physician should order a Mantoux TB skin test. In this test, purified protein derivative (PPD) from the TB bacillus is injected intradermally. It takes 48 to 72 hours for the immune system to react to the PPD substance. A positive test is characterized by **induration** or hardness of the area where PPD was injected. Redness is NOT a feature of a positive test.[5] For the person with no risk factors for TB infection, the size of a positive induration is 15 mm. For clients in a high-risk group for TB, a positive test is variable (5 to 10 mm depending on the risk factors). If the skin test is positive, the physician will order a chest X-ray. The chest X-ray is used to determine the evidence of pulmonary infection.

DETERMINING NONINFECTIOUS STATE IN CLIENT

The CDC suggests that a client who has been treated for active TB is no longer contagious if three criteria are achieved. Medical treatment must render the client to:

1. Not be in the coughing stage.
2. Have three consecutive negative sputum smears taken on three separate days.
3. Have taken effective anti-TB drugs for at least 2 weeks (Box 2-1).[5]
4. Have a negative sputum culture.

The physician should verify successful treatment by ordering a culture after 3 weeks of drug treatment to ensure that the disease is not resistant to the antimicrobial agents used. The client who contracts multiple drug-resistant TB is more difficult to treat and remains contagious longer. The client with active TB will take three to four anti-TB drugs for 6 to 12 months, depending on the client's risk group or coinfection with HIV. However, when drugs to which the TB bacillus is sensitive are taken for 3 weeks, the client is not contagious. The success of medical therapy is verified with laboratory culture results.

MEDICAL CONSULTATION FORM

A medical consultation form should be prepared by the dental office that identifies the signs of active TB (e.g., persistent cough, cough that produces blood). The form should request the physician to notify the dental office when the disease is noninfectious and the client is not contagious. The returned consultation form should be placed in the client's permanent record. In summary, for the client who has completed medical evaluation and who does not have active TB, dental treatment can be provided with no risk of transmitting TB to the clinician. For the client who received a diagnosis of active TB, the three criteria for noninfectiousness should be verified by the physician in a signed medical clearance document before oral health care is provided (see Box 2-1). Web sites for information on TB are included in Box 2-2. Samples of medical consultation forms can be found on the POINT site accessible by purchasers of this text.

WORKPLACE SCREENING

The CDC has recommended that all health professionals have routine screening skin tests for TB.[2] In the dental office, this should be part of the annual IC program, and the frequency should be determined on the basis of the prevalence of TB in

Box 2-1

Criteria for Noninfectiousness in Active Tuberculosis

- Effective anti-TB drugs taken for 2 weeks or longer.
- Three consecutive negative sputum smears taken on different days are documented.
- Client is not in coughing stage.
- Negative sputum cultures

(Reprinted with permission from Core Curriculum on Tuberculosis: What the Clinician Should Know. 2013.)

Box 2-2

Web Sites for Tuberculosis Information

- CDC Division of Tuberculosis Elimination: www.cdc.gov/tb/
- Guidelines for Preventing the Transmission of *Mycobacterium tuberculosis* in Healthcare Settings, 2005: www.cdc.gov/mmwr/PDF/rr/rr5417/pdf
- Guidelines for Infection Control in Dental Healthcare Settings, 2003: http://www.cdc.gov/OralHealth/infectioncontrol/guidelines/.
- World TB Day: www.cdc.gov/tb/WorldTBDay/default.htm

the community the dental office serves. The local public health office is the official agency that keeps the TB prevalence data for the local community. This agency can make IC recommendations (outlined by the CDC) to the dental office based on the degree of risk for TB being introduced in the dental office. If one of the dental staff tests positive for TB infection and active disease is ruled out, the physician may order the person to take a single anti-TB drug to prevent disease from developing. Generally, it is recommended that isoniazid (INH) be taken for 6 months, although other preventive drug regimens may be used. The staff worker with a positive Mantoux skin test and no symptoms of active disease is not contagious to other members of the dental office and cannot transmit TB.

Self-Study Review

7. Redness is not a sign of a positive Mantoux skin test. Induration at the skin test site is a sign of a positive test.
   a. Both statements are true.
   b. Both statements are false.
   c. The first statement is true, and the second statement is false.
   d. The first statement is false, and the second statement is true.

8. A client diagnosed with active TB taking appropriate medications, should not be treated by a dental provider for 6 months because this level of drug therapy is needed to ensure that the disease is not resistant to the antimicrobial agents and that the client is no longer contagious.
   a. Both the statement and reason are correct and related.
   b. Both the statement and reason are correct, but NOT related.
   c. The statement is correct, but the reason is NOT.
   d. The statement is NOT correct, but the reason is correct.
   e. NEITHER the statement NOR the reason is correct.

9. An office staff worker who has a positive Mantoux skin test and no symptoms of active TB disease is:
   a. not contagious and can continue working.
   b. not contagious, but cannot work for 3 weeks.
   c. is contagious and cannot work for 3 weeks.
   d. is contagious and may not work until the disease is controlled.

CHAPTER SUMMARY

Items on the ADA Health History Form are discussed regarding the relevance for their inclusion on the history form. This chapter highlighted screening questions and follow-up questions related to TB. Types of TB and dental management considerations were presented to identify individuals who may be infectious to others. Implications for oral HCWs who test positive on the screening test for TB were presented. Chapter 3 will include information on the next section of the ADA Health History Form that deals with the dental health history and current oral problems.

Review

1. Differentiate between TB infection and active TB disease.
2. List the screening questions to identify active TB recommended by the CDC.
3. Identify three etiologies of persistent cough.
4. Describe the criteria for determining noninfectious status in clients with active TB.

Case Study

Case A

Mr. Cameron, rehabilitation aide working at a local long-term care facility for the elderly and disabled, presents for a prophylaxis. During completion of the medical history, he approaches the reception desk and reports that he often has episodes of frequent coughing. He denies coughing of blood or having flu-like symptoms.

1. What follow-up questions would you ask to determine more information about the significance of this finding?
2. If the client reports night sweats and occasional temperature of 99°F to 100°F, would you proceed with dental treatment?
3. If the client was then tested and diagnosed with active TB, what protocol would you use for determining when oral health care could be performed?
4. If the client was then tested and diagnosed with TB infection, what protocol would you use for determining when oral health care could be performed?

Case B

Mary Myers presents to work having attended an Occupational Safety and Health Administration (OSHA) continuing education program. She is excited about what she has learned and suggests that the office staff have a screening test for TB. To her surprise, one of the receptionists tests positive on a Mantoux skin test.

1. If active disease is ruled out, is further treatment needed?
2. If medication was prescribed, list the most likely agent(s) and what would the duration have been?
3. When can the employee resume working?

Chapter Three

The Dental History

Objectives

After completing the self-study chapter the reader will be able to:

- Identify appropriate information needed from the client as it relates to the Dental Information section of the 2007 American Dental Association (ADA) Health History Form.
- Apply didactic information to determine treatment modifications based on responses provided by the client during the health history interview or from conditions found during the intraoral examination.
- Describe stress-related emergencies that can occur in treatment and management procedures to prevent or to resolve the emergency situations.

Key Terms

Blood dyscrasia: an abnormal condition where components of the blood contain an overabundance of certain cells, immature cells, or inadequate quantities of cellular elements, such as in leukemia or hemophilia.

Chief complaint: the client's current oral health problem, generally the reason for the client seeking oral health care

Crepitation: a clicking or popping sound as the jaw is opened

Dental caries: dental decay, a cavity

Etiology: the cause of any condition or disease

Historical information: information related to the past experiences in health care; often provides clues for causes of past problems

Hyperventilation: excessive intake of oxygen and exhalation of carbon dioxide; fast breathing often precipitated by anxiety

Periapical pathology: disease at the apex of the tooth (e.g., abscessed tooth)

Postural hypotension: reduction in blood pressure, usually as a result of a drug side effect; leading to loss of consciousness due to cerebral ischemia

Subluxation: movement of the condyle out of the normal maxillary joint space

Syncope: fainting; temporary loss of consciousness due to cerebral ischemia

Tetany: sharp flexion of the wrist and fingers, muscle twitches caused by a decrease in the concentration of extracellular calcium

TMJ: temporomandibular joint

Vasodepressor syncope: fainting

MEDICAL CONDITION

INTRODUCTION

The dental information section of the American Dental Association (ADA) Health History Form asks specific questions about the client's oral care history, access to fluoridated water, and the reason for the current dental appointment. Questions in this section relate to oral problems which may need treatment. However, one of the questions concerns problems with previous dental treatment. This question is intended to identify the client who may be at risk for a stress-related emergency situation. The discussion that follows each item from the ADA Health History Form includes appropriate follow-up questions, information on common stress-related emergencies that may occur during a dental appointment, and management procedures to prevent or to resolve them. This chapter will discuss the relationship of these questions to planning treatment for the oral care appointment.

DENTAL INFORMATION

It is important to consider information related to the client's perceived dental problems and past experience with oral care. The following questions on the ADA form provide an opportunity to (1) identify problems that may be related to oral disease, (2) develop a perception of the client's value for the teeth and regularity of oral health examination, and (3) determine problems experienced in the past during dental treatment. The information may prompt the clinician to look for oral conditions related to the questions asked; for example, "bleeding gums" prompts the clinician to assess gingival tissues and plaque control and design an individualized oral health education program. This information is also used to identify appropriate treatment modifications. In some cases, client responses may help the clinician to determine factors for client motivation that can be used to influence changes in the client's oral hygiene practices. Because of these issues, the discussion of a positive or "yes" response to questions in the dental information section of this text will include clinical application information. The reader should refer to clinical textbooks for a complete discussion of clinical issues related to the dental questions as it is not the purpose of this text to provide a complete discussion of clinical techniques and procedures. However, in those situations in which the question on the ADA History Form identifies appropriate modifications to the oral healthcare treatment plan, those modifications will be included.

"Do your gums bleed when you brush or floss?"

This question may identify bleeding associated with poor plaque control, the most common reason for bleeding gingiva. It is an excellent reason to support oral health education related to control of microbial plaque. In Maslow's hierarchy of needs, the statement "a satisfied need does not motivate" is made. When the client reports an unsatisfied need (bleeding gums), the clinician may be more successful in influencing a behavioral change to practice plaque control techniques. Follow-up questions might include "For how long have your gums been bleeding? Do you know why your gums bleed? Are you concerned about it? What have you done to resolve the condition?" The client may be persuaded to follow recommendations for more effective biofilm removal if the following question is used "Do you realize you have a bacterial infection affecting your gums?"

Application to Practice

Obviously, a positive answer to this question will cause the clinician to consider client responses to questioning and examine the periodontium for factors related to gingival bleeding. There are other, less common, reasons for bleeding gingivae, unrelated to bacteria. These may include pharmacologic reasons (taking anticoagulant medication or aspirin), traumatic injury to the soft tissues, or the presence of a systemic disease, that involves a **blood dyscrasia**. The clinician should search for reasons for the bleeding, while gathering historical information and clinical data related to possible causes during the periodontal examination.

"Are your teeth sensitive to cold, hot, sweets, or pressure?"

Sensitivity is a sign associated with the following conditions: caries, fractured teeth, **periapical pathology**, and exposed dentin.

Application to Practice

Ask the client to identify the specific area or tooth (teeth) involved, and investigate the area for etiologic factors. Percussing the cusp tips in an apical direction with the blunt end of an instrument, such as the mouth mirror handle, is often used to identify inflammation in the periodontal ligament of a tooth. Clinical examination of the occlusal, buccal, and lingual surfaces may identify caries, enamel fractures, or exposed root surfaces; all possible factors in sensitivity. Radiographs may be needed to evaluate periapical or alveolar bone tissues. Recent restorative treatment may have resulted in "high spots" that need attention. The clinician becomes a dental investigator to determine the cause of the pain. Additionally, exposed dentin on the root can be sensitive. A desensitizing dentifrice can be helpful to reduce dentin sensitivity and, when exposed root surfaces are present, is the appropriate oral health recommendation.

"Does food or floss catch between your teeth?"

Open embrasures or proximal tooth contacts promote food accumulation between teeth. This can develop from restorative procedures that do not restore normal anatomy of the contact area. Another common factor is pathological tooth movement (migration) following periodontal disease and loss of clinical attachment. Food impaction can occur, leading to additional trauma to periodontal fibers and bone loss. When floss catches between the teeth, the most likely **etiology** is an overhanging restoration. Extensive caries can be another potential cause.

Application to Practice

A positive response to this item indicates a need to determine the etiology of the issue. If restorative treatment is the causative factor, the client should be appointed for a dental examination and correction of the open contact area or replace the restoration, and thereby restoring the interproximal contact area. If periodontal disease has caused pathological migration, periodontal care should be recommended.

"Is your mouth dry?"

Dry mouth (also known as xerostomia) can develop from a variety of situations. The most common etiological factors are drug therapy and systemic diseases or disorders (e.g., diabetes mellitus, Sjögren syndrome). More than 400 medications can affect the salivary glands, causing them to produce less saliva. Radiation to the head and neck area can damage salivary gland function, leading to chronic dry mouth (xerostomia). Cancer treatment can reduce serous secretions, making mucoid secretions prevail and saliva thicker, causing the mouth to feel dry. Dry mouth can cause difficulties in tasting, chewing, swallowing, and speaking. It can lead to increased **dental caries** and oral fungal infection (candidiasis), resulting in oral discomfort. Dry mouth can be a sign of disease. The condition is associated with a burning sensation of mucosal tissues, possibly a manifestation of candidiasis. Saliva does more than keep tissues lubricated; it helps digest food, it helps control bacterial growth and fungal overgrowth in the mouth, it replenishes the minerals in the enamel, and it assists in chewing and swallowing.

Application to Practice

Dry mouth is not a normal part of aging and should be investigated for causative factors and associated oral effects. Chronic xerostomia often results in root caries. If increased dental caries is found, a home fluoride program should be recommended to reduce the risk for dental caries. Research reports the primary anticaries strategies are fluoride, sealants, and dietary practices that reduced the risk for caries.[1] Xylitol gum is an adjunctive recommendation for individuals at high risk for caries, as the noncariogenic sweetener has been shown to stimulate salivation, to reduce the levels of *Streptococcus mutans*, and to reduce the risk for caries.[1,2]

Research has shown that the root surface caries can be successfully treated with a chlorhexidine/thymol varnish.[1]

If the salivary glands are hyposecreting, the dentist can prescribe a medication to increase secretions (e.g., pilocarpine, cevimeline). These agents can be used for radiation-associated xerostomia and for managing discomfort from Sjögren syndrome. Artificial salivary agents are another option for the client with xerostomia.

Additionally, frequent sips of water to moisten oral tissues can be helpful.

"Have you had any periodontal (gum) treatments?"

A positive response to this question will identify the client with a history of periodontal disease. Periodontal disease can result in a loss of bone and gingival tissue. Exposed root surfaces can result after periodontal treatment. It is important to learn what the client knows about the causes of periodontal disease, oral hygiene measures to resolve the condition, and the need for frequent maintenance to keep the disease arrested or prevent further inflammation.

Application to Practice

During the periodontal examination the clinician will determine whether periodontal disease is arrested or has reoccurred. In addition, the clinician has the opportunity to learn what the client knows about the etiology of periodontal disease and the strategies to control the disease. After asking the client to explain his or her understanding of the disease process, the clinician can "fill in the gaps" and provide additional oral health information. An assessment must be made of the client's ability and desire to remove biofilm (also called plaque) on a daily basis. This is an excellent time to establish rapport, gain the trust of the client, and gather valuable information about the client's value for oral health.

"Have you ever had orthodontic (braces) treatment?"

This question provides information for consideration during the examination of the periodontium, assessment of the occlusion, and related effects on the temporomandibular joint (TMJ) area. A systematic review of studies to assess the effects of orthodontic therapy suggested that orthodontic therapy is associated with gingival recession, small amounts of alveolar bone loss, and increased pocket depth when compared to no treatment.[3] Follow-up questioning would include "Have your appliances been removed? Do you have a permanent lingual bar? Are any teeth loose?" The responses to these questions might affect the clinical treatment plan.

Application to Practice

A positive response to these questions requires the consideration of several issues related to wearing orthodontic appliances. These include:

1. Assessing periodontal health, including gingival inflammation, gingival recession, clinical attachment loss, and exposed root surfaces.
2. Examining the occlusion, noting missing teeth, and assessing **TMJ** function.
3. Determining whether decalcification is present and implementing strategies to address clinical features, such as fluoride therapies, sealant application, the use of selective polishing for stain removal, and selection of appropriate nonabrasive polishing agents.
4. Assessing aids needed for personal plaque control.
5. Formulating alterations in instrumentation techniques, if appliances are present; or taking radiographs to determine effects of tooth movement on the tooth root.
6. Determining how all these factors can be used in an oral health education plan individualized to the client's specific needs (Box 3-1).

Box 3-1

Clinical Considerations of Orthodontic Treatment

- Examine occlusion, missing teeth, TMJ dysfunction
- Gingival recession, exposed root surfaces
- Decalcification, fluoride therapy, selective polishing, low abrasive polishing agents
- Plaque removal aids
- Instrumentation alterations, radiographic assessment
- Oral health education topics individualized to needs

Orthodontic treatment is intended to result in optimal occlusion; however, all clients may not achieve this goal. There may be a variety of changes in the dentition as a result of wearing orthodontic appliances. These changes listed below may need to be addressed in therapy.

DISCUSSION OF CLINICAL CONSIDERATIONS

1. Assessing gingival features, recession, clinical attachment level, and exposed root surfaces: Difficulty in removing biofilm from orthodontic brackets, wires, and appliances may

influence the development of chronic gingival inflammation, leading to attachment loss. A thorough periodontal assessment must be completed following placement of orthodontic appliances and monitored periodically with probing. Gingival recession involving mandibular anterior teeth may be present if teeth were moved out of the facial bone during orthodontic movement. Clinical issues include enamel demineralization, root caries, and sensitivity of root surfaces. Exposed root surfaces are at increased risk for root caries, and a fluoride program or placement of chlorhexidine/thymol varnish should be recommended to reduce this risk.[1] Exposed dentin is often sensitive. The client should be questioned regarding the locations of sensitive areas and care taken to avoid instrumenting these areas until a desensitizing agent has been applied. A desensitizing dentifrice may be helpful to reduce dentin sensitivity. Exposed root surfaces should not be polished with an abrasive prophylaxis paste and rubber cup polishing as tooth structure can be abraded and removed. Additionally, a nontraumatic toothbrushing method with a dentifrice having a low abrasion particle size should be recommended to prevent abrasion on exposed root surfaces.

2. Examining the occlusion, missing teeth, and TMJ function: The occlusion should be classified and checked for bruxism and occlusal irregularities, such as an open bite or anterior overbite. First premolar teeth are often removed in orthodontic treatment to make room for the remaining dentition. Missing teeth may result in occlusal irregularities. During TMJ examination, the clinician may find abnormal movements of the mandibular condyle as it moves forward in the fossa (**subluxation**) or a clicking sound may be heard as the client opens and closes the mouth (**crepitation**). The etiology of these signs is often related to abnormal occlusion or occlusal irregularities. When these signs occur and no pain associated with them is reported, generally no treatment is recommended. If pain occurs, referring the client to a dentist who specializes in correcting occlusal irregularities and abnormal TMJ function should be considered.
3. Determining whether decalcification is present: Examine the teeth for white areas of decalcification where appliances were placed. When decalcification is found, a fluoride program should be recommended that includes an in-office fluoride treatment and a daily home fluoride product.[4] Currently new dental products are being investigated that involve increased remineralization of enamel with amorphous calcium phosphate products. These products are not recommended by the ADA for caries prevention.[1] In-office fluoride products have a higher concentration of fluoride and are used sporadically, whereas the home fluoride products have a low concentration of fluoride and are used more frequently. Oral health education information should include the role of decalcification in the etiology of dental caries and the role of fluoride in reversing this demineralization. Decalcified areas should not be polished with a rubber cup and abrasive polishing agent because more enamel is removed from decalcified areas with this procedure. A selective polishing technique is indicated to avoid further harm to decalcified areas.
4. Assessing plaque control aids: Daily plaque removal around orthodontic appliances may be tedious for the client and require innovative oral hygiene aids. Toothbrushes are available with a reduced bristle height in the midline of the brush head to accommodate orthodontic wires. Interproximal brushes can be used around bands and arch wires. Floss threaders may be helpful to assist interproximal cleaning. Oral irrigation (Waterpik) was originally designed for the orthodontic client. Gingival health must be monitored for gingivitis and gingival hyperplasia caused by chronic irritation from bacterial plaque.
5. Treatment plan alterations for instrumentation and radiographs: Orthodontic appliances may require alterations in the adaptation of instruments during hard deposit removal. The design of the band and wire placement used in orthodontics may require a change in the polishing technique used to remove stains. The type of band adhesive must be considered when selecting a product for the topical fluoride application at the end of the appointment. If a bonding technique is used to attach bands to teeth, a neutral sodium fluoride is recommended. Other in-office fluoride products, such as sodium fluoride varnish, might be indicated. The current ADA recommendation is to use fluoride varnish for professionally applied fluoride treatment in children younger than 6 years.[4] Either varnish or gel (either APF or NaF) is appropriate for children aged ≥ 6 years who are at moderate to

high risk for caries. Radiographic examination might reveal external resorption of roots that occurs when teeth are moved too quickly. This results in shortened, "ice cream cone"–shaped roots that makes the tooth loose. The client who has had orthodontic treatment may experience some of the conditions described above.

6. Individualize the oral health education plan according to the needs of the client: Using the data obtained during the clinical examination for the items listed on previous page, the clinician will develop a care plan that addresses the specific needs of the client. When planning oral health care for the orthodontic patient, this self-study reference guides the reader to find official guidelines for various issues and supplements clinical practice textbooks.

Self-Study Review

1. From the following list, identify the four reasons for gingival bleeding during toothbrushing.
   a. Poor plaque control
   b. Periodontal therapy
   c. Orthodontic treatment
   d. Daily use of aspirin therapy
   e. Trauma
   f. Blood dyscrasia
   g. Fluoride therapy
   h. Root caries
2. Xerostomia is a common finding associated with the aging process. This condition often results in an increase in caries.
   a. Both statements are true.
   b. Both statements are false.
   c. The first statement is true, and the second statement is false.
   d. The first statement is false, and the second statement is true.
3. A client presents with exposed root surfaces in the maxillary right posterior sextant. This finding most likely represents:
   a. a past history of periodontal surgery.
   b. evidence of dental decay.
   c. a need for oral health education.
   d. fear of dental treatment.
4. It is safe to use a rubber cup and polishing agent in areas that are decalcified because plaque removal will promote remineralization of the enamel.
   a. Both the statement and reason are correct and related.
   b. Both the statement and reason are correct, but NOT related.
   c. The statement is correct, but the reason is NOT.
   d. The statement is NOT correct, but the reason is correct.
   e. NEITHER the statement NOR the reason is correct.
5. From the following list, identify the clinical findings associated with orthodontia.
   a. Enamel demineralization
   b. Tooth sensitivity
   c. TMJ dysfunction
   d. External root resorption
   e. Root caries
   f. Bruxism
   g. Gingival recession
   h. Xerostomia

"Have you had any problems associated with previous dental treatment? If so, explain."

This question may identify the client at risk for a stress-related medical emergency during treatment. Those clients having anxiety or fear of dental treatment are most likely to fail to use dental services, often have more severe oral disease, and are at an increased risk to have an emergency situation during oral health care.[5] This is the only question on the Dental History section of the ADA Health History Form that may identify a risk for an emergency during treatment. Stress-related medical emergencies are the most common emergency situations to occur in the dental office. If the problems described by the client involve something the clinician can avoid, such as avoiding the application of compressed air on sensitive dentin (and the subsequent pain), the necessary precautions should be taken. Whatever information the client provides must be considered, and plans made to avoid repeating the problem. The most common emergencies experienced during dental treatment involve **syncope**, **hyperventilation**, and **postural hypotension**. Both syncope and hyperventilation are associated with anxiety and fear and will be discussed in association with this dental history item. There are other causes of syncope that may involve other factors. When syncope occurs and the precipitating factors are unknown, after recovery, the client should be advised to seek medical evaluation. Postural hypotension is most often related to drug side effects and will be discussed in the section of the ADA History Form that involves current medications that are taken. The next section will discuss possible emergency situations related to fear and anxiety and the appropriate management for each emergency.

STRESS-RELATED EMERGENCIES

Stress plays a significant role in precipitating medical emergency situations during dental treatment. Clients may fear having oral procedures or they may fear the possibility of suffering pain during procedures. Clients who have a history of requesting dental appointments only for emergency treatment, or those who often cancel or do not meet scheduled appointments, may do so because of anxiety or a stress disorder. This possibility should be investigated during the follow-up of this medical history question. If the clinician can gain the confidence and trust of the client, and help the client relax, this may reduce the anxiety level. Other stress reduction strategies include

1. Discussion of client interests during treatment (distraction strategy) and relaxation.[6]
2. Use of careful technique or a local anesthetic to prevent pain or injury.
3. Nitrous oxide sedation to provide analgesia and promote relaxation.
4. Prescription of antianxiety drugs (Box 3-2).

Box 3-2

Stress Reduction Strategies

- Discuss topics that occupy client's mind
- Ensure adequate pain control
- Consider nitrous oxide conscious sedation
- Prescribe an antianxiety drug

Stress Reduction Strategies

In some cases, talking with the client about personal interests (hobbies, vacations, children, and so forth) during the oral procedure is enough to keep the client's mind occupied from the treatment, facilitating a coping mechanism for anxiety. In addition, relaxation methods have been shown to reduce anxiety in moderate to highly anxious dental patients.[6] *It is essential that pain control and gentle technique be used to supplement "occupation of the mind" strategies.* Nitrous oxide is a gas that relaxes an individual and has been used with success to reduce anxiety. It also reduces pain sensation and is called "conscious analgesia." It requires specialized equipment that is not found in all dental offices. Antianxiety drugs are commonly used to reduce stress-related emergency situations. A dentist can prescribe an antianxiety drug to clients who are very anxious or fearful and seem to be at risk for a stress-related emergency. These strategies are used to prevent emergency situations in the client identified as "at risk"; however, the health history may not always identify the client who will experience a stress-related emergency. Clients may not reveal having a fear of dental treatment. The clinician must be a keen observer of client behavior indicating anxiety. Rapid breathing, pale facial color or perspiration, or hands clutching the arms of the chair are signs of anxiety. When evidence of anxiety is observed, oral treatment should be delayed. This is a sign to talk with the client about the cause for anxiety. It may help to reassure the client that it is permissible to stop treatment procedures at any time. Pain control options, such as nitrous oxide analgesia, topical anesthesia, or injectable local anesthesia, should be offered. The client needs to believe that the clinician has empathy for the client's feelings.

Vasodepressor syncope (often referred to as fainting) and hyperventilation are two common stress-related emergencies that can be experienced in the healthy dental client.

Vasodepressor Syncope

The most common emergency in the dental office is syncope or fainting[7]. It involves a brief loss of consciousness due to a lack of oxygenated blood flow to the brain (cerebral ischemia) that results after a loss of blood pressure. There are several types of syncope; however, this discussion will include the syncopal episode that most often occurs in the dental office. The most common precipitating event is stress and anxiety, often as a result of fear of a local anesthetic injection.[7] *Syncope associated with dental treatment always occurs when the client is in an upright position.* The situation starts with a response of the sympathetic nervous system, as part of the "flight or fight" response. Sympathetic response causes a vasodilation in skeletal muscles, and blood is diverted to this area. If the skeletal muscles are used (e.g., walking, running), the blood returns normally to the heart and is oxygenated, and cardiac output supplies adequate oxygen to the brain. In this situation, unconsciousness is avoided. For the client seated in a dental chair and not using skeletal muscles, the blood pools in the extremities and venous blood return to the heart is significantly reduced (less blood to be oxygenated in the lungs). This reduction leads to a compensatory slowing of the heart rate (bradycardia), reduced cardiac output, and vasodilation of blood vessels. This vasodilation and associated events lead to hypotension and inability of the cardiovascular system to push oxygenated blood to the brain.[8] It usually can be resolved easily by placing the client in a prone position so that gravity promotes the brain receiving oxygenated blood and by assuring an open airway. Having the client lift the feet and push on a stable surface (e.g., your hands) to promote skeletal muscle activation will assist in venous return of blood to the heart (Fig. 3.1).

Predisposing Factors

There are two predisposing factors that may result in syncope during oral care. The most common factor is due to psychogenic reasons, such as fear and anxiety. The other factor relates to placing the client in an upright position for treatment. The dental procedure most likely to result in syncope is receiving an injection of local anesthetic.[7] Observing the facial color (pale, perspiration) and body posture (clutching arms of chair, trembling) may identify a nervous, anxious individual. The "white knuckle syndrome" is characterized by grasping the arms of the dental chair tightly and exhibiting either fast, incessant talking or unusual silence. Psychogenic factors include such things as feeling fearful or anxious, experiencing sudden and unexpected pain, and the sight of blood. A common contributing factor for syncope is being placed in an upright position for treatment. The risk for syncope is increased in an anxious client seated in the upright position.[7] Other nonpsychogenic reasons include standing for long periods of time, lack of food or hunger, hypoglycemia, poor physical condition, and hot environments. These are infrequent reasons for syncope during oral health care. Syncope during oral health care is most likely to occur in men and in the young adult age group, as they may be trying to hide their fear. Children and elderly clients are less likely to experience syncope during oral health care as they are unlikely to suppress anxious feelings. Children will cry and act out their anxiety, whereas older adult or elderly patients are more likely to inform the clinician of their apprehensions.[7]

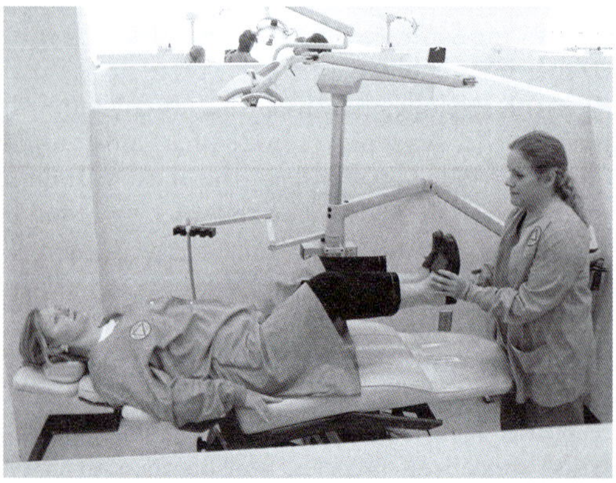

Figure 3.1 ■ Clinical photograph of positioning for syncope management.

Stages of Syncope

Stages of syncope include the pre-syncope period, the loss of consciousness in the syncope event, and the post-syncope stage. Signs and symptoms of the *pre-syncope* period include facial paleness, perspiration and feelings of warmth, possible feelings of nausea, and an increased pulse rate. If the clinician observes these signs and quickly places the client in a supine position, loss of consciousness can be averted. Signs and symptoms immediately before unconsciousness from syncope can include yawning, dilated pupils (indicating cerebral ischemia), feeling cold, dizziness, and experiencing hypotension.[9] After the client loses consciousness, supine positioning of the client and elevating the feet to assist venous return of blood to the heart usually promotes a return to consciousness within 1 to 2 minutes. Both the pulse rate and blood pressure will be low. During the post-syncopal period, the client may experience facial pallor, nausea, weakness, and disorientation. As the client recovers, the blood pressure and heart rate slowly return to normal (Box 3-3).

Strategies for Prevention

In clients who have a history of fainting during local anesthetic administration, a preventive strategy might include placing the client in a supine position for local anesthesia administration. In addition, management should include behaviors to avert the client's mind from "having a shot," such as shaking the individual's cheek during the injection. The client may be thinking, "Why is she shaking my cheek?" then the clinician says, "Well,

Box 3-3

Signs of Vasodepressor Syncope

Pre-syncope:	Facial paleness Perspiration, feelings of warmth Nausea Increased pulse rate
Syncope:	Yawning Dilated pupils Feeling cold Dizziness Hypotension Low pulse rate
Post-syncope	Facial pallor Nausea Weakness Disorientation

that's over, are you doing okay?" The client will be surprised and delighted the injection is over and he or she did not even know it was being given! This is a comforting thought to anxious clients. Some offices offer headsets so the client can listen to music, as a strategy to divert attention from the injection. As described in the discussion of syncope, the clinician must be observant for signs that precede syncope and place the client in a supine position to avert loss of consciousness.

Management

For the client who faints while seated in an upright position, the chair back should be lowered and the client placed in a supine position, while elevating the legs.[8] In the past a position with the head lower than the heart, called the *Trendelenburg position*, was used. However, it was found that this position can restrict respiration and diminish the effectiveness of breathing.[7] The Trendelenburg position is more appropriately used to manage airway obstruction.[7] Basic life support should be provided (e.g., monitor airway, breathing, and circulation). Oxygen is administered, as needed. Ammonia inhalants can be used to stimulate consciousness if recovery seems prolonged. Consciousness should return quickly (Box 3-4). Ammonia causes a burning of the nasal mucosa, resulting in a rapid return to consciousness. Monitor vital signs and, following recovery, record this information in the treatment record along with a description of the emergency, the dental procedure that precipitated it, and how the situation was resolved. On recovery, it is essential to determine whether treatment can continue. The client should remain in a supine position until recovery is complete, as the client has an increased risk of fainting again. In some instances, the client may not feel like continuing with treatment, and the appointment will need to be rescheduled. Occasionally, the client will ask to continue with treatment. When normal vital sign levels return, there is no contraindication to continuing with dental hygiene treatment; however, the clinician should observe client behavior for signs of a recurrent episode of syncope. Should this occur, treatment should be suspended, the client placed in a supine position for recovery, and the appointment rescheduled. For future appointments, the clinician should consider whether the client would benefit from oral antianxiety medication, for example, diazepam (Valium). When the dentist prescribes antianxiety medication, instructions should be given to the client, including:

Box 3-4

Management of Syncope

- Place client in supine position with feet raised
- Monitor vital signs, assure open airway, breathing, and circulation
- Observe for recovery
- Administer oxygen or ammonia stimulants for prolonged recovery

1. To have someone drive him or her to and from the dental appointment.
2. To refrain from making important business or personal decisions.
3. To refrain from operating hazardous equipment during the day the medication was taken.

After any adverse event with a dental client, the clinician should make contact to ensure the client recovered. This can be done by calling the client at home the evening after the appointment.

Hyperventilation

Hyperventilation, also referred to as hyperventilation syndrome, is characterized by rapid breathing that results in excessive loss of carbon dioxide and inspiration of too much oxygen, disrupting the CO_2–O_2 balance in the blood. This CO_2–O_2 imbalance causes a transient respiratory alkalosis. The client remains conscious until the late stages of the event, if not reversed. It represents the second most common stress-related medical emergency to occur in dentistry.

Predisposing Factors

Fear and anxiety are common precipitating factors in the dental setting. The release of adrenalin as part of the flight or fight response of the sympathetic nervous system plays a role.[10] *A previous history of hyperventilation during dental treatment is a clue in anticipating this emergency.* The period after receiving an injection of a local anesthetic is the most common time for initiation of signs of hyperventilation.[10] Similar to individuals predisposed to syncope, generally, the young adult is most likely to experience hyperventilation. The client who admits to fear and anxiety is least likely to experience hyperventilation, for example, children or older clients.[7]

Signs and Symptoms

Some clients have obvious symptoms of increased respiration when suffering a "panic attack." Others have more subtle signs. The client may complain of lightheadedness or dizziness, altered consciousness, chest discomfort, or nausea. Trembling, sweating, and heart palpitations may be reported. These signs result from the sympathetic stress response. Numbness of the face and **tetany** of the fingers commonly result. Clients may gasp for breath as respirations approach levels of 60 breaths per minute.[10]

Prevention

When an overly anxious client is identified, management procedures to prevent hyperventilation include:

1. Talking with the client to reassure and build confidence.
2. Offering pain control options, such as those identified in the syncope discussion.
3. Offering antianxiety medication [diazepam (Valium)] prior to future appointments.

The same signs of stress, as were identified in the syncope discussion, apply to identifying the client at risk for hyperventilation (e.g., talkative or very quiet, nervous, white knuckle syndrome).

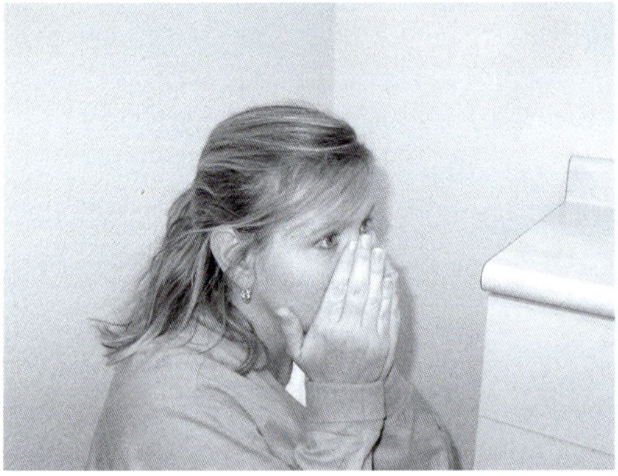

Figure 3.2. ■ Clinical photograph of positioning for hyperventilation management.

Management

The client should be placed in an upright position and instructed to cup the hands over the mouth to rebreathe the expired carbon dioxide gas (Fig. 3.2). Verbal instructions to consciously try to slow the rate of breathing and to try to relax may be helpful to the client. Have the client breathe as you count and follow your guidance slowing the breathing rate. An alternative procedure to cupping the hands over the mouth is to have the client breathe into a paper bag.[9] This would not be done if the client has COPD, or cardiac disease as the symptom may be unrelated to stress, and a manifestation of a cardiac disorder. *Do not administer oxygen during this emergency because the client is getting excessive amounts of oxygen with increased respiration.* After normal breathing patterns are achieved, vital signs should be measured and values recorded in the treatment record; along with a description of the emergency, when it occurred in the treatment sequence, how it was managed, and how long before normal breathing was restored (Box 3-5). When breathing has returned to normal levels, a discussion should follow with the client regarding whether treatment should continue or be postponed to another day. The dentist may decide to delay the appointment and prescribe antianxiety medication. If this is the decision, safety instructions, described above regarding the antianxiety medication, should be provided.

"Is your home water supply fluoridated? Do you drink bottled or filtered water? If yes, how often—daily, weekly, occasionally?"

This item provides a basis for fluoride recommendations.

Box 3-5

Management of Hyperventilation

- Raise chair back to upright position, reassure client
- Guide client to try to slow the rate of breathing
- Have client cup hands over mouth
- Instruct client to rebreathe expired air
- Monitor vital signs and record values in treatment record
- Record description, duration, and description of management information of emergency

Application to Practice

In situations in which there is adequate community water fluoridation, and the client reports drinking water from the community supply, additional fluoride is not indicated in treatment. In individuals who have a low risk for caries, additional fluoride supplementation may not be beneficial. Fluoridated water and fluoride dentifrice may provide adequate caries prevention in the low-risk category.[4] On the other hand, both children and adults who are at a moderate to high risk for caries may benefit from additional fluoride, both in drinking water and in topically applied products (e.g., dentifrice, gels, rinses). Fluoride supplementation guidelines are available from the ADA.[11] Prenatal fluoride supplements and fluoride supplements for children/adolescents are not recommended, except for older children in low water fluoridated areas.[12]

"Are you currently experiencing dentally related discomfort?"

This item may relate to the reason the client is seeking oral care. The client's chief concern should always be addressed early in the treatment plan.

Application to Practice

Follow-up questioning would identify the type of pain being experienced and the area(s) involved. Based on a clinical examination and the experience of the clinician, a collection of possible findings would be provided and used to determine how to manage the discomfort. In some instances, especially if the discomfort relates to periodontal inflammation or obvious caries, the clinician would be able to identify the etiology of the discomfort and provide adequate direction to resolve the condition.

"Do you have headaches, earaches, or neck pains?"

When a positive response is made, an appropriate follow-up question is "Do you know what is causing the pain?" Responses such as "osteoarthritis" or "migraines" are common reasons for head and neck pain, but the cause could be dental infection, muscle spasm associated with bruxism, or other reasons.

Application to Practice

In situations in which the client does not know the cause of head or neck pain and no obvious dental infection is found, occlusion-related problems, such as bruxism and TMJ muscle hypercontraction, should be considered. During the examination of the occlusion, the centric relationship should be noted; as well as open bites, cross bites, and lateral excursion interferences. The muscles of mastication should be palpated for pain and examined clinically. A prominent masseter muscle may signify frequent bruxing or clenching of teeth. A client having these problems should be referred to a dentist with experience in treating occlusion abnormalities. Earaches and neck aches can have a variety of etiologies, so the clinician should examine the mouth and radiographs for evidence of periapical pathology, such as an abscessed tooth, especially in the mandibular area of the side affected. In this instance, the infection may move from the periapical area into the adjacent structures. This event can manifest as pain in the neck and ear area.

"Do you have any clicking, popping, or discomfort in the jaw?"

This item on the health history relates to malocclusion, and associated oral problems; or to osteoarthritis, generally found in older individuals.

Application to Practice

Questioning should include when the clicking event occurs (often referred to as crepitation) and factors that promote the occurrence. As was discussed previously in the item related to orthodontic appliances, occlusal irregularities should be investigated. Whatever information is discovered in the questioning and examination of the TMJ should be provided to the dentist for management.

"Do you brux or grind your teeth?"

Clenching and bruxism (e.g., grinding of teeth) are other signs of malocclusion.

Application to Practice

Follow-up questioning should include if the client bruxes during the night. A common solution for nocturnal bruxism is for the dentist to fabricate a night guard to wear during sleep. This appliance prohibits tooth to tooth contact and opens the bite so that the muscles to the TMJ are not traumatized. This item should be associated with other questions that involve malocclusion, including "headaches, earaches, and tooth sensitivity."

"Do you have sores or ulcers in your mouth?"

A positive response for this item should be followed up by identifying the lesion.

Application to Practice

Oral herpetic vesicles or ulcerations may contraindicate continuing with treatment. Oral herpetic lesions in the prodromal stages, the vesicular stage, or in the crusted stage signify a contraindication to continuing with oral care because they are infectious. The viral organisms within the lesion can be a source for operator infection (e.g., ocular herpetic infection, herpetic whitlow) when barrier protection fails.

"Do you wear dentures or partials?"

A positive response requires oral examination related to the type of removable appliance. The appliance should fit and function properly to allow for eating various foods.

Application to Practice

The clinician should determine how well the appliance fits and examine the teeth and soft tissue under the appliance for pathology. Two common pathologic conditions associated with an ill-fitting removable partial denture include dental caries (where clasps contact tooth surfaces) and a soft tissue fungal infection and tissue response (papillary hyperplasia). Figure 3.3 shows the clinical appearance of this soft tissue condition. If soft tissue pathology consistent with papillary hyperplasia is found, the client should be informed and referred to a dentist,

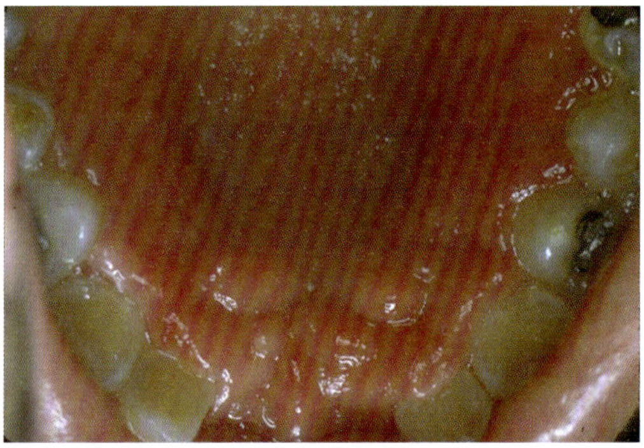

Figure 3.3 ■ Clinical photograph of papillary hyperplasia and candida infection under removable partial.

as generally the appliance must be relined or reconstructed to resolve the condition. The dentist will prescribe an antifungal agent to treat the soft tissue and to kill the fungal organism on the removable appliance. Oral health information includes

1. Warning the client to take the appliance out of the mouth every day and let them choose which time of day works best. Some authorities suggest appliances should be removed while sleeping.
2. Instructions on cleaning the appliance and abutment teeth.
3. Instructions to use a home fluoride product (rinse or gel) to prevent caries on abutment teeth.
4. If the client has missing teeth NOT replaced by a dental appliance, the oral health education program should include the benefits of replacing missing teeth with a dental appliance or an implant.

"Have you ever had a serious injury to your head or mouth?"

This item has a variety of possible clinical implications, depending on the severity of the event. The most obvious clinical implication is missing teeth from a traumatic blow to the mouth. Other traumatic events could involve a broken jaw and associated oral problems. The complete history related to the event should be elicited from the client and communicated to the dentist. A clinical examination for oral issues would be included.

"Date of your last dental examination."

The clinician should consider the dental habits of the client. If the client has not had regular, annual dental examinations, it is likely that there will be extensive dental disease. As was discussed earlier, fear of receiving oral care may be a reason for lack of using dental care.[5] During the oral health education program, the client should be informed that more frequent oral examinations might identify disease early. Early treatment allows the condition to be treated more easily, with less discomfort and with less cost than allowing the disease to become advanced. Advanced dental disease may require more costly treatment (endodontics, crown and bridge preparation, implants, or prosthetic appliance fabrication). Many clients will want to have nonpainful, low-cost dental treatment, so these may be strong influential factors to use when stimulating client motivation.

"What was done at that time?"

The clinician would examine the areas treated and provide the client with indicated follow-up care. This **historical information** also may provide information that may be important in treatment planning. For example, if fixed bridgework was placed, the clinician would want to inspect the appliance and assess the client's ability to clean abutment teeth. Another example relates to reports of previous treatment for oral cysts, tumors, or malignancies. In this situation, the area treated should be examined to determine if recurrence has developed.

"Date of last dental X-rays."

The need for dental radiographs is based on an evidence of need following a clinical examination.[13] Although a recent systematic review of the evidence[13] no longer recommends routinely taking radiographs without first completing a clinical examination, knowledge of when the most recent radiographs were taken can be useful. For example, if the client reports having a full series of radiographs within the past year that were taken at another facility, the clinician should try to get a copy of the films to use in oral evaluation. This reduces the radiation exposure to the client. If the client reports several years since dental radiographs were taken, and the oral examination reveals dental disease or suspicious dental disease, there is adequate rationale for exposing the client to radiation for dental purposes. If the client is new to the dental practice and has not had dental radiographs for several years, but no evidence of oral disease is present, the dentist may decide dental radiographs are necessary. This establishes baseline information to be used as a basis for comparison with future situations that might develop. The risk of exposing the client to ionizing radiation and whether it is in the client's best interests should be a major consideration in determining a need for radiographs. Box 3-6 summarizes patient selection criteria for dental radiographs.

BOX 3-6

Patient Selection Criteria for Dental X-Rays

- A clinical examination should precede the decision to take dental X-rays.
- Exposures should be limited to the fewest number needed for diagnosis.
- Factors to consider: age, dental developmental stage (primary dentition, transitional dentition, adolescent with permanent dentition, dentate adult, partially edentulous adult or edentulous adult).
- Clinical circumstances (symptomatic or asymptomatic)
- New patient or continuing care (recall) patient
- Risk factors for caries or dental disease.

"What is the reason for your dental visit today?"

This portion of the ADA Health History provides information related to the client's dental problem, sometimes referred to as the chief complaint. This should be described in the client's own words to reflect the oral concerns as the client perceives them.

Application to Practice

The clinician should address the chief complaint early in the treatment plan, generally during the initial appointment. Occasionally the clinician may find other oral disease that should be addressed before resolving the problem reported by the client. When this happens, the clinician should explain the logical sequence of treatment and identify which part of the treatment plan will address the client's **chief complaint**.

"How do you feel about your smile or appearance of your teeth?"

The dialog associated with this question may provide a clue to the client's value of oral and dental health. The answer may depend on the client's perception of what is being asked and why. One client may reply, "They are too yellow," revealing a value for outward appearance and a desire to whiten the teeth. The unsatisfied need is to have whiter teeth to look better, identifying this client's motivational factor. Others may say, "I have cavities and my teeth hurt," revealing they know there is disease present.

Application to Practice

The motivational factor for this client may be in oral health behaviors that will reduce pain in the future. Whatever the client reports, the clinician should attempt to analyze the unsatisfied need and determine to what extent the client values oral health. These factors should be used to influence client motivation toward good oral health and dietary practices. Eliminating between meal snacks and having fermentable carbohydrates only at mealtimes have been shown to reduce the risk for caries.[14] The clinician can follow up information provided with questions, such as "Do you hope to keep your teeth all your life?" The answer may provide an opportunity for oral health education on how to maintain teeth for the lifetime.

Self-Study Review

6. The most common emergency in the dental office is:
   a. airway blockage.
   b. hypertension.
   c. hyperventilation.
   d. syncope.
7. All of the following techniques may be used to reduce stress during oral health treatment EXCEPT one. Which one is the EXCEPTION?
   a. Distraction
   b. Antianxiety medication
   c. Postpone the procedure
   d. Conscious analgesia
8. Should a client experience syncope:
   a. place in an upright position with the head between his/her knees.
   b. lower the chair back and place the client in a supine position.
   c. place the client in the Trendelenburg position.
   d. raise the chair so the client's head is higher than the heart.
9. Facial pallor, nausea, and disorientation are signs of which type of syncope?
   a. Pre-syncope
   b. Syncope
   c. Syncope just before loss of consciousness
   d. Post-syncope
10. The client most likely to experience hyperventilation during an oral health appointment is the:
    a. child.
    b. teenager or young adult.
    c. mature adult.
    d. older adult.
11. A prominent masseter muscle usually indicates:
    a. bruxism.
    b. ear infection.
    c. neoplasia.
    d. previous orthodontia.
12. What is the term that refers to the client's reason for his/her dental or dental hygiene visit?
    a. Dental problem
    b. Chief complaint
    c. Unsatisfied need
    d. Motivational influence

CHAPTER SUMMARY

This chapter discusses items related to the dental history and experiencing problems with previous dental procedures. Identification and management of common stress-related emergencies, including syncope and hyperventilation, were discussed with the dental history question related to identifying previous stress-related emergency situations. The importance of recognizing anxiety and offering stress reduction protocols was emphasized as a means of preventing stress-related emergencies. The importance of the dental history and criteria for selecting patients for receiving dental X-rays are identified. The next chapter will begin the examination of medical information and the client's current health situation.

Review

1. Define the following terms: hyperventilation and vasodepressor syncope.
2. Explain why oxygen is contraindicated when managing hyperventilation.
3. Describe the significance of the client's chief complaint.
4. Identify three strategies for reducing a client's stress during oral health treatment.
5. List the signs and symptoms of pre-syncope, syncope, and post-syncope.
6. List the patient selection criteria for dental radiographs.

Case Study

Case A

Harry Carpenter, a 13-year-old client, presents to the dental office for a prophylaxis. The client grips the arms of the dental chair tightly during the oral examination and while radiographs are performed. As the dental hygienist begins the prophylaxis, she notices that John's breathing is rapid and shallow. His pulse is 80 bpm, respiration is 40 breaths/min, and blood pressure is 100/60 mm Hg, sitting, right arm.

1. What is the most likely diagnosis for the rapid breathing of the client?
2. If the rapid breathing is left untreated, what condition may result next?
3. List two techniques for treating this client's condition.
4. Describe what information should be placed in the dental record regarding this emergency situation.

Case B

Bradford Johnson, a 35-year-old client, presents for periodontal treatment. Initial vital signs include pulse 76 bpm, respiration 22 breaths/min, and blood pressure 120/80 mm Hg, right arm, sitting. A graft procedure is planned for the mandibular facial incisor area. As the dentist begins to apply a topical anesthetic in preparation for administration of local anesthesia, he notices that the client has become pale, is perspiring, and is breathing rapidly. The dentist inquires whether the client is anxious about receiving an injection, and the client responds in the negative. The dentist proceeds to pick up the needle, turns to the client, and notices that the client has lost consciousness.

1. What is the name for the loss of consciousness the client experienced?
2. What is the most likely cause of this loss of consciousness?
3. What is the physiologic cause of this loss of consciousness?
4. What emergency treatment would you provide given this situation?
5. Why is the Trendelenburg position contraindicated for treatment of this condition?

Chapter Four

Medical Information and Current Drug Therapy

Objectives

After completing the self-study chapter the reader will be able to:

- Identify the types of information needed to determine the client's physical health status.
- Discuss the importance of obtaining significant recent health information concerning illnesses and hospitalizations.
- Discuss the reasons for investigating drug therapy as part of the health history review.
- Identify the clinical relevance of effects of pharmacologic products to the oral healthcare treatment plan.
- Identify the side effects of medications that pose a risk for medical emergencies.
- Identify the five elements that must be considered when evaluating the types of prescription and nonprescription medications or supplements clients are taking.
- Describe prevention and management procedures for side effects that are likely to result in a medical emergency during oral health care.

Key Terms

Aggregation: process of clumping together, as in platelets forming a clot

Agranulocytosis: an acute disease characterized by a dramatic decrease in the production of granulocytes, causing pronounced neutropenia and leaving the body defenseless against bacterial invasion; often caused by a sensitization to drugs or chemicals that affect the bone marrow and depress the formation of granulocytes

Blood dyscrasia: an alteration in blood cell levels, can include white blood cells, red blood cells, or platelets

Leukopenia: reduction in the number of leukocytes (white blood cells) in the blood with the count being 5,000 or less

Neutropenia: a diminished number of neutrophils in the blood

Postural hypotension: reduction in blood pressure that results from drug-induced vasodilation

Thrombocytopenia: a decrease in the number of platelets in circulating blood

MEDICAL CONDITION

INTRODUCTION

The medical information section includes questions related to current medical therapy and the client's perception of his or her current health status. In the chapters that follow, each medical condition in the American Dental Association (ADA) Health History Form will be discussed and the clinical implications identified. For those medical conditions that could involve a medical emergency, the emergency will be identified along with a discussion regarding steps the clinician should take to prevent the emergency. Should the emergency situation develop, in spite of the clinician's efforts, the management for the emergency will be provided.

"Are you now under the care of a physician? If yes, what condition is being treated?"

A positive response to this item requires determining the medical condition for which the client is receiving care. The dialog described by the client should be considered in terms of:

1. The risk for medical problems arising during dental treatment.
2. Potential adverse side effects from medications prescribed to treat the condition and drug interactions with agents to be used during oral care.
3. The potential for cross-contamination in the dental office from the medical condition.

This item is followed by an area to provide the physician's name and contact information including the office phone and address. Although the ADA health history form does not include space for the office fax phone number, getting this information from the medical office can facilitate receiving information, such as medical consultation forms.

Drug side effects that may predispose the client to a medical emergency will be discussed later in this chapter, in the section in which current medications are listed. Drug-disease interactions when a local anesthetic is planned; and more importantly, the vasoconstrictor used in combination with the local anesthetic; is the most common interaction to be investigated. Others might include oral analgesic recommendations (acetaminophen, ibuprofen, etc.).

"Are you in good health?"

This question on the ADA Health History Form relates to the client's perception of his or her current health status. If a client responds negatively, this implies the need for further questioning, such as *"What is the cause of your poor health?"* Depending on the response, the clinician may need a physician consultation. This question should be considered in conjunction with the other items in the medical information section of the health history form.

"Has there been any change in your general health within the past year?"

A positive response should require follow-up questions investigating changes that occurred and the medical care received. Depending on the response, the clinician must determine how the condition may influence oral health care and whether a medical consult is needed. Refer to Chapters 9 to 14, which discuss specific medical conditions for clinically relevant information.

"Date of last physical examination"

It is relevant to determine whether the client regularly monitors the general health status. This is commonly done by having a physical examination. Asking the client for the findings of the physical examination can alert the clinician to medical problems within the past year. This question should be correlated with physical evidence of disease, such as abnormal vital signs, and to disease further identified in the later specific medical section of the health history form. For example, when blood pressure is elevated, has the client had a physical evaluation within the past year and was blood pressure elevated at that time? What treatment was recommended? The hypertensive dental patient should be seeking routine medical care to evaluate treatment success. If extensive dental treatment is needed, and vital signs indicate abnormal values, medical evaluation should be considered before treatment to determine whether the client can withstand the stress of the dental procedure and if a vasoconstrictor limitation is appropriate.

"Have you had a serious illness, operation, or been hospitalized in the past 5 years? If yes, what was the illness or problem?"

The information provided by the client should be considered in terms of potential risks during oral healthcare treatment. Having a 5-year interval for serious medical conditions provides a reasonable amount of time for consideration of relevant medical information. For example, this interval provides information that can be used when deciding whether antibiotic prophylaxis should be considered before treating a client who received a total joint replacement. Recently, the ADA collaborated with the American Society of Orthopaedic Surgeons (AAOS) reviewing the science on the efficacy of antibiotic prophylaxis prior to oral procedures and the subsequent risk of dental treatment on prosthetic joint infection (PJI).[1] The call for prophylaxis during the first 2 years following placement of the prosthetic joint was dropped. There is insufficient evidence that prophylaxis prevents PJIs; however, only one qualified study was found directly relating to this issue. The recommendation reflected this finding but was given a "limited" level of support. Practitioners were advised that following a recommendation of such low level of scientific support is risky. Practitioners were advised to follow professional judgment. Given this, orthopedic surgeons may recommend to patients receiving prosthetic joints to take antibiotic prophylaxis prior to dental treatment when special circumstances exist (such as having a compromised immune system). Another example would be identifying the client with a heart attack within the past month. Both situations require special consideration. The ADA and the AAOS's joint policy on antibiotic prophylaxis after total joint replacement is based on a variety of factors that could increase the risk for PJI, but the guidelines note there is no evidence to support giving antibiotic prophylaxis prior to dental procedures as a measure to prevent PJI.[1] No elective dental treatment is recommended for a client who has had a myocardial infarction (heart attack) for 1 month after the event.[2] For a client who has suffered a stroke—the recommendation is to have no elective dental treatment for a 6-month period after recovery from the stroke.[2] Appropriate follow-up questions would be based on specific diseases or medical treatments reported and official guidelines for the medical issue. The chapters in this self-study that deal with specific medical conditions include relevant historical questions for a wide variety of medical conditions.

Self-Study Review

1. If a client indicates that he/she has experienced a change in general health within the past year, the clinician should:
    a. ask follow-up questions regarding the health change.
    b. determine how the client's condition affects oral health care.
    c. determine whether a medical consult is warranted.
    d. all of the above.
2. What interval of time is used on the ADA Health History Form for evaluating serious medical conditions?
    a. 3 years
    b. 5 years
    c. 7 years
    d. 10 years
3. When is it appropriate to treat clients with a recent history of myocardial infarction?
    a. 4 weeks
    b. 6 weeks
    c. 2 months
    d. 6 months

MEDICATION HISTORY

The next portion of the ADA Health History Form includes questions related to prescribed or over-the-counter medications or supplements being taken by the client. Investigation of drug actions, precautions, side effects, and possible interactions with agents used in oral health care is essential to identify potential risks in treatment. Common drug side effects that may influence oral treatment are identified in this chapter. The risks involved during treatment from drug actions or side effects and the clinical implications are discussed.

"Are you taking or have you recently taken any prescription or over-the-counter medicine(s)? If so, please list all, including vitamins, natural or herbal preparations, and/or diet supplements."

Any pharmacologic agent taken by the client should be investigated using a drug reference text before initiating treatment. Serious adverse drug events (ADEs) and medication errors in the

United States have increased 2.6-fold from 1998 to 2005.[3] ADEs can be minor (e.g., lichenoid drug reactions on oral mucosa) or major (death). When investigating drugs reported on the medical history, it is important to know:

1. The action of the drug (What does the drug change in the body? Does this affect healing or increase bleeding? In what ways will the treatment plan be affected?).
2. The dose the client is taking (high doses may result in increased side effects).
3. Side effects relevant to oral changes or to treatment modifications (dry mouth, candidiasis, gingival hyperplasia, increased blood pressure, postural hypotension, gastrointestinal [GI] complaints or nausea, increased bleeding, leukopenia, and neutropenia are examples of side effects with a clinical relevance to oral healthcare procedures).
4. Interactions between the client's drug and drugs used during oral health care or interactions between a disease the client reports and a drug likely to be used or recommended by the clinician (e.g., most nonsteroidal anti-inflammatory agents, like ibuprofen, are contraindicated when antihypertensive medications are taken; aspirin is contraindicated in gastric ulcer disease).
5. Dental treatment considerations exist for the medical condition that requires drug use, interactions with drugs used in dentistry, and relevant side effects of the drug.

There are several drug reference resources. The most commonly used drug references include the *Physician's Desk Reference* and other drug references that focus on dental implications for drugs, such as LWW's *Dental Drug Reference with Clinical Implications,* Mosby's *Dental Drug Reference*, and *Drug Information Handbook for Dentistry*. These resources can be used to investigate drug effects and indicated clinical considerations. Drug side effects associated with a risk for a medical emergency or modifications during treatment include[3]:

1. Postural hypotension
2. Anticoagulant effect or increased bleeding
3. Hypertension
4. Arrhythmia
5. Nausea, vomiting, or GI reflux disease
6. **Blood dyscrasias**, such as **leukopenia**, **neutropenia**, or **thrombocytopenia**

Herbal, Vitamin, or Dietary Supplement Use

The current ADA medical history includes a question on herbal and nonherbal supplement use. Use of these types of products has increased to such an extent that it is very likely the client may be self-medicating with herbs. Reports of adverse effects from herbal supplements that can be relevant to oral health care include **postural hypotension** (niacin), interference with sedative drugs (kava, valerian, St. John's wort), hypertension, arrhythmia and tachycardia (ephedrine, goldenseal), and increased bleeding (ginkgo, ginseng, garlic, high doses of vitamin E).[4] This is an area that is currently being investigated, and other adverse effects are likely to be reported in the future. Most herbal products should be discontinued 1 to 2 weeks prior to surgical procedures.[4]

Self-Study Review

4. Drug side effects associated with a risk for medical emergencies include all of the following EXCEPT one. Which is the EXCEPTION?
   a. Postural hypotension
   b. Bleeding
   c. Vomiting
   d. Gingival hyperplasia

5. Postural hypotension is associated with the use of which supplement?
   a. Niacin
   b. St. John's wort
   c. Ginseng
   d. Ephedrine

6. Tachycardia is an adverse effect associated with the use of which supplement?
   a. Niacin
   b. St. John's wort
   c. Goldenseal
   d. Ephedrine

POTENTIAL EMERGENCY SITUATIONS AS A RESULT OF SIDE EFFECTS FROM PHARMACOLOGIC OR HERBAL PRODUCTS

The side effects discussed below represent the more common effects likely to result in a medical emergency during oral care. A complete study of drug effects and adverse effects will be presented during a pharmacology course later in the curriculum. It would be premature to present more in-depth pharmacologic information than is needed to identify the situations that would

Table 4.1 Drug Side Effects and Treatment Indications

Postural hypotension	Raise back of chair slowly Have client sit upright for few minutes before standing Measure blood pressure before dismissing patient As patient leaves the dental chair, stand nearby for support as needed
Bleeding	Apply digital pressure to encourage clot formation Use local hemostatic agents as needed
Hypertension, arrhythmia	Monitor vital signs for normal limits, inform client if excessive Do not provide treatment when values are ≥ 180/110 mm Hg and over 100 bpm
Nausea, vomiting, GI reflux	Position in semiupright position for treatment
Leukopenia, thrombocytopenia	Observe for increased infection, reduced healing Monitor for excessive bleeding that does not clot Request complete blood count if blood dyscrasia is suspected and procedures involving bleeding are planned

most likely result in an emergency situation. Therefore, this discussion will include only the most common side effects likely to result in a medical emergency, strategies to prevent the emergency situation, and management of the emergency should it occur. Oral side effects such as dry mouth, candidiasis, and gingival hyperplasia would not result in an emergency situation and are managed with caries reduction agents (fluoride, xylitol gum), salivary stimulants, antifungal agents, and strict plaque control. These preventive strategies will be included in future courses in the curriculum that deal with preventive dentistry concepts. Drug side effects and appropriate treatment modifications are discussed below and summarized in Table 4.1.

Postural Hypotension

Postural hypotension (also called orthostatic hypotension) is a common cause of unconsciousness in dental settings.[5] To understand changes from normal blood pressure to those seen in postural hypotension, the following description is provided.

Normal Physiologic Response

When a client is placed in the supine position, blood flow to the brain requires less blood pressure. The body adapts to the reduced blood pressure needed to supply oxygenated blood to the brain by dilation of blood vessels. This vasodilation results from the action of baroreceptors in the nervous system that sense the change in orthostatic position. A physiologic blood pressure reduction, or hypotensive effect, results. When the client assumes an upright position, it takes a certain period of time for the blood vessels to adapt to the change and constrict to increase the blood pressure. As blood pressure is increased, the blood flow needed to supply the brain is established.

Abnormal Response

Orthostatic hypotension occurs when the client is changed from the supine position to the upright position and the physiologic response to increase blood pressure is delayed. It is most likely to occur in elderly clients,[2] and the most common etiologic factor is hypotension as a result of a drug or supplement side effect. It is rarely associated with stress, unlike unconsciousness from vasodepressor syncope. Other factors that may result in postural hypotension include prolonged periods in a prone or supine position, prolonged periods standing "at attention," standing in hot temperatures, late-stage pregnancy, varicose veins, and several rare disease syndromes. With the exception of long appointments in a prone or supine position, most of these situations are unlikely to occur during oral procedures. Unconsciousness associated with pregnancy will be discussed with the question on the ADA Health History Form related to being pregnant. Although it is a form of postural hypotension, it occurs from a different mechanism than that described above.

Drug Side Effect Implications

When the client takes a medication with a side effect of "postural hypotension," it is likely that the normal physiologic blood pressure reduction described in this page that occurs in the supine chair position, combined with the hypotensive drug side effect, can result in low blood pressure. Antihypertensive drugs used to lower blood pressure frequently include postural hypotension as a potential side effect. When these drugs are taken it is not unusual for the blood pressure to drop even more when the client is changed from the supine position to the upright position. A decline of 20 mm Hg or more in the systolic blood pressure and a decline of 10 mm Hg or more in the diastolic blood pressure are signs of impending postural hypotension.[6] It is during this brief period after repositioning the client that a loss of consciousness from inadequate blood flow to the brain can occur. The client is likely to lose consciousness after standing to leave the dental chair because blood pressure may not have increased quickly enough to force oxygenated blood to the brain. The heart rate generally remains within normal limits and is affected very little in postural hypotension; however, the pulse may increase up to 30 bpm after the individual stands.[5]

Prevention of Emergency

Individuals who have experienced postural hypotension in the past are more likely to experience the effect. For this reason when the drug has a potential side effect of "postural hypotension," the appropriate follow-up question is "Have you ever lost consciousness after getting up due to low blood pressure?" or "Have you experienced postural hypotension while taking this drug?" This may identify the client at an increased risk for the emergency.

The management strategy to prevent a loss of consciousness from hypotension is to raise the back of the dental chair slowly and to allow the client to sit upright for a few minutes before leaving the dental chair while the practitioner stands nearby in case of a complication. The baroreceptors in the nervous system recognize the positional change, causing a vasoconstriction of blood vessels, and blood pressure is elevated. The increased pressure supplies oxygenated blood to the brain. A short period of time is needed for these changes to occur before allowing the client to arise from the dental chair. An additional strategy to reduce the risk of the client losing consciousness from postural hypotension after dismissal from the dental chair is to reposition the chair to an upright position as described above and measure the blood pressure before allowing the client to stand. Pressures below 80/60 mm Hg indicate the client should remain seated until blood pressure increases above that level.

Management of Unconsciousness

If the client **loses** consciousness because of postural hypotension, place the individual in a supine position, making sure the airway is open. The feet can be elevated slightly to assist in venous return of blood to the heart. Provide basic life support as recommended in any cardiopulmonary resuscitation (CPR) course. This includes assessing an open airway, assuring breathing, and assessing circulation. Administer oxygen by face mask or nasal cannula at 4 to 6 L/minute. Measure the blood pressure and record values in the treatment record. The client who has just experienced postural hypotension will recover within a few minutes if the airway is open because breathing and circulation are not affected in this emergency situation. After recovery, measure the blood pressure again and record the values in the treatment record along with a description of:

1. When during the appointment the event occurred.
2. The management procedures provided.
3. Events observed during the recovery period.

Allow the client to recover in a semi upright position in an appropriate area of the dental facility (Box 4-1). Most patients recover uneventfully and, after resting and regaining normal blood pressure levels, can drive themselves home. If there is any question regarding whether the client has achieved a full recovery, ask the client whom to call to take the client home. Note in the client's chart whether or not someone escorted the client home, and who took charge of the client.

Box 4-1

Prevention and Management of Postural Hypotension

Prevention

- Raise dental chair back slowly
- Remain in upright position for 2 to 3 minutes before dismissing client
- Measure blood pressure before leaving dental chair

Management

- Place in supine position
- Assure airway is open, breathing and circulation are present
- Observe for signs of recovery while measuring blood pressure
- When blood pressure is above 80/60 mm Hg, client can stand

Record events of emergency in treatment record

Increased Bleeding

Any drug, vitamin, or supplement that has a side effect of "increased bleeding" requires monitoring of bleeding and poor clotting during oral procedures. Drug side effects related to increased bleeding include platelet inhibition (aspirin results in bleeding due to this mechanism of action), reduction of the formation of clotting factors (called anticoagulant effect), and a rare side effect of thrombocytopenia (a situation in which reduced number of platelets are formed in the bone marrow).

Self-Study Review

7. Examples of causes of postural hypotension include all of the following EXCEPT one. Which one is the EXCEPTION?
   a. Running in place
   b. Standing for a long period of time
   c. Pregnancy
   d. Varicose veins
8. Signs of impending postural hypotension include:
   a. a decline in blood pressure.
   b. a decline in respirations.
   c. loss of consciousness.
   d. an increase in blood pressure.
9. When a client is placed in a supine position, blood flow to the brain is increased by baroreceptors in the nervous system. The client will experience a subsequent decrease in blood pressure when returned to an upright position.
   a. Both statements are true.
   b. Both statements are false.
   c. The first statement is false, and the second statement is true.
   d. The first statement is false, and the second statement is true.

Drug Side Effect Implications

Most of the drugs or supplements that cause increased bleeding do so by reducing the ability of platelets to stick together normally (called platelet **aggregation**), thereby reducing clot formation. An over-the-counter drug with this effect that many people take is aspirin. It can increase bleeding by the same mechanism. Another common prescription-only drug, warfarin (Coumadin), acts by a different mechanism that involves reducing the formation of vitamin K–dependent clotting factors. Coumadin is taken by clients who have a medical condition in which blood clots form and move within the circulatory system. It is frequently taken when the client has had a stroke. Clients who have heart valve replacements take warfarin to decrease clot formation around the artificial valves. If warfarin is listed on the medication section, special management procedures are indicated and are discussed below.

Prevention of Uncontrolled Bleeding: Antiaggregation Effect

The clinician cannot prevent increased bleeding from occurring when the client is taking a pharmacologic product with this action; however, the clinician should monitor the degree of bleeding that results from oral procedures. If excessive bleeding is observed, stop the procedure and apply digital pressure to the involved area. Some clinicians have observed increased bleeding in clients taking a low-dose aspirin product and have questioned whether this presents a clinically significant event when the planned treatment would result in bleeding. A clinical study reported that one 100-mg aspirin a day does not increase bleeding to the extent that it causes an emergency bleeding episode after dental treatment.[7] In this study, bleeding time in the group taking 100 mg/day aspirin was within acceptable bleeding time limits (less than 20 minutes). A local application of pressure was sufficient to control bleeding, and no episodes of uncontrolled bleeding occurred. Other widely used drugs with the antiplatelet effect are clopidogrel (Plavix) and ticagrelor (Brilinta). These drugs are indicated for many cardiovascular patients, particularly **following placement** of coronary artery stents. The ADA has developed a joint policy with the American Heart Association, the American College of Cardiology, the Society for Cardiovascular Angiography and Interventions, and the American College of Surgeons advising healthcare providers who perform invasive or surgical procedures, such as those associated with oral care, to contact the cardiologist and discuss patient management before discontinuing antiplatelet drugs.[8] The risk for intravascular clot formation is greater than the risk for hemorrhage, so discontinuing antiplatelet agents prior to oral procedures is not recommended.

Prevention of Uncontrolled Bleeding: Anticoagulant Effect

For the client taking an anticoagulant medication (also called a blood thinner), such as warfarin

(Coumadin), that reduces the formation of clotting factors, a different preventive strategy is recommended. The clinician must obtain laboratory data on the degree of anticoagulation caused by the client's dose. As stated above, high doses result in increased anticoagulant effects. Increased bleeding that results can develop into an emergency situation. The laboratory report that identifies the degree of anticoagulation effect is called a **prothrombin time (PT)**. A more accurate test is an international normalized ratio (INR). The clinician should request the most recent PT or INR data from the client or the client's physician. Medical management goals are to keep the client in a range of 2 to 3, with the exception of the cardiac valve replacement where the INR is maintained at 3.5. An INR level of 3.5 or less is acceptable for dental hygiene procedures that result in bleeding, without a risk of hemorrhage.[2] If the INR is higher, the clinician must ask the physician for a recommendation regarding prevention of hemorrhage during treatment. However, after physician consultation, elective oral healthcare procedures may need to be delayed until the INR/PT is in an acceptable range. If the procedure is necessary and cannot be delayed for weeks, the physician may decide to lower the dose of the anticoagulant for a short time before the dental procedure. After the dose reduction, it is recommended to wait at least 3 days before appointing the client for oral procedures to allow time for the liver to form the necessary clotting factors. After the treatment procedure, the client will resume the normal dose of the anticoagulant medication. It is during this time of dose reduction that the client must be monitored for other adverse effects, such as clot formation, leading to myocardial infarction or stroke. Reducing the dose is risky in some clients. The physician following the client's cardiovascular care makes the decision on the protocol to follow and the postoperative follow-up care. Occasionally, when the client is questioned about the PT levels taken at the most recent maintenance visit, the client will have been told the levels were "OK." This generally means the laboratory test revealed expected INR levels. If the laboratory test revealed too high or too low INR levels, the medical practitioner would change the client's dose of warfarin. In the case described above, not having an official INR/PT number, the clinician must consider the treatment planned and the potential risk for uncontrolled bleeding. If only minor bleeding is expected, the clinician must monitor the clotting frequently (after treating two to three teeth) while treatment, such as oral prophylaxis, is provided. Treatment should be stopped if excessive bleeding develops. Digital pressure may initiate clotting. Do not dismiss the client until bleeding has been controlled.

During the pharmacology course that occurs later in the curriculum, more information related to normal limits of bleeding time and coagulation time will be provided. For this discussion as part of the preclinical education, the focus will be on preventing and managing the potential emergency situation.

Blood Dyscrasia (Thrombocytopenia)

This is a rare side effect in which the drug inhibits the bone marrow formation of platelets. The function of platelets is to cause a clot to form. It makes sense that if a client has a significantly reduced number of platelets, clotting will be reduced. Identifying the client with this side effect is difficult. When thrombocytopenia is listed as a potential side effect in the drug profile, the best way to prevent hemorrhage (bleeding that does not stop) is to monitor bleeding frequently during treatment, ensure that clot formation has occurred, and institute local measures described below to stop uncontrolled bleeding.

Management of Uncontrolled Bleeding

When uncontrolled bleeding is observed, the clinician must stop the dental procedure. For the client taking a product that has an antiaggregation effect (such as aspirin, gingko, or garlic), the clinician must assess the degree of bleeding. If clotting does not occur within a few minutes, digital pressure using the thumb and forefinger should be applied to the area to stimulate clot formation. For the client taking anticoagulant medications, locally applied hemostatic agents may induce a clot. Local hemostatic agents that can be used when digital pressure does not stop bleeding include applying agents, such as absorbable gelatin sponge (Gelfoam), or having the client rinse with tranexamic acid (Cyklokapron). Gelfoam is found in most dental offices, but tranexamic acid must be secured from a pharmacy and is not often a part of dental inventory. Injection of a local anesthetic with 1:50,000 epinephrine may reduce uncontrolled bleeding via the vasoconstrictor action of epinephrine. Tannic acid, which is the active ingredient in tea bags, is sometimes recommended after tooth extraction to control bleeding. It is not usually used after other oral procedures. These strategies are usually successful in controlling bleeding. If bleeding is not controlled, the client must be evaluated in a medical facility where intravenous agents, such as platelet infusions or clotting factors, can be administered to stop bleeding.

Hypertension, Hypotension, Tachycardia, and Arrhythmia

These side effects would be listed in the cardiovascular category of side effects. When they are listed for a medication, the clinician should evaluate the blood pressure and pulse values and qualities. If the medication has the potential side effects listed but the client's vital signs are within normal limits, the side effects do not apply to the client being seen and can be disregarded. Not all clients experience drug side effects. Some medications would be expected to affect the vital signs. For example, antihypertensive medications and decongestants are two groups likely to affect vital signs. If antihypertensives are effective, blood pressure would be reduced, and there is a risk for postural hypotension. Decongestants often increase the heart rate, but the rhythm should not be affected.

Drug Side Effect Implications

If blood pressure values are not within normal limits, the client should be informed. The client should be advised to report the condition to the prescribing physician. If blood pressure is below 80/60 mm Hg, there is a risk for a hypotensive episode during treatment. The pulse quality and value are considered when "tachycardia or arrhythmia" is listed. It is the clinician's responsibility to assess the vital sign values and determine whether a complication exists. When abnormal values or rhythm is found, the client should be informed. The clinician must determine whether there is a risk in continuing with treatment.

Prevention of Emergency

It is logical that when blood pressure values are seriously elevated (see Chapter 1, Table 1.2), oral healthcare treatment should be avoided and the client referred for medical evaluation. Generally, hypertension is a sign of a systemic disease rather than a result of a drug side effect. Very low blood pressure levels should be managed according to recommendations in the discussion of postural hypotension. Vasoconstrictors in local anesthetic agents can increase blood pressure levels; however, the use of epinephrine in local anesthetic solutions is not contraindicated in hypertension. For clients with cardiovascular disease, it is recommended to limit vasoconstrictor concentrations in local anesthetic preparations to low concentrations, such as no more than two cartridges of 1:100,000 or four cartridges of 1:200,000.[9] When arrhythmia occurs, there is a potential for a heart attack. In fact, arrhythmia is the most common sign preceding a heart attack. Determining whether the abnormal vital sign is a drug side effect or a sign of cardiovascular disease is not possible when reviewing the medical history. The client with a fast, irregular heartbeat and blood pressure above normal limits should be referred for medical evaluation and treatment delayed until the cardiovascular system is stabilized.

Management

Severe hypertension can result in adverse cardiovascular events, such as a stroke. When BP levels are ≥180/110 mm Hg, oral procedures are contraindicated and the client should be referred for immediate medical evaluation.[2,6] If cardiovascular events occur during oral therapy, they are managed by basic life support procedures learned in the CPR course and, in some cases, by calling for emergency medical services (EMS) through the 911 system. These will be more fully discussed in Chapter 11, which deals with cardiovascular disease.

Nausea, Vomiting, and GI Reflux

When the client takes a drug that has the side effects listed above, the follow-up is to determine whether any of the side effects have occurred. In most situations, the side effects would have caused the client to change to another medication with less problematic side effects. An exception would be taking an antibiotic that can cause nausea. The client would generally expect the side effect to occur during the short course of treatment.

Drug Side Effect Implications

Esophageal and stomach pain are reported to occur with a wide variety of drugs. When this side effect occurs, the client may take other medications to control the discomfort of the side effect. For example, the client may take cimetidine (Tagamet) to reduce the GI pain associated with taking naproxen (Naprosyn) for arthritis. Usually if a drug results in vomiting, the client stops taking the drug. GI reflux can be both a disease condition and a side effect from some medications. In this condition, the stomach acids enter the esophagus and pharyngeal area, creating discomfort and burning to the client.

Prevention and Management

If GI pain, reflux, and nausea are a problem, treatment is best completed with the client in a semiupright position. This minimizes the possibility of reflux occurring. Many clients report greater comfort during oral procedures if placed in a semi-upright position for treatment. When the client does not report experiencing these side effects, the supine position can be used. The clinician should monitor the client in the supine position in case GI side effects develop during treatment.

Leukopenia, Agranulocytopenia, and Neutropenia

These blood dyscrasias are rare side effects listed with a wide variety of drugs. They occur either as an inhibition of bone marrow function, where blood elements are formed, or as a hypersensitivity reaction to the drug.

Drug Side Effect Implications

Leukopenia is defined as a reduced number of white blood cells and can result in increased infection and reduced healing. **Agranulocytosis** is a significant reduction in polymorphonuclear leukocytes (the first line of immune defense) and results in increased infection. Neutropenia is a term to describe a reduction in neutrophils. All of these conditions can result in increased infection and reduced healing.

Prevention and Management

The clinician should examine the tissues to determine whether there is evidence of increased oral infection above that expected from the amount of microbial biofilm present. If increased infection is observed, the client should be referred to the physician who prescribed the medication for a complete blood count to determine whether a blood dyscrasia has occurred. No oral health care that could result in the creation of a wound should be attempted. Treatment should be delayed until laboratory work determines that the blood count is within acceptable limits. This is a rare side effect, and it is unlikely to be seen.

Nonemergency Oral Side Effect: Xerostomia

A variety of drugs result in a reduction of salivary flow. This side effect would not relate to a medical emergency, but it has significant oral implications. When a drug resulting in xerostomia is taken every day for weeks to years, a chronic reduction of saliva can result in oral disease. Chronic dry mouth is associated with increased caries and candidiasis. Oral health education should include home fluoride products, chewing xylitol gum, and, if needed, use of salivary substitutes. An antifungal medication (usually nystatin, an oral rinse) is commonly prescribed by the dentist for oral candidal infection.

Self-Study Review

10. The most common drug causing platelet inhibition is:
- a. aspirin.
- b. acetaminophen.
- c. atenolol.
- d. atorvastatin.

11. In cases of increased bleeding during treatment, the first treatment the clinician should try is:
- a. observing the client until the bleeding stops.
- b. applying clot-forming medication to the sites.
- c. applying digital pressure.
- d. activating the emergency response system.

12. If a client presents with symptoms of reflux and nausea, treatment is best completed in a prone position because the chance of reflux is decreased and the client will be more comfortable.
- a. Both the statement and reason are correct and related.
- b. Both the statement and reason are correct, but NOT related.
- c. The statement is correct, but the reason is NOT.
- d. The statement is NOT correct, but the reason is correct.
- e. NEITHER the statement NOR the reason is correct.

13. Leukopenia and neutropenia may cause:
- a. increased infection and reduced healing.
- b. increased infection and bleeding.
- c. bleeding and reduced healing.
- d. increased plaque formation and reduced healing.

CHAPTER SUMMARY

This chapter provided an overview of medical history questions related to the current health status, contact information for the client's physician, and recent hospitalizations, followed by a request for prescription and nonprescription medications taken by clients. New guidelines regarding antibiotic prophylaxis to prevent PJI are summarized. Common side effects and drug actions were discussed, and prevention and management strategies for side effects that could result in a medical emergency during oral health care were presented. The clinician has an opportunity to use the medical history to discuss all forms of medications with the client, including supplements and herbal products, as a means of identifying potential risks for a medical emergency during treatment.

Review

1. Explain the significance of the medical history questions "Are you now under the care of a physician?" and "Have you had a recent hospitalization?"
2. Define the following terms: thrombocytopenia, leukopenia, agranulocytosis, and neutropenia.
3. List the major types of side effects that can represent a risk for medical emergencies.
4. Identify examples of supplements and herbal medications that can cause adverse effects during oral health care.
5. List five criteria used to investigate prescription and nonprescription medications.
6. Describe how vital signs can be used to determine side effects of medications.

Case Study

Case A

Mr. Garcia, a 59-year-old client, presents to the office for a routine prophylaxis. On review of the medical history, the client reports that he is 3 weeks after placement of two stents in his heart as a result of a myocardial infarction. The client states that he is participating in a cardiovascular rehabilitation program and takes Plavix, antihypertensives, and anticholesterol medications daily. In addition, Mr. Garcia notes that his recent health experience has caused him to start taking multivitamins, one "baby" aspirin, and ginseng to improve his health. The client denies any other medical problems, reports he can now return to running and physical activities, and denies any oral health complaints. His vital signs are pulse 70 bpm, respiration 18 breaths/min, and blood pressure 146/86 mm Hg, right arm.

1. Is it safe to perform a prophylaxis at this time?
2. Is there a need to obtain laboratory values prior to treatment?
3. After consulting a dental drug reference, what adverse effects, if any, would you expect to find with the medications the client is using? What about those being used to self-treat?
4. On completion of treatment, the client is seated upright and asked to remain in that position for several minutes. What is the rationale for this recommendation?

Case B

Mrs. Berkowski, a 45-year-old client, presents for restorative dental care. She reports that she recently underwent an endoscopy procedure and was diagnosed with erosive esophagitis and a hiatal hernia. Nexium 40 mg daily for 4 weeks was prescribed. The client notes that she has had some improvement with this medication, but still experiences episodes of nausea and reflux, particularly in the morning and at bedtime. To help relieve these symptoms, the client states that she sleeps with the upper portion of the bed elevated and drinks ginger tea as needed. This client's vital signs are pulse 72 bpm, respiration 15 breaths/min, and blood pressure 118/70 mm Hg, right arm.

1. What chair position would most likely provide comfort to the client?
2. After consulting a dental drug reference, what adverse effects, if any, would you expect to find with the medication the client is taking?
3. If on examination you note that the client has evidence of moderate to severe gingivitis with minimal plaque present and had a healthy clinical presentation at the previous appointment, what adverse drug reaction would you suspect?

Chapter Five

Total Joint Replacement and Potential Effects of Bisphosphonates

Objectives

After completing the self-study chapter the reader will be able to:

- Explain the rationale for requiring clients to wear safety glasses during treatment.
- Identify elements of professional 2012 joint guidelines related to prescribing antibiotic prophylaxis prior to oral procedures for the client who has received a total joint replacement.
- Identify information to provide when bisphosphonate medication is planned, currently being administered or in those who received bisphosphonates in the past.

Key Terms

Antibiotic prophylaxis: use of antibiotics to prevent infection in cardiac valves caused by bacteremia

Bacteremia: the presence of bacteria in the circulation; capable of being transferred to distant sites within the body

Hematogenous: spreading via the bloodstream

Immunosuppression: a condition characterized by a reduced immune response, resulting in reduced healing and increased risk of infection

Innocuous: harmless

Total joint replacement: replacement of a joint, such as a hip, knee, elbow, finger, or ankle

MEDICAL CONDITION

INTRODUCTION

The next section from the American Dental Association (ADA) Health History form continues the discussion of medical information and includes conditions related to wearing contact lenses, determining the need for **antibiotic prophylaxis** in selected clients with a **total joint replacement** (TJR) prior to oral procedures, and possible adverse effects of taking bisphosphonate (BIS) medications. The clinical significance for identifying the client wearing contact lenses begins the discussion.

"Do you wear contact lenses?"

This question relates to offering safety glasses for use during oral health care. It has no relationship to medical problems, but alerts the clinician to provide safety glasses and be aware of the need to protect the eyes from aerosols and spatter during oral procedures. Issues related to wearing contact lenses follow.

CLINICAL MANAGEMENT ISSUES

Eye covering will prevent splashing materials into the eyes. Contaminated particles can cause an eye infection and related discomfort in the eyes. Dark-tinted lenses will help lessen glare from intense overhead dental lights directed toward the oral cavity. Wearing contact lenses makes the eye sensitive to any foreign particle, no matter how small. Spatter from polishing or toothbrushing may be deflected into the eyes, increasing the risk for eye infection from translocation of oral microorganisms. The client can remove the contact lenses during treatment or wear safety glasses with side shields for maximum protection. It is a common practice to offer protective eye covering throughout treatment, regardless of whether or not contact lenses are worn.

TOTAL JOINT REPLACEMENT

"Have you had an orthopedic total joint (hip, knee, elbow, finger) replacement? Date:"

In 2012, the ADA and the American Academy of Orthopaedic Surgeons (AAOS) published a joint policy identifying issues for consideration when the client with a TJR seeks dental care.[1] The joint policy includes conditions posing an increased risk for prosthetic joint infection (PJI) but does not recommend routine antibiotic prophylaxis for individuals with hip or knee prosthetic joints prior to dental care. The only recommendation states "The practitioner might consider discontinuing the practice of routinely prescribing prophylactic antibiotics for patients with hip and knee prosthetic joint implants undergoing dental procedures." The recommendation is founded in evidence that dental procedures are unrelated to PJI, there is no proof that **bacteremia** causes PJI, and that subsequent antibiotic prophylaxis does not reduce the risk for PJI.

Since no recommendation was made for antibiotic prophylaxis, no specific antibiotics to prescribe were included. The joint policy statement applies only to hip and knee replacements since the single study used to support the suggestion that antibiotic prophylaxis might be discontinued is based on only one case–control study of good quality. The guidelines reaffirm that patients with pins, plates, or screws do not need antibiotic prophylaxis before dental procedures. It also clarified that the recommendations were not to be considered a "standard of care" nor used as a substitute for clinical judgment when determining whether antibiotics are indicated in the client with a TJR. The policy advised clinicians to use professional judgment, including patient values, when making the decision regarding antibiotic prophylaxis. In some instances, clients with immunocompromised defense systems **(immunosuppression)** may benefit, although no study has been completed to investigate this issue. The guidelines did not recommend use of antibacterial rinses (such as chlorhexidine) to prevent PJI. Good oral hygiene was recommended by consensus since it is **innocuous**. Prophylactic antibiotics might be considered in selected clients with specific medical histories who are at an increased risk of joint infection when a bacteremia occurs.[1,2] There is limited evidence that some immunocompromised clients with TJRs may be at a higher risk of late joint infection from bacteremia. The medical conditions considered to be at greatest risk are listed in Box 5-1.[1] In the past, specific dental procedures involving bleeding were recommended for antibiotic prophylaxis, but this was not included in the 2012 guidelines as science did not support the practice.[3] In the joint ADA/AAOS policy, it was noted that routine brushing/flossing and other daily procedures have been shown to produce bacteremia. However, there is no recommendation for antibiotic prophylaxis prior to those events.

Box 5-1

Conditions Indicating Increased Risk for Infection after Total Joint Replacement

- Time after joint replacement
- Immunocompromised or immunosuppressed patients (e.g., rheumatoid arthritis, systemic lupus erythematosus, or drug- or radiation-induced **immunosuppression**)
- Insulin-dependent (type 1) diabetes mellitus
- Previous prosthetic joint infections, multiple implants
- Bisphosphonate therapy
- Hemophilia
- HIV infection
- Malignancies

(Adapted from AAOS/ADA Clinical Guidelines, Appendix II Causal Pathway, December 2012.)

Although the risk of bacteremia is much greater in inflamed gingivae than in healthy gingivae, there is no proof that gingival health would prevent PJI. High-level evidence (randomized controlled trials) suggests that antibiotic prophylaxis reduces the incidence of postdental procedure related bacteremia, but there is no evidence that bacteremia increases the risk of PJI.[2]

Subsequent research revealed that some activities of daily living, such as brushing, flossing, and chewing, can result in formation of a significant bacteremia,[3] and that bacteremia can occur both in individuals with healthy periodontal tissues and those with gingivitis or periodontitis.[4] In addition, more recent evidence indicates that prophylactic antibiotics do not eliminate the formation of bacteremia.[5] The former rationale for antibiotic prophylaxis was based on the premise that bacteremia in the bloodstream may infect spaces in the area of a joint replacement and the most critical period is within the first 2 years after joint replacement surgery. However, a literature review reported that there is not one documented case of a PJI from a dental treatment-induced bacteremia.[6] In addition, a recent systematic review of evidence related to the effectiveness of antibiotic prophylaxis to prevent infection following TJR reported that there is no scientific basis for the use of prophylactic antibiotics before dental procedures in individuals with hip, knee, and shoulder prosthetic joints.[7] Antibiotic prophylaxis guidelines (AAOS/ADA, 2012) are based on limited evidence or are consensus-based, and it is possible that some physicians may still require antibiotic prophylaxis prior to oral procedures.

DATE OF TOTAL JOINT REPLACEMENT

This part of the question is intended to identify the client whose joint replacement surgery occurred within 2 years before the oral healthcare appointment. It should be remembered, however, there is no proof that dental procedures are related to PJI and no proof that antibiotic prophylaxis prevents PJI, so the increased risk during the first 2-year period is unfounded. In addition, the client with TJR who develops an infection in the prosthetic joint (even after the initial 2-year period) is among the increased risk group and the same lack of scientific support applies. In essence, most patients will follow the recommendation of the orthopedist even though more rigorous studies are needed to answer the clinical question.

"If you answered yes to the above question, have you had any complications?"

COMPLICATIONS OR DIFFICULTIES WITH JOINT REPLACEMENT

This question is intended to identify the TJR client who may have had an infection or other problems during the joint replacement postoperative period. It is speculated that a bacteremia associated with an acute dental infection has the potential to infect the joint implant space. Therefore, acute oral infection should be treated and the source of the infection eliminated (incision and drainage, endodontics, extraction). It is helpful to know the signs of joint infection. The signs of joint infection include fever, swelling, pain, and a joint that is warm to the touch.

One complication making the client with a TJR at risk for a **hematogenous** joint infection is hemophilia. It is speculated that bleeding into the joint space with microorganism-containing blood may increase the risk of PJI, although no DNA verified case reports exist within this medical group following dental procedures. Potentially infectious bacteremia is likely to enter the joint space in a hemophiliac because of the increased bleeding relative to the disease condition. Antibiotic prophylaxis before oral healthcare procedures has been shown to reduce the magnitude of bacteremia but bacteremia still formed.[8] The 2012 joint guidelines include three recommendations: (1) to discontinue routinely prescribing antibiotics prior to dental treatment for individuals with a hip or knee joint replacement, (2) no recommendation for or against the use of topical antimicrobials was made, due to no evidence of effectiveness to reduce PJI, and (3) to maintain good oral hygiene to promote oral health.[1]

DECISION-MAKING TOOL

For the first time, guidelines include a shared decision-making tool—a template designed to be used by both orthopedic surgeons and dentists with the patient—was developed to accompany the guideline. Shared decision-making is a collaborative process that enables patients and their healthcare providers to make treatment decisions together, taking into account both the best scientific evidence available and the patient's values and preferences. The tool supplements, but does not replace, informed consent procedures.[1]

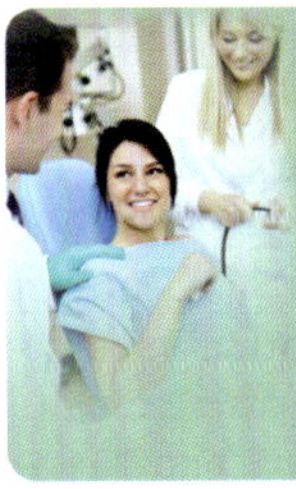

Follow-up Questions

"Have you been told to take antibiotics prior to having dental work? If so, who advised prophylaxis? Provide name and contact information. Are you allergic to any antibiotics?"

Clinical Application

It is important to identify the client who has been advised to take prophylactic antibiotics before dental treatment. The ADA/AAOS guidelines stress that the health professional must use professional judgment before deciding whether antibiotic prophylaxis is indicated. One issue to consider is taking antibiotics unnecessarily adds to the rising incidence of antibiotic resistance. The dental professional may determine some clients could benefit from antibiotic prophylaxis, such as a client who is immunosuppressed. In this situation, the client may have a poor host response to fight infection and a reduced healing response. In the joint ADA/AAOS policy recommendation, those clients with diseases that make them immunocompromised (such as type 1 or 2 diabetes mellitus, taking immunosuppressive drugs, HIV infection, malignancy) may be at a higher risk for joint infection and may benefit from antibiotics before oral procedures. Immunosuppressive agents which may be taken include prednisone, hydrocortisone, and antirejection drugs taken after an organ transplant. Radiation treatments may suppress the immune response and are identified as a risk factor in clients with TJR.

The ADA/AAOS addresses the issue of using professional judgment by encouraging the clinician to consult with the physician to determine whether there are special considerations that might affect the decision on whether or not to premedicate with antibiotics. The clinician is encouraged to share a copy of the guidelines with the physician before the consultation to ensure the physician is aware of the guidelines. After the consultation, the decision can be made (or not) to follow the physician's recommendation. All consultations should be followed up with a letter summarizing the issues discussed and decisions made. A copy of this correspondence should be placed in the client's medical record.

Self-Study Review

1. The ADA/AAOS guidelines state that there is no evidence to support the routine use of prophylactic antibiotics in patients with prosthetic hip and knee implants. Oral health professionals should use professional judgment and limit the use of antibiotics for patients who are immunosuppressed or have had a prosthetic joint placed within 1 year of the dental hygiene appointment.
   a. Both statements are true.
   b. Both statements are false.
   c. The first statement is true, and the second statement is false.
   d. The first statement is false, and the second statement is true.
2. The ADA and the AAOS joint guidelines specify that patients with pins, plates and screws need antibiotic prophylaxis prior to dental procedures. This recommendation is considered a standard of care for the profession.
   a. Both statements are true.
   b. Both statements are false.

c. The first statement is true, and the second statement is false.
d. The first statement is false, and the second statement is true.

3. To date, how many cases of a PJI having occurred from dental treatment-induced bactermia have been documented?
a. 0
b. 3
c. 5
d. 10

4. Clients with a history of TJR who are immunocompromised may have:
a. poor host response to infection but increased healing response.
b. poor host response to infection and a reduced healing response.
c. improved host response to infection but a reduced healing response.
d. improved host response to infection and increased healing response.

"Are you taking, or scheduled to begin taking either of the medications, alendronate (Fosamax) or risedronate (Actonel) for osteoporosis or Paget disease? Are you taking any antiresorptive drug (denosumab)?"

In May 2005, the drug company Novartis Pharmaceuticals sent a letter to dentists across the United States to warn them of reports of an adverse drug reaction described as osteonecrosis of the jaw (ONJ) in some individuals who received intravenous (IV) BIS. A literature review following the sequence of reports identified subsequent reports of ONJ in some individuals who received the oral doseforms: *Fosamax* and *Actonel.*[9] It has been determined that the associated adverse drug effect (ONJ) is more prevalent with the IV doseforms of this class of drugs and is rarely associated with the oral doseforms.[10] In fact, most reports of cases that included oral doseforms revealed the number of cases to be significantly fewer than those related to IV doseforms.[11,12] When the ONJ condition was first reported it was linked to drugs in the BIS class. Since that time other antiresorptive drugs have been developed. One new agent, denosumab (a human monoclonal antibody), has been linked to ONJ so the new ADA guidelines refer to the condition as "antiresorptive agent-induced ONJ" (ARONJ).

One study reported an association between implant failure in subjects who took BIS therapy compared with individuals who received dental implants but did not receive BIS.[13] Recently, the ADA published guidelines for management of individuals who have received any form of BIS or antiresorptive drug.[10]

MECHANISM OF ACTION OF BISPHOSPHONATES

The mechanism for the necrosis of bone in the jaw is unknown, but several authors describe that an oversuppression of bone turnover from the antiresorptive drugs, such as BIS and a newer drug, denosumab, is probably the primary mechanism for the development of this condition, although there may be contributing comorbid factors. These agents are powerful inhibitors of osteoclastic activity. Prolonged use of antiresorptive agents may suppress bone turnover to the point that microdamage occurs and accumulates with subsequent doses. Antiresorptive agents are excreted by the kidneys without normal metabolism in the liver and have a high attraction for hydroxyapatite of the bone. They are remarkably persistent drugs and do not leave the bone for up to 12 years, possibly longer.[10] Those BIS that contain a nitrogen side chain in the chemical structure are the most potent form of the class of drugs (Table 5.1). It is this long persistence within the skeleton that adds to the precaution for those who

Table 5.1 Nitrogen-Containing Bisphosphonate Drugs

Generic Drug Name	Brand Name of Drug	Route of Administration
Alendronate	Fosamax	Oral, once weekly
Risedronate	Actonel	Oral, once weekly or once a day
Ibandronate	Boniva	Oral, once a month
Pamidronate	Aredia	IV, various 4–12 times/yr
Zoledronic acid	Zometa	IV, various 4–12 times/yr

have taken or are currently taking drugs in the class. It is thought that individuals who have taken oral BIS for 2 years or longer are at the greatest risk for developing ONJ.[10]

"Since 2001 were you treated or are you currently scheduled to begin treatment with the IV bisphosphonates (Aredia or Zometa) for bone pain, hypercalcemia, or skeletal complications resulting from Paget disease, multiple myeloma, or metastatic cancer? Date Treatment began:____"

The IV doseforms of BIS are administered as a part of cancer chemotherapy when the malignancy has metastasized to bones (see Table 5.1). ARONJ is more prevalent in individuals with a malignancy.[10] ARONJ has developed in both the mandible and the maxilla, although the mandible is the most common oral location. The anatomical area most commonly involved is the mylohyoid ridge on the lingual of the mandible.

RISK FACTORS FOR ARONJ

While many cases of ARONJ have been associated with an invasive dental procedure such as tooth extraction, ARONJ also occurs spontaneously or in patients with minor mucosal irritation such as those who wear dentures.[10] The condition can occur spontaneously, but is more commonly associated with specific medical and dental conditions, including dental procedures or conditions that increase the risk for bone trauma. ARONJ is associated with invasive bone procedures such as dental extractions. Older age (over 65 years), periodontitis,[14] prolonged use of BIS (more than 2 years), smoking, denture wearing, and diabetes have been associated with an increased risk for ARONJ.[10]

Much is unknown about risk factors for the condition and so little is known about the causative factors that it is unknown how to prevent the condition. Because the current recommendations are not based on randomized studies of the condition, but rather on the experience of a variety of oral surgeons who have managed numerous cases, or from health databases, management is consensus based and may change as more information becomes available.

The most important predisposing factors for the development of ARONJ involve the form of the drug administered and the duration of therapy; plus a history of trauma, oral surgery, or oral infection. Trauma to oral tori is also associated with ARONJ. Periodontal disease has been associated with the development of ONJ in patients who received IV BIS therapy.[14] This is a strong factor in favor of maintaining a healthy periodontal and dental condition. A troubling feature of some reports, however, is of ARONJ developing in clients with no dental disease or recent oral surgery, and who took BIS or antiresorptive therapy.

Signs and Symptoms

Patients may be considered to be diagnosed with ARONJ if they have three characteristics: they are currently receiving, or have received BIS in the past; exposed bone, necrotic bone in the jaw area that has persisted for more than 8 weeks is present; and there is no history of radiation therapy to the jaws.[10,15] A similarly appearing jaw necrosis has been reported to follow high doses of radiation to the head and neck area, called osteoradionecrosis of the jaw.

The clinical features of the patient who presents with ARONJ include a spontaneous exposure of bone of the jaw or a surgical or extraction site that fails to heal (Figs. 5.1–5.4). ARONJ can remain asymptomatic for weeks, months, or years and can result in pain or a nonpainful exposed maxillary or mandibular bone.[15] Pain is a feature when the bone becomes infected and antibiotics along with irrigation with chlorhexidine antibacterial solution are recommended. Signs and symptoms that can occur before clinically detectable ONJ include pain, tooth mobility, mucosal swelling, erythema, and ulceration of the overlying mucosa. Radiographic changes are not evident until there

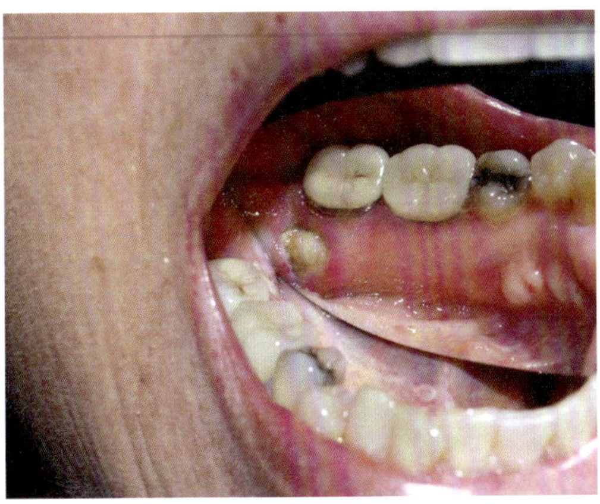

Figure 5.1 ■ Spontaneous ARONJ. (Courtesy of Sal Ruggiero, DMD, MD.)

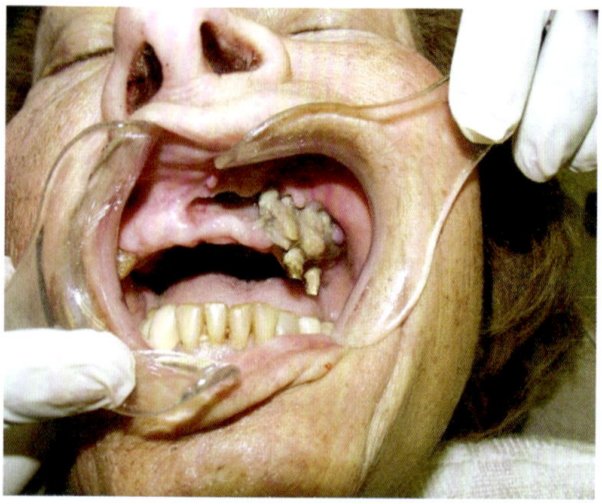

Figure 5.2 ■ ARONJ following implant placement. (Courtesy of Sal Ruggiero, DMD, MD.)

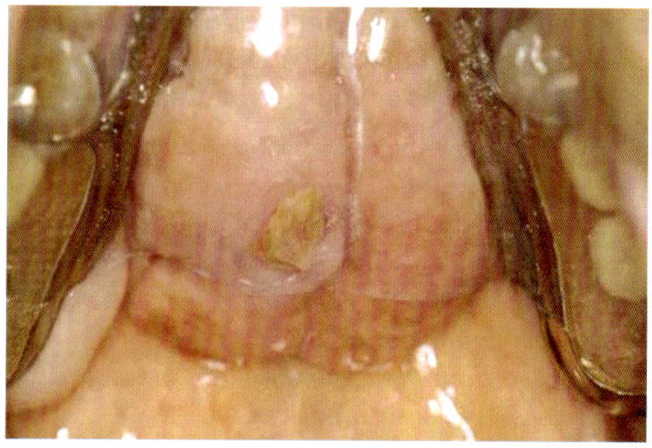

Figure 5.4 ■ ARONJ following local trauma. (Courtesy of Sal Ruggiero, DMD, MD.)

is significant bone involvement, so individuals who are in the early stage of the disease cannot be identified with a full series of radiographs. Radiographic changes resemble classic periapical radiolucency or regions of mottled bone similar to that of diffuse osteomyelitis. Widening of the periodontal ligament space has been reported with some cases. In some individuals on long-term BIS therapy, osteosclerosis of the bone may be noted radiographically, especially in the lamina dura surrounding teeth.

MANAGEMENT FOR ARONJ

Oral and maxillofacial surgeons have been responsible for counseling, managing, and treating a majority of those with ONJ.[15] A task force was appointed by the American Association of Oral and Maxillofacial Surgeons (AAOMS) to develop guidelines and a staging system to assist practitioners in managing ONJ cases. The expert panel formed by ADA considered strategies to be relevant, based on information reported in the literature and reflect clinical observations of the task force members. Because of a paucity of clinical data on the dental management of patients on antiresorptive therapy, these recommendations primarily are based on expert opinion.[10] They stress that as the knowledge base evolves and experience indicates successful treatment, that modifications and refinements will be made in the recommendations.[10]

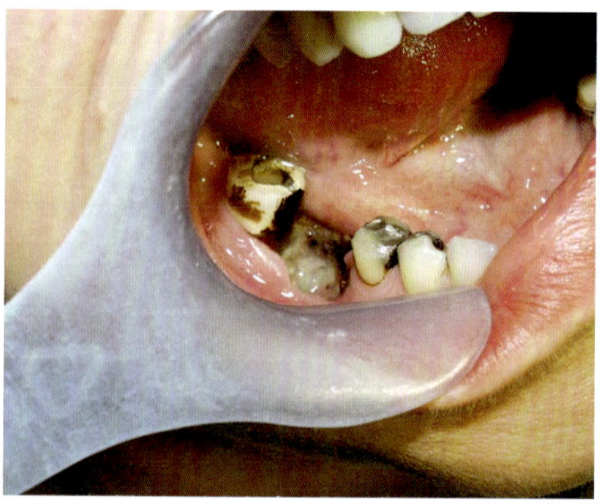

Figure 5.3 ■ ARONJ following tooth extraction. (Courtesy of Sal Ruggiero, DMD, MD.)

Prevention

Although there are no proven strategies to prevent ARONJ, patients who are considering starting antiresorptive therapy should report to the dentist the specific agent taken and have a thorough oral examination early in the therapy. Any unsalvageable teeth should be removed, any periodontal inflammation treated and resolved, and dental health restored. The client should be instructed on how to achieve and maintain optimal oral health and hygiene and warned of a small risk for developing ONJ (oral doseform) or an increased risk for ONJ (IV doseforms). Patients taking antiresorptive agents should be instructed to contact their dentist if any problem develops in the oral cavity.

In this group, oral procedures can be performed with no other restrictions. Routine dental therapy is not contraindicated when antiresorptive agents are taken.[10] Individuals should be informed of the possible risk of developing ARONJ but that oral treatment needed should be completed as a measure to possibly prevent the condition. Any recommendation regarding delaying antiresorptive therapy is done in consultation with the physician.

For the individual who is about to initiate IV BIS therapy the above applies and, if surgical removal of teeth or surgery to remove large tori was necessary, the dentist should consult with the client's oncologist and advise waiting to start BIS therapy until the area has reestablished mucosa over the surgical site. The treatment objective is to minimize the risk of developing ARONJ.

For the client who is currently receiving an oral BIS and who is asymptomatic for ARONJ but who needs an extraction or surgical procedure, the recommendation is there is no evidence that delaying therapy will reduce the risk for ARONJ and endodontics or removing the crown at the gingival margin and allowing the roots to exfoliate may be the best method.[10]

In general, oral antiresorptive agents have less severe manifestations of ARONJ and those affected respond better to treatment. There is evidence that BIS do not need to be continued after 5 years of use because the risks outweigh the benefits.

For the client who is currently receiving IV administered BIS or who has received IV BIS therapy in the past, and who is asymptomatic for ARONJ, maintaining effective oral hygiene and preventing oral disease is of paramount importance. Avoiding the need for surgical procedures in the oral cavity is essential. Placement of implants carries minimal risk according to the ADA guidelines.[10] A new IV doseform of zoledronic acid (Reclast) has been approved by the Food and Drug Administration for osteoporosis and is given once yearly. At this time, based on a 3-year study that reported no cases of ONJ developed, this doseform and infrequent dose schedule (once yearly vs. once monthly or weekly) may be safer than more frequent administration.[16]

Management

For patients with an established diagnosis of ARONJ the goal is to eliminate pain, control infection of the soft and hard tissues, and minimize the progression or occurrence of bone necrosis.[10] Surgical debridement may or may not help resolve symptoms. This has been proposed to be due to difficulty in finding viable bone (bone that has an established circulation can bleed) as the entire jawbone has been affected by the BIS, which is especially persistent. In those who need oral surgery to eliminate necrotic bone or infected teeth in the area of necrotic bone, tooth removal is recommended as it is unlikely to exacerbate an already established process. Areas of necrotic bone that are a source of soft tissue irritation can be removed. Loose segments of bony sequestrum (dead bone that has migrated to the surface) can be removed without exposing uninvolved bone. Elective dental surgical procedures in seemingly unaffected bone should be avoided because these surgical sites may result in additional areas of exposed necrotic bone. Hyperbaric oxygen therapy, which is successful in establishing healing in bone damaged from radiation therapy (osteoradionecrosis), has been tried with variable success. However, a clinical trial has been funded to establish the efficacy of hyperbaric oxygen therapy in treating BRONJ and early reports reveal a promise of success in some patients.[17]

The AAOMS has a staging recommendation for established ARONJ and this is available online in the ADA guidelines.[10]

Role of the Dental Hygienist

Box 5-2 summarizes patient information to be provided when antiresorptive agents are reported on the health history. The guidance provides general information on dental treatments during therapy and is designed to prompt discussion between the oral health professional and the patient about treatment options. The dental hygienist can play a major role in providing this information and ensuring the client understands the importance of maintaining oral health and seeking regular oral examinations to identify disease early, so that the need for surgery does not develop. Two online Web resources are provided following the references. These can be accessed for additional information.

Clinical Application

The items on the ADA Health History Form serve as the follow-up questions for the client with a history of receiving antiresorptive medications. The clinical applications involve examining the oral cavity for evidence of exposed bone. There are cases that were asymptomatic and were discovered by the oral care professional. All clients with the history of antiresorptive therapy should be told about the potential for the adverse drug effect and given information regarding the need to report any oral problems. A summary of the information provided to the patient should be recorded in the dental record.

Box 5-2

Patient Education on Risks of Antiresorptive Therapy Include

- Antiresorptive therapy for low bone mass use places them at low risk for developing ARONJ (the highest prevalence estimate in a large sample is 0.10%).
- The low risk for developing ARONJ can be minimized but not eliminated.
- An oral health program consisting of sound oral hygiene practices and regular dental care may be the optimal approach for lowering the risk for developing ARONJ.
- There is no validated diagnostic technique currently available to determine which patients are at increased risk for developing ARONJ.
- Discontinuing bisphosphonate therapy may not eliminate any risk for developing ARONJ. However, discontinuation of bisphosphonate therapy may have a negative impact on the outcomes of low bone mass treatment. Therefore, significant dental risks need to be present to consider cessation of antiresorptive therapy for low bone mass, cancer, or other off-label therapies. Discussion with all members of the healthcare team is recommended prior to discontinuing therapy.
- The patient should be informed of the dental treatment needed, and alternative treatments.

Self-Study Review

5. ONJ is more prevalent in those taking the IV doseform of BIS. The primary mechanism of this ONJ response is oversuppression of bone turnover.
    a. Both statements are true.
    b. Both statements are false.
    c. The first statement is true, and the second statement is false.
    d. The first statement is false, and the second statement is true.
6. BIS do not leave the bone for up to:
    a. 3 years.
    b. 6 years.
    c. 9 years.
    d. 12 years.
7. Within what time frame are individuals who have taken oral BIS at the greatest risk for developing ONJ?
    a. 6 months
    b. 1 year
    c. 2 years
    d. 5 years
8. ARONJ is most prevalent in individuals with osteoporosis because they are more likely to be exposed to IV BIS.
    a. Both the statement and reason are correct and related.
    b. Both the statement and reason are correct, but NOT related.
    c. The statement is correct, but the reason is NOT.
    d. The statement is NOT correct, but the reason is correct.
    e. NEITHER the statement NOR the reason is correct.
9. All of the following conditions represent an increased risk for ARONJ EXCEPT one. Which one is the EXCEPTION?
    a. Older age
    b. Perimenopausal
    c. Smoking
    d. Diabetes mellitus
10. ARONJ begins with bone pain. Fortunately, this condition can be prevented by practicing good oral health.
    a. Both statements are true.
    b. Both statements are false.
    c. The first statement is true, and the second statement is false.
    d. The first statement is false, and the second statement is true.
11. The anatomic area most commonly involved with BRONJ is the:
    a. maxillary tuberosity.
    b. mandibular condyle.
    c. mandibular mylohyoid ridge.
    d. hard palate.

12. Signs and symptoms of ONJ include pain, mobility, and ulceration of mucosa. Early radiographic changes of ONJ show mottled bone and widening of the periodontal ligament.
   a. Both statements are true.
   b. Both statements are false.
   c. The first statement is true, and the second statement is false.
   d. The first statement is false, and the second statement is true.

CHAPTER SUMMARY

This chapter provided an overview of the indications for antibiotic prophylaxis when previous surgery to replace a joint is reported. In addition, issues related to the client who has been referred for an oral examination as a prerequisite for receiving BIS medication, and the features associated with this possible adverse drug effect are explained. Chapter 6 will address concepts related to allergic reactions.

Review

1. Define the following terms: bacteremia, immunosuppression, innocuous.
2. Explain the reason for placing safety glasses on clients during treatment.
3. Describe the recommended regimen for antibiotic prophylaxis prior to dental treatment for the client who is 18 months posthip joint replacement.
4. List the characteristics for diagnosis of ARONJ.

Case Study

Case A

Mr. Gibson, a 60-year-old client in good health, presents for a routine oral prophylaxis. He reports that 3 months ago he underwent a right knee total joint replacement (TJR). The client states that he is feeling terrific and is able to resume golfing and walking activities. His vital signs are pulse 74 bpm, respiration 16 breaths/min, blood pressure 120/70 mm Hg, right arm, sitting.

1. Is the client considered at risk for infection during oral health care?
2. Is prophylactic antibiotic therapy recommended for this client?
3. If the client had a history of hemophilia, would antibiotic prophylaxis be indicated? If so, why?
4. If Mr. Gibson stated that his orthopedic surgeon recommended he have antibiotic premedication prior to dental or dental hygiene treatment, what steps would you take to address his concern?

Case B

Olivia Rosenfeld presents for a dental examination. She is a 59-year-old client who has a medical history of osteoporosis. Treatment for this condition has consisted of weekly oral doses of Fosamax over a 3-year period of time. Her yearly dexa scan has shown improvement with her status changing from profound osteoporosis to osteopenia. Mrs. Rosenfeld has no oral complaints or other significant health concerns. Her vital signs are pulse 80 bpm, respiration 18 breaths/min, and blood pressure 110/60 mm Hg, right arm, sitting.

1. What other aspect of the medical history would you review to determine other risk factors for ONJ?
2. Upon examination, the dentist recommends that the client have an erupted wisdom tooth extracted. Should treatment be delayed?
3. If this client did develop ARONJ, what treatment options are available?

Chapter Six

Allergies to Drugs, Environmental Substances, Foods, and Metals

Objectives

After completing the self-study chapter the reader will be able to:

- Identify precautions during treatment when the client reports a history of allergy.
- Compare signs of mild with severe allergic reactions.
- Identify appropriate historical questions to gain appropriate information and apply sound judgment related to preventing emergency situations caused by allergic reactions.
- Describe management procedures for clients who have symptoms of anaphylactic shock and for those with symptoms of localized skin or mucosal allergic reactions.

Key Terms

Acute allergic reaction: an immediate response or symptoms appearing within a few hours

Allergen: a substance that can produce a hypersensitive response in the body

Anaphylactic shock: a severe, and sometimes fatal, allergic reaction characterized by respiratory distress and hypotension, leading to cardiovascular collapse

Anaphylactoid reaction: idiosyncratic reactions that occur on the initial exposure to a particular drug or agent rather than after sensitization

Atopy: having a genetic predisposition to develop an allergy to a substance; usually allergy to several substances is present

Complement: an enzymatic serum protein that causes lysis of a cell

Dyspnea: labored or difficult breathing

Erythematous: having a red appearance, caused by dilation of superficial blood vessels

Hypersensitivity: an abnormal condition characterized by an excessive reaction to a particular stimulus, such as allergy

Hypersensitivity reaction: an inappropriate and excessive response of the immune system to a sensitizing antigen; an antigen–antibody reaction; an allergic reaction

Innocuous: harmless

Sensitization: an acquired reaction in which specific antibodies develop in response to an antigen

Stomatitis: ulcerations within the mouth

Urticaria: skin reactions characterized by itching, elevation of tissues (hives) with well-defined erythematous margins

Vesicles: small fluid-filled blisters

MEDICAL CONDITION

INTRODUCTION

The questions in this section of the American Dental Association (ADA) Health History Form involve a variety of substances likely to be used as part of oral health care that may cause an allergic reaction. Local anesthetics (LA) are the most common drug used in dentistry, and a history of allergy to any LA presents a potential clinical problem, although allergy to the ester type of LAs has the greatest risk. The most common allergic reactions include reactions to antibiotics. Oral infections are managed by debridement (removing infectious debris), by draining, and, in some cases, with penicillin-based antibiotics or other antimicrobial agents. Other substances used during oral procedures associated with causing severe allergic reactions include latex products. Dental products composed of latex should be selected only after determining the client has no latex **hypersensitivity**.

"Are you allergic to or have you had a reaction to the following?"

1. LA
2. Aspirin
3. Penicillin, antibiotics
4. Barbiturates, sedatives, sleeping pills
5. Sulfa drugs
6. Codeine, or other narcotics
7. Metals
8. Latex (rubber)
9. Iodine
10. Hay fever or seasonal allergy
11. Animals
12. Food
13. Others

To yes responses, specify type of reaction.

Most of the drugs and substances identified above are likely to be used during oral procedures. Identification of substances that could precipitate an allergic reaction is essential to preventing serious **hypersensitivity reactions** during treatment. In addition, identifying the client with an increased risk for an allergy to substances likely to be used as part of oral procedures, such as the client with **atopy**, is important. Hay fever or seasonal allergy, allergies to animals, and allergies to food are included because clients with a positive history of any allergy are at an increased risk for having an allergy to products used as a part of oral health care.[1] Allergy to metals must be considered before using metal instruments in the client's mouth and also before selecting restorative materials. The length of time between being exposed to an allergenic substance and the development of signs of allergy can alert the healthcare professional to the risk of life-threatening emergency situations. Usually the more rapidly the signs develop, the more dangerous the situation. Rapid onset of signs of allergy must be responded to immediately to prevent medical complications (bronchoconstriction and asphyxia) leading to death.

PATHOPHYSIOLOGY OF ALLERGY AND HYPERSENSITIVITY

Hypersensitivity reactions are a result of the body's immune system responding to an allergenic substance. The allergenic substance (drug, food, metal) acts as an antigen and stimulates the immune system to form antibodies against it. Generally, no observable reaction occurs on this initial exposure, called **sensitization**. For an allergic reaction to occur, the ingested or inhaled substance is metabolized to a reactive hapten by the host immune response.[2] The hapten acts as an antigen after combining with proteins in the body. The antigen stimulates the production of antibodies by plasma cells in the humoral pathway of the immune system. Plasma cells are a type of B lymphocyte, and a small number of these can develop into memory cells, which are responsible for the secondary immune response after re-exposure to the antigen.[3] On re-exposure to the **allergen**, antibodies detect the offending substance and bind to it in an attempt to neutralize it. The result is called an antigen–antibody reaction and is followed by observable signs of allergy. Skin reactions, such as hives, **erythematous** rash, and local swelling, are the most common signs. If the allergic response continues the bronchioles constrict and blood vessels dilate, causing the blood pressure to fall. These are serious signs of allergy and lead to suffocation and shock. When the oral cavity and pharynx are affected, a condition called angioedema can occur. Angioedema is characterized by swelling of the lips, tongue, and, in some cases, the larynx. This leads to inability to breathe, or **dyspnea**. Unlike skin reactions, the tissue is normal in color and does not manifest as hives or itching. If the swelling extends to the larynx, the airway can be obstructed, leading to asphyxiation. The antigen–antibody reaction is neither dose dependent nor predictable (on the first experience); hence, it does not represent an overdose (or toxic) adverse reaction. In fact, only a small amount of a substance will result in an antigen–antibody response in a previously sensitized individual. An exception to this is an unusual response, called an anaphylactoid response, that causes a reaction on the initial exposure.[1] An **anaphylactoid reaction** does not appear to be associated with an immunologic response, and the cause of the response is unclear.

Box 6-1

Signs of Allergy

Mild	Skin rash, erythema Hives, raised area Urticaria (itching)
Severe	Bronchiolar constriction (narrow airway) Asphyxiation, dyspnea Reduction of blood pressure (shock) Cardiovascular collapse

Types of Hypersensitivity Reactions

There are four types of hypersensitivity reactions:

Type I: Type I (immediate) reactions are caused by immunoglobulin E (IgE) antibodies. When the antibody binds to the antigen, a group of immunologic substances are released. These include histamine released by degranulation of mast cells. Mast cells are part of the immune cell system that also includes B and T lymphocytes. B lymphocytes are associated with humoral immunity, and T lymphocytes are associated with cell-mediated immunity. Other substances released include leukotrienes and prostaglandins. These three immunologic chemicals produce vasodilation, edema, and other signs of allergy. In Type I reactions, the target of these chemicals includes the skin, resulting in hives, redness, and itching, a condition known as **urticaria**. Less commonly, the bronchioles of the lungs and the blood vessels are affected, resulting in constriction of the airway and hypotension. These signs lead to cardiovascular collapse (Box 6-1). Reactions affecting the respiratory system can also cause symptoms of rhinitis and asthma. Because Type I reactions occur relatively quickly after exposure to the allergen (seconds to minutes), they are known as immediate hypersensitivity reactions. **Anaphylactic shock** is an acute, life-threatening allergic reaction characterized by hypotension, bronchospasm, laryngeal edema, and cardiac arrhythmias. Drugs used in dentistry that have caused fatal anaphylaxis include the penicillins, the ester class of LAs (such as benzocaine topical [Hurricaine®], tetracaine injectable [Pontocaine®]), and aspirin products.[1,2] Products used in dentistry that have caused anaphylaxis include latex products (gloves, tubing, polishing cups, others).

Type II: Type II reactions are described as cytotoxic because they result in lysis of host cells. They are complement-dependent reactions that involve immunoglobulin G (IgG) and immunoglobulin M (IgM) antibodies. The antigen–antibody complex attaches to circulating red blood cells and lyses the cells, resulting in hemolytic anemia.

Type III: Type III reactions, also called Arthus reactions, are caused by IgG. These reactions cause **complement** to be deposited in the vascular endothelium (inner lining of blood vessels). The reaction is manifested as serum sickness with symptoms of arthralgia, arthritis, lymphadenopathy, fever, and urticarial skin lesions. This reaction has occurred after injection of the hepatitis vaccine series and also can occur after penicillin administration.

Type IV: Type IV reactions are described as delayed reactions that generally occur several days after coming in contact with the allergen. This reaction is mediated by T lymphocytes and macrophages. When these cells contact the allergen, an inflammatory reaction is produced through the release of immunologic chemicals called lymphokines. An example of a Type IV reaction is allergic dermatitis after use of topical products, such as metals, drugs, or soaps. Some latex allergies manifest as a Type IV reaction rather than a Type I immediate reaction. Poison ivy produces a Type IV reaction. Type IV reactions are managed by avoiding the substance in the future. Antihistamines, such as Benadryl®, or topical corticosteroids can be used if the symptoms are uncomfortable.

Self-Study Review

1. An allergic substance acts as a(an):
   a. antibody.
   b. antigen.
   c. complement.
   d. toxic reaction.
2. The most common allergic reaction is:
   a. hypotension.
   b. vesicles.
   c. hives.
   d. stomatitis.
3. Anaphylactoid reactions:
   a. are classic antigen–antibody reactions.
   b. affect the lips, tongue, and larynx.
   c. cause an allergic response with initial exposure.
   d. are not life-threatening.
4. From the following list, identify those that can cause an anaphylactic reaction in dentistry:
   a. Aspirin
   b. Latex gloves
   c. Saliva ejector
   d. Benzocaine topical
   e. Penicillin
   f. Polishing cups
   g. Curet
   h. X-ray film
5. Anaphylactic shock represents which type of hypersensitivity reaction?
   a. Type I
   b. Type II
   c. Type III
   d. Type IV
6. Allergic dermatitis is an example of which type of hypersensitivity reaction?
   a. Type I
   b. Type II
   c. Type III
   d. Type IV
7. Serum sickness is an example of which type of hypersensitivity reaction?
   a. Type I
   b. Type II
   c. Type III
   d. Type IV

PRODUCTS USED IN ORAL CARE RELATED TO ALLERGY

The ADA Health History section for allergy lists various drugs and products likely to cause an allergic reaction. Many latex products are used during the provision of oral health care, and reports of latex hypersensitivity are increasing. Nonlatex products are available to avoid this problem. Allergy-related conditions included within the history questionnaire include hay fever or seasonal allergy and allergy to animals or foods.

Local Anesthetic Reactions

There are two main classifications of LA agents, esters and amides. The most common allergy related to LA agents involves those from the ester category. There are no longer any injectable LA agents in the ester category. The examples in the ester group of topical anesthetic agents are benzocaine (Hurricaine) and tetracaine (Pontocaine). Benzocaine is the most common topical anesthetic agent used in dentistry and is considered very safe, unless the client has an allergy to the ester group of anesthetic drugs. Allergy to the amide group of LAs is rare, and products in this group (lidocaine [Xylocaine®], prilocaine [Citanest®], mepivacaine [Carbocaine®], articaine [Septodont®]) are among the most widely used in dentistry. There is no cross allergenicity among the amide LAs; therefore, if the client shows an allergy to one product in the group, another product could likely be used. The client would need to be medically evaluated by an immunologist to determine whether an allergy exists to any of the other amide LAs. Allergic reactions to LAs range from a mild skin rash to severe anaphylaxis.

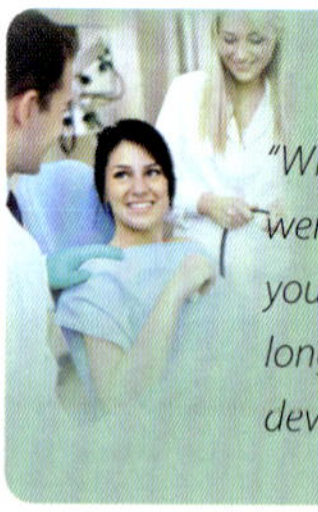

Follow-up Questions

"What LA caused your reaction? What were the symptoms that made you think you were allergic to the anesthetic? How long after the injection did the signs develop?"

If the client marks "yes" to this drug group, determine the specific LA that precipitated the allergic reaction, the type of reaction that resulted, and how quickly the signs developed. It is well known that fear and anxiety related to having a "shot" can result in syncope and loss of consciousness. If this is the type of reaction described by the client, then it is logical to assume that the client suffered an anxiety-related syncope, rather than a true allergy. If the client has a true allergy to the ester type of LAs, benzocaine would not be used as a topical anesthetic. An amide topical, such as lidocaine (Xylocaine®), should be selected. It is uncommon, although still possible, to have an allergy to both esters and amides. If the client reports that signs of allergy developed quickly (within a few minutes) of the dental injection, the risk is high for the client to have an anaphylactic reaction. If another LA agent is used, the client should be monitored closely for signs of an allergic reaction.

Aspirin Reactions

Allergy to aspirin is uncommon in the general population. Symptoms range from mild skin reactions (erythema, rash, hives, itching) to anaphylaxis. Bronchospasm is the chief allergic sign in most people with aspirin allergy.[1] Clients with asthma have a greater incidence of allergy to aspirin and aspirin-related products, such as nonsteroidal analgesics or nonsteroidal anti-inflammatory drugs (NSAIDs) (e.g., ibuprofen, naproxen). It is estimated that between 15% and 19% of asthmatics are allergic to aspirin. This means that most asthmatics may take aspirin with no problems; however, the client should be questioned to determine whether an aspirin allergy exists. Serious systemic reactions involving constriction of the bronchioles (resulting in asphyxiation) and loss of blood pressure, leading to cardiovascular collapse, can occur.

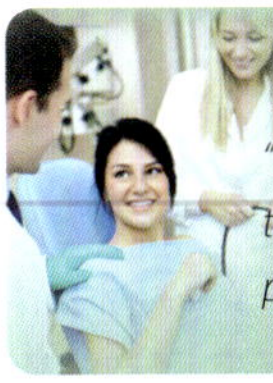

Follow-up Questions

"What were your symptoms? Do you take NSAIDs or acetaminophen for pain?"

If the client specifies "yes" to aspirin allergy, have the client describe the symptoms experienced to determine whether the response represents a true allergy. In the asthmatic client, aspirin sensitivity can also cause increased mucous secretion in airway passages. This results in exacerbation of asthma symptoms and an "asthma attack." For those aspirin-sensitive clients who need an analgesic for oral pain, acetaminophen (Tylenol®) is an effective mild analgesic. If the client reports an allergy to aspirin but has taken an NSAID, such as ibuprofen, suggest an NSAID for oral pain. Some common brand names for NSAIDs are listed in Box 6-2.

Box 6-2

Common Nonsteroidal Drug Products

Generic Name	Brand Name
Ibuprofen	Advil, Excedrin IB, Midol IB, Motrin IB, Nuprin, Pamprin IB
Naproxen	Naprosyn, Anaprox, Aleve
Aspirin	Ecotrin, Empirin, Arthritis Foundation Pain Reliever

(Adapted from Pickett F, Terezhalmy G. Lippincott's Dental Drug Reference. 2011.)

Penicillin or Other Antibiotics

Penicillin is the most allergenic drug. Reactions range from mild skin reactions described above to systemic anaphylaxis, a life-threatening reaction. Injections of penicillin are responsible for the majority of severe anaphylactic reactions; however, the topical application of penicillin is the most likely route of administration to sensitize the individual. Because 90% of oral infections are sensitive to narrow-spectrum antibiotics (penicillin, erythromycin), dentists frequently use them as first-choice therapy in treating oral infections. For clients with penicillin allergy, either erythromycin (or one of the other antibiotics in the macrolide class) or clindamycin can be used for oral infections requiring antibiotics.

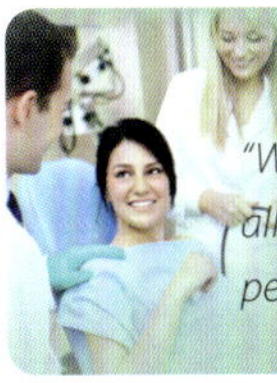

Follow-up Questions

"What were your signs of allergy? Are you allergic to any other antibiotic besides penicillin?"

As in the previous discussion, ensure that the signs described represented allergy. Nausea (often reported as a sign of allergy by clients) is usually a drug side effect, not an allergic reaction. Multiple antibiotic allergies can occur; however, many clients with multiple allergies can take other antibiotic products. Information gained with these

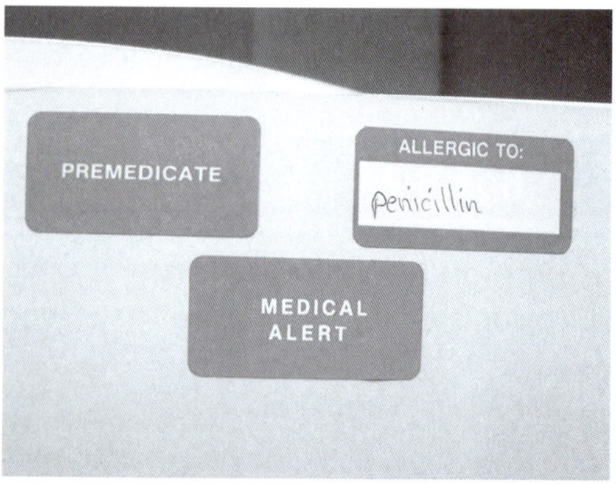

Figure 6.1 ■ Medical alert chart. (Adapted from the Medical Arts Press Catalog.)

follow-up questions will assist the dentist to select the appropriate antibiotic for the client. *It is imperative to mark the chart section alerting the dentist to a penicillin allergy as this antibiotic is commonly prescribed in dentistry.* A variety of medical alert chart systems are available to identify serious medical conditions (Fig. 6.1). When the client reports a positive response to drug allergy questions, determine what antibiotics have caused adverse effects and what signs occurred. To protect the privacy of the client, keep the chart available only to those who are intended to see the client information.

Barbiturates, Sedatives, or Sleeping Pills

These three drug types are widely used as part of a stress reduction protocol in clients unable to respond to stress or who are fearful of having dental treatment.

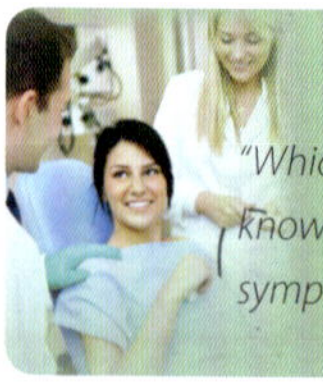

Follow-up Questions

"Which drug caused the reaction? Do you know the dose prescribed? Describe your symptoms."

The clinician should investigate which category of drugs caused the reaction and determine whether the symptoms described are allergenic in nature or may be related to other causes. Dose-related side effects, such as nausea or dizziness, are often reported. The client may believe these reactions are signs of allergy. It is important to use critical thinking skills when listening to client information. Correlating the description of the symptoms experienced with scientific information for signs of allergy allows the clinician to discern drug side effects from a true allergic reaction. Using a sedative in a lower dose or selecting a sedative less likely to cause the reported side effect, such as nausea and vomiting, may be useful to manage drug effects.

Sulfa Drugs

These drugs are commonly indicated for urinary tract infections and are not likely to be prescribed by the dentist. There are no chemically related anti-infective agents used for dental infections. However, there are reports of anaphylaxis occurring after taking a drug that includes sulfa-containing binding agents in the preparation. For clients who report a "sulfa" allergy, drugs with components determined to contain sulfa should not be prescribed.

Codeine or Other Narcotics

A positive response to this question is not uncommon. Many clients confuse an allergy to codeine (and other narcotic products, such as hydrocodone) with common side effects of codeine, such as nausea, vomiting, and gastrointestinal complaints. Codeine and non-narcotic analgesic combination drugs (Tylenol 1®, Tylenol 2®, acetaminophen/hydrocodone, and so forth) are frequently prescribed for oral pain. These products use a small dose of the narcotic plus a normal dose of the non-narcotic analgesic to get additive pain relief. Using a low dose of the narcotic is thought to cause fewer side effects. However, allergy is an adverse effect that is NOT related to dose. Giving a very small amount of this drug will excite an allergic reaction in the truly codeine allergic client. The practitioner must determine whether symptoms represent a true allergy to codeine, as the codeine combination products would be contraindicated in the client who is allergic to codeine.

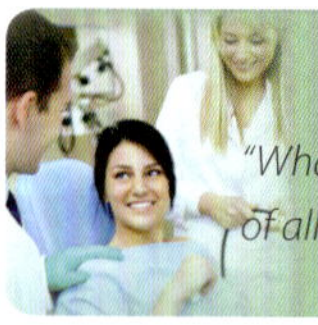

Follow-up Questions

"What specific narcotic drug caused signs of allergy? What were your symptoms?"

For the client who reports "rash, hives, and itching" after taking codeine, codeine-containing analgesics are contraindicated. Clients often confuse the side effect of nausea, commonly reported with codeine, with a drug allergy. When the client experiences a side effect of nausea, using a lower dose of codeine (or using hydrocodone which has less risk for nausea) combined with a non-narcotic analgesic is a common practice. For example, the combination of hydrocodone and acetaminophen has been consistently within the list of the top 10 most common drugs prescribed in the United States in recent years. Side effects are dose related, and the low-dose opioid and non-narcotic combinations help reduce nausea. Dental use of these agents to relieve pain is for a short term, usually up to 5 days. These narcotic combination analgesics, due to the narcotic component that is a controlled substance, can produce drug dependence if taken for long periods of time. Death due to overdose of hydrocodone is increasing and practitioners are encouraged to properly instruct patients on how to take the drug safely.[4] Hydrocodone combinations with acetaminophen, aspirin, or ibuprofen are commonly prescribed and are in schedule III for drugs with abuse potential. It has been recommended to move these combination agents with hydrocodone to schedule II.[4] If this is approved, the action would prevent the dentist from calling in a prescription for the hydrocodone combination product.

Self-Study Review

8. From the following list, identify the two anesthetic agents most likely to cause an allergic reaction.
   a. Lidocaine
   b. Procaine
   c. Benzocaine
   d. Mepivacaine
   e. Propoxycaine
   f. Tetracaine
   g. Articaine
9. Clients reporting a history of asthma have an increased risk of allergy to:
   a. acetaminophen.
   b. aspirin.
   c. codeine.
   d. penicillin.
10. The most allergenic drug is:
    a. aspirin.
    b. codeine.
    c. sulfa.
    d. penicillin.
11. The drug least likely to be used in dentistry is
    a. Aspirin
    b. Codeine
    c. Sulfa
    d. Penicillin

Latex Allergy

A study conducted as part of the ADA's annual health screening program found that 6.2% of the dentists, hygienists, and assistants, who participated tested positive for Type I hypersensitivity of natural rubber latex.[5] In 1992, the U.S. Food and Drug Administration reported that between 1988 and 1992 it received reports of 1,118 injuries and 15 deaths attributed to latex products.[6] Because of the increased use of latex products in health care and the increasing incidence of true latex allergy, a positive response to this question has significant management implications. It is essential to determine whether signs experienced by the client represent signs of allergy. The exposed skin presents with a dermatitis that can become dry, reddened, and develop vesicle formation followed by crusted lesions, as well as itching. Many items in the dental armamentarium contain latex. These include rubber tubing, gloves used in treatment, elastic on masks, rubber polishing cups, the rubber seal on LA cartridges, and rubber dam latex (Box 6-3).

Box 6-3

Dental Products Containing Latex

- Rubber tubing on unit, stethoscope, blood pressure cuff
- Gloves, latex barriers, elastic on face mask
- Rubber polishing cup
- Rubber dam
- Rubber on LA cartridge

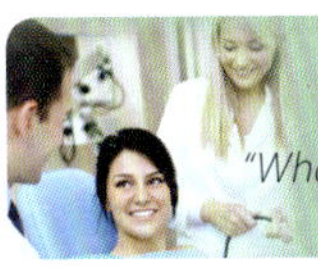

Follow-up Question

"What were your symptoms?"

If allergenic skin reactions or difficulty in breathing are reported after coming into contact with a latex product, the client may have a latex allergy.

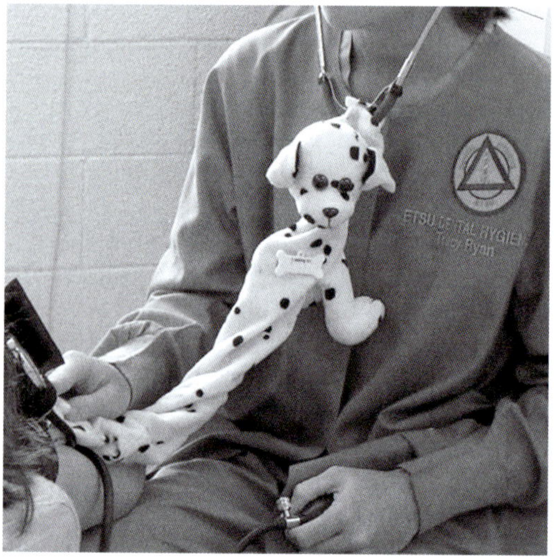

Figure 6.2 ■ Barrier covering on latex tubing of stethoscope.

It is vital that the dental office have available NONLATEX products to use when treating a client with a latex allergy. The practitioner, as well as the client, must be considered and barriers applied to prevent contact with products that are only available in latex (e.g., the stethoscope).

Prevention of Latex Allergy

Practitioner

The oral healthcare practitioner can cover the stethoscope latex tubes with a barrier, such as fabric (Fig. 6.2).

Vinyl gloves or nonlatex gloves (Nitrile®) should be available for use during treatment. Masks that tie on are available to avoid the latex elastic that secures most masks. When hands are covered, touching items that contain latex presents no problem to the practitioner with a latex allergy. The powder lining latex gloves contains latex protein. This causes a potential for latex allergens to become airborne. When others in the office put on or take off latex gloves, proteins are aerosolized, increasing the risk for an allergic reaction in the latex-sensitive clinician or client. A safe protocol to follow for the office that employs staff with latex sensitivity is to purchase only nonlatex gloves. Another prevention strategy is to use non-powdered latex gloves.

Manufacturers have introduced latex-free products to assist in reducing the risk for latex allergy events. Latex-free injectable LA cartridges and latex-free polishing cups are available. When ordering supplies, catalogs will identify those products which are latex-free.

Client

When the client reports a latex allergy, the clinician must mark the chart with a LATEX WARNING label illustrated in Figure 6.1. Products selected for use must be carefully considered. It is helpful for the office to have a prepackaged tray setup for the latex-sensitive client. Items to consider for the packet include nonlatex rubber polishing cup, nonlatex gloves, nonlatex barriers, covers for dental unit hoses (if hoses are latex), and covers for stethoscope tubing. Applying a nonlatex barrier (plastic, cellophane) to the arm before placing the blood pressure cuff should provide adequate protection to the client. Metal napkin chains and alternatives for any latex product that may cause an allergic reaction should be selected. Appointment planning should include early morning appointments (the first appointment in the day) when the room air is unlikely to be contaminated with latex protein particles. If the office is closed on a weekend day, appoint on Monday when airborne particles are less likely to occur. Because allergy is an adverse reaction that is not dose related, breathing in a small amount of latex-contaminated air (in a latex-sensitive person) can incite a reaction. There are reports of anaphylaxis and death as a result of a latex allergic reaction.

Iodine Allergy

This question relates to iodine-containing dental products that may be used within the oral cavity, such as Betadine® antiseptic solution. In the past, disclosing solutions containing iodine were used, but erythrosine dye products have replaced these products. Some anti-infective hand soaps used for presurgical scrubs contain iodine. Surface disinfection solutions may contain iodine (iodophors).

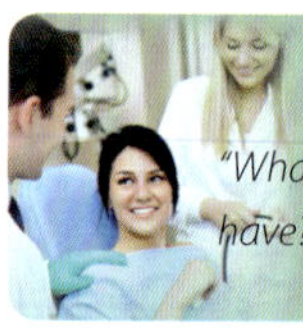

Follow-up Questions

"What product was used? What signs did you have?

Question the client to determine whether signs of allergy developed after use of the iodine product. The clinician and auxiliary must consider product ingredients used in the office and take care to select noniodine products for the client who reports an allergy to iodine.

Hay Fever or Seasonal Allergy, Animals, Food, and Metals

Hay fever is considered to be a risk factor for having an allergy to products used during oral procedures. When multiple allergies are reported (food, antibiotics, other substances), in addition to hay fever, the risk for allergy significantly increases and the client should be monitored whenever any product is placed in the mouth. For example, in the atopic client, the use of topical fluoride (a rare product to cause an allergic reaction) can incite an allergic reaction. A history of allergy to metals must be followed up because the most common dental restorative material (amalgam) contains metal. In addition, metal instruments are used routinely in the client's mouth.

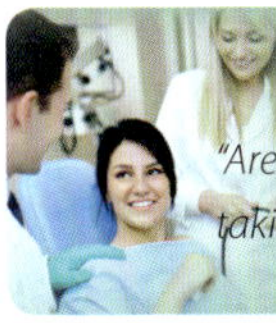

Follow-up Questions

"Are you having symptoms today? Are you taking any medications for hay fever?"

Appropriate follow-up questions should attempt to identify the specific item that causes allergic symptoms.

If the client is having postnasal drainage, the semisupine chair position should be used. Placing a symptomatic client in a supine position is likely to result in coughing or choking. Medications used to alleviate symptoms of hay fever include antihistamines, decongestants, or the combination of these products. Significant side effects can include dry mouth (if taken for several consecutive days), increased blood pressure, and tachycardia. A home fluoride product should be recommended if chronic xerostomia is suspected. Monitoring vital signs will identify whether cardiovascular side effects are produced. Many clients do not have these side effects. Comparison of blood pressure values with the normal limits of vital signs should determine whether a client is affected. This is another example of using critical thinking when assessing risks for emergency situations and modifying treatment to prevent potential problems. Plastic instruments are available that can be used for deposit removal. There is also a plastic covering for the ultrasonic insert tip that is available for purchase. These plastic instruments were developed for use on dental implants.

It is well known that the client who reports allergy to one substance is often allergic to other substances, such as cats, dogs, or various foods. This places the client at an increased risk for allergy to products used in oral healthcare treatment as discussed above. It is appropriate to question the client about previous experience with products to be used during the current treatment, such as disclosing solution, fluoride, or toothpastes.

"To yes responses, specify type of reaction."

SIGNS OF ADVERSE OR ALLERGENIC REACTIONS

It is not unusual for a client to indicate having an allergy to a drug that has caused a side effect. For this reason, the request to describe the reaction will assist the clinician in determining whether the symptom experienced by the client represents a true allergic reaction. Signs of acute allergy include erythematous skin rash, hives (raised lesions), urticaria (itching), and, in some cases, bronchiolar constriction resulting in wheezing, respiratory difficulty with poor oxygen exchange, development of cyanosis, as well as hypotension.

Application to Practice

When the client reports allergy to a drug or product likely to be used in the dental appointment, *the official chart or dental record should be marked to call attention to the allergy* (Fig. 6.1).

Follow-up questions should relate to the symptoms that occurred after taking the drug or using the product to determine whether a true allergy exists or whether the adverse effect was related to another cause, such as a drug side effect. Oral healthcare workers must be careful to avoid using a product to which the client reports an allergy. Even a condition as common and seemingly **innocuous** as hay fever or seasonal allergy is thought to be an indicator to identify the client at risk for an allergic reaction to an oral product. Those clients who report multiple allergies are at a significant risk for allergy to products used during treatment and must be monitored for signs of an **acute allergic reaction** during treatment (hives and an erythematous, itching rash are common signs). *Immediate hypersensitivity reactions are considered the most dangerous reactions.*[1] An immediate reaction is characterized by airway constriction and falling blood pressure called anaphylactic shock.

Management of Anaphylactic Shock

Anaphylactic shock (anaphylaxis) is a potentially fatal allergic reaction and must be managed immediately by a dentist or the client who can inject epinephrine

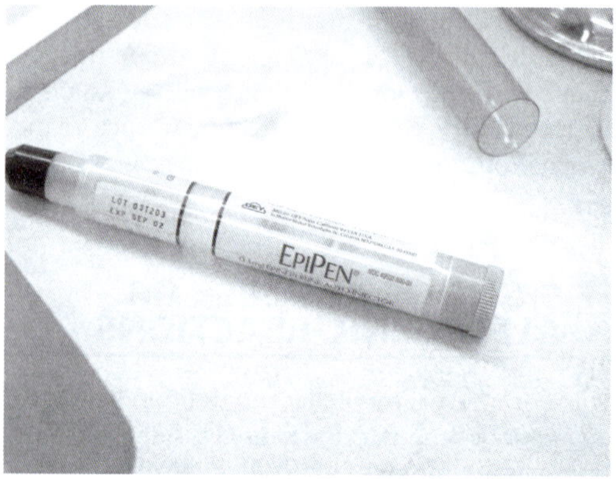

Figure 6.3 ■ EpiPen device.

sublingually (dentist) or intramuscularly (client) in an effort to reverse bronchiolar constriction and hypotension that characterize this condition. The dose is 0.3 to 0.5 mg of a 1:1,000 concentration for adults and 0.1 to 0.3 mg or 0.01 mg/kg for children.[3] If the client has brought an autoinjectable epinephrine device to the appointment, assist the client in securing the device and allow the client to administer the medicine (Fig. 6.3). Symptoms usually begin with an immediate onset of skin reactions, progress to other areas, such as the respiratory system, and end with effects of the cardiovascular system. After identifying signs of anaphylaxis, reposition the client to an upright position and provide 100% oxygen.[1] Call 911 to summon the emergency medical system. After summoning the emergency response team, closely monitor the victim's vital signs and airway.[3] Monitor and record vital signs every 5 minutes. If respiratory or cardiac arrest occurs, begin resuscitation efforts. Recently, the cardiopulmonary resuscitation (CPR) procedures were modified to include cardiac compression only while awaiting emergency medical services (EMS) support, if the rescuer is unable or unwilling to provide rescue breaths.[7] Although in the United States the administration of emergency drugs is not within the purview of drugs allowable within dental practice acts to be administered by dental hygienists (with the exception of oxygen), the hygienist can secure the emergency kit and bring it to the area of patient management so the dentist can quickly retrieve the specific drug needed.

Management of Other Signs of Allergy

Fortunately, the most common allergic reactions associated with using allergenic products during oral health care are less dangerous than anaphylaxis.[3] These reactions are characterized by formation of **vesicles** that break to form small ulcers, development of erythema, rash, itching, or causing stinging and tissue sloughing. When these signs occur on the oral mucosa the condition is called contact stomatitis. It is usually a delayed hypersensitivity reaction. The management strategy for contact stomatitis is to refrain from using the agent that precipitated the allergy. If the reaction is severe and the client has increased discomfort, a topical corticosteroid to help alleviate symptoms can be prescribed by the dentist. This can be followed with oral ingestion of an antihistamine product, such as Benadryl®.

Self-Study Review

12. Items in the dental armamentarium that contain latex include all of the following EXCEPT one. Which is the EXCEPTION?
   a. Rubber tubing
   b. Polishing cups
   c. Tie-on masks
   d. Stethoscope

13. Clients reporting a recent onset of hay fever with postnasal drip should be placed in which position for oral health care?
   a. Supine
   b. Semisupine
   c. Upright
   d. Prone

14. Allergic reactions are typically dose dependent. Practitioners should monitor amounts of LA administered to avoid an allergic reaction.
   a. Both statements are true.
   b. Both statements are false.
   c. The first statement is true, and the second statement is false.
   d. The first statement is false, and the second statement is true.

CHAPTER SUMMARY

This chapter described the types of hypersensitivity reactions and reviews the items on the medical history related to allergic responses. This information will help clinicians distinguish between allergic reactions and adverse effects of medications. Management strategies for addressing allergic reactions were provided to enable the oral healthcare professional to appropriately address situations that arise in the dental office setting.

Review

1. Define the following terms: anaphylactic shock, hypersensitivity reaction, and sensitization.
2. List the signs of a mild allergic reaction and the signs of a severe allergic reaction.
3. If a client reports that she is allergic to local anesthesia, what follow-up questions should you ask?
4. Identify at least five items of the dental armamentarium that can cause a latex allergy.

Case Study

Case A

A female child, 9 years of age, presented for dental treatment. The chief complaint was "my back tooth hurts." The child had never been to a dentist. Medical history was noncontributory except for allergy to tomatoes, strawberries, seafood, and erythromycin antibiotics. When asked whether the child had received any local anesthetic (LA) drugs, the mother said the child had never had a dental anesthetic before. Oral examination revealed a large carious lesion in tooth number 30; radiographs revealed no evidence of loss of tooth vitality. To be safe the dentist selected lidocaine for local anesthesia. Within minutes after the injection, the dental assistant noticed erythema on one side of the child's face, and the child seemed anxious and reported difficulty breathing. It was clear that immediate medical intervention was necessary.

1. What was the most likely source for the child's symptoms?
2. What type of allergic reaction does this case represent?
3. What management strategies should be used to treat this adverse reaction?
4. What management strategies should be used to prevent this allergic reaction from recurring in the dental office setting?
5. If the client reported that she felt sick to her stomach, should this be considered part of an allergic reaction?

Case B

A 49-year-old woman presents for a dental hygiene continuing care appointment. The client relates a chief complaint of recent onset of soreness and ulceration of her mouth. Examination reveals multiple small ulcers of the buccal mucosa and a sloughing of the gingiva. The dental hygienist questioned the client regarding changes in oral products used, and the client indicated that she recently switched toothpastes to a new tartar control brand.

1. What is the name for the oral condition described in the examination?
2. What is the most likely cause of this condition?
3. What management strategies would be recommended for this client?

Chapter Seven

Substance Abuse (Controlled Substances, Tobacco Use, Alcohol)

Objectives

After completing the self-study chapter the reader will be able to:

- Describe the clinical relevance associated with clients who abuse controlled substances, alcohol, and other substances.
- Identify drugs used in oral care procedures that interact with controlled substances or alcohol.
- Describe a tobacco cessation plan when the client is interested in stopping a tobacco habit.

Key Terms

Bidis: filterless cigarettes from India and Southeast Asia, containing nicotine, but sold in a variety of flavors

Coanalgesia: using more than one drug for pain relief

Controlled substances: narcotics or drugs affecting the central nervous system that lead to addiction; these drugs are controlled by the Drug Enforcement Administration (DEA) and can only be prescribed when a DEA number has been received by a prescriber

CVD: cardiovascular disease

Hemostasis: procedures to stop bleeding or encourage clot formation

IE: infective endocarditis

MI: myocardial infarction (heart attack)

Substance abuse: the overuse of substances to modify or control mood or state of mind in a manner that is illegal or harmful to oneself or others

Sympathomimetic: having actions of the sympathetic nervous system, stimulation results in increased blood pressure and increased heart rate

MEDICAL CONDITION

INTRODUCTION

The American Dental Association (ADA) Health History continues with questions to identify the client who may be abusing **controlled substances**, alcohol, or other substances, including tobacco. Currently an estimated 43 million Americans (16% of the population) suffers from chemical dependence, alcohol abuse, or both. Drug use is highest among adults 18 to 25 years of age with over 54 million Americans reporting participating in binge drinking in the previous 30 days. Sixteen million Americans are considered to be heavy drinkers of alcohol. Although there is no question regarding a history of participating in an "addiction recovery" program, this history is also important. There are significant dental implications for clients with these histories, some of which relate to an increased risk for an emergency situation as well as in prescribing medication for pain. The dental team must be more alert to recognize individuals who need special care and referral for alcohol, tobacco, and other addiction services. Confidentiality is essential to protect client medical information.

"Do you use controlled substances (drugs)?"

Substance dependency is characterized by three features: the tendency to use more substances during the addiction period, physiological and psychological changes leading to bizarre behavior when the substance is withdrawn, and an overwhelming desire to continue using the substance despite negative consequences. **Substance abuse** affects all age groups, the young, the middle aged, and the older adult, and affects individuals in all income levels. Marijuana is a common drug of abuse in the United States, followed by cocaine. Cocaine accounted for the illicit drug that led to the most hospital emergency visits. According to the 2004 National Survey on Drug Use and Health, approximately 14% of people 12 years of age or older in the United States have tried cocaine at least once (34 million individuals) and those aged 18 to 25 years have the highest rate of cocaine use, with males having more than twice the rate of female users. Approximately 2 million people in the United States have participated in some form of Alcoholics Anonymous or Cocaine Anonymous programs. According to the National Center on Addiction and Substance Abuse at Columbia University, the demand for alcohol and drug treatment has increased since the September 11, 2001, terrorist attacks. Stress is considered a high risk for relapse to alcohol, drug abuse, and smoking. When substance abuse is suspected and the client does not mark "yes" on the question related to use of controlled substances, the practitioner should question the client more thoroughly, explain the signs observed that lead one to be suspicious of substance abuse, and make appropriate referrals for medical help to get the client in recovery. Establishing a trusting relationship and concern, as well as ensuring the confidentiality of medical information is very important in helping a client to seek medical help for substance abuse. Clients may express concerns to the dental office staff, such as the dental hygienist, rather than the dentist, therefore being educated on an appropriate response to issues of substance abuse is essential. Screening for substance abuse can include a brief verbal interaction that focuses on potential harms of using controlled substances on oral tissues and possible serious interactions with drugs commonly used during oral care.

Significant issues related to substance abuse (including prescribed narcotics) include

- The deleterious oral effects of drug abuse.
- Medical problems related to drug abuse.
- Participation in a recovery program, or a history of being in a recovery program.
- Interactions between some controlled substances and drugs used as part of oral care, illegal drugs, and agents used commonly in dentistry.
- Appointment control issues, such as missed appointments or excessive complaints, during the appointment.

Specific oral complications of drug use include xerostomia, mucosal injuries, rampant caries, and rapidly progressive periodontal disorders.[1] Periodontal disease is high among drug abusers, often due to neglect in oral cleaning complicated by use of tobacco. However, one report suggests marijuana (cannabis) users who do not smoke cigarettes (or otherwise use other tobacco products) have a high risk for developing periodontal disease.[2] Rampant caries is associated with use of methamphetamine (meth mouth).[3]

Systemic effects associated with substance abuse include cardiovascular disease (**CVD**; myocardial infarction [**MI**] or heart attack, infective endocarditis [**IE**]), bloodborne communicable diseases, liver dysfunction, and immunosuppression. For the client who is recovering from substance abuse in the past, these medical problems can be lifelong and need follow-up to determine the degree of control over the organs affected. Effects of CVD can result in hypertension and an increased demand for oxygenated blood by blood vessels supplying the cardiac muscle. The regular monitoring of vital signs for individuals with a history of substance abuse is a method to identify poorly controlled systemic disease. For individuals with a history of endocarditis, the current recommendation for antibiotic prophylaxis prior to oral procedures (such as oral prophylaxis, periodontal probing, etc.) can be applied. In addition, liver dysfunction can predispose the substance abuser to increased bleeding problems and poor metabolism of drugs in general (clotting factors are formed in the liver and most drugs are metabolized and inactivated by the liver).

For clients in a recovery program, inadequate pain relief can be a trigger to take pain-relieving narcotics. In this instance, it is important for the dentist to consult with the client's physician regarding recommendations for pain medication. Dental personnel should make oral product recommendations that avoid alcohol-containing mouthrinses and non-narcotic analgesics.

In addition, marijuana, amphetamines, and cocaine have **sympathomimetic** effects and are reported to interact with vasoconstrictors in local anesthetics. Administration of local anesthetics containing epinephrine or use of gingival retraction cords impregnated with epinephrine may enhance tachycardia and increase blood pressure values caused by the combination of epinephrine with these drugs.

Substance abusers often have a history of missed appointments, dramatic unexpected complaints related to oral care, and repeated requests for narcotic prescriptions. Drug-seeking behavior has been described as a "new patient" who comes to the dental office close to the end of the day with excruciating pain. The client wants a prescription to get them through the night and may make an appointment for dental treatment the next day. The tolerance that develops to pain-relieving medications may make it difficult to relieve pain adequately with a local anesthetic during the appointment. While the client is in the operatory, the office prescription pads should be in a secure area. Assurance of confidentially with regard to information related to substance abuse is mandatory. The client should be questioned about an interest in stopping substance abuse to demonstrate motivation prior to a referral for medical help for recovery programs.

ETHICAL CONSIDERATIONS FOR THE SUBSTANCE-ABUSING CLIENT

The ADA has a section within the journal that discusses a situation posed by a dentist with the question, "What should I do when I suspect a patient may be abusing prescription drugs?"[4] The dentist describes a situation in which a patient was seen recently on an emergency basis the previous month and was referred for extraction of a tooth previously treated with an endodontic procedure that fractured at the gumline. The history revealed the client was a patient of record for 2 years but did not follow-up with preventive maintenance visits and, on the most recent visit, had not completed the referral for the extraction. The client continued to call the dentist after office hours for narcotics to relieve pain. The client has a history of rescheduling dental appointments and avoiding oral care. The dentist suspected the client of abusing prescription narcotic medication and was seeking advice on how to deal with the situation.[4]

The issue was addressed by a member of the ADA Council on Ethics, Bylaws and Judicial Affairs and referred the dentist to the ADA Principles of Ethics and Code of Professional Conduct. The dentist's most important obligation is competent and timely delivery of dental care within the bounds of the clinical circumstances. The suspicions of the dentist and the client's failure to have the necessary care warrant caution before continuing to prescribe narcotics. The Ethics committee member reminded the dentist that drug addiction is a disease, and it may result in personal failings and unfortunate circumstances. The symptoms of drug abuse (numerous caries, tooth fracture, decreased response to local anesthetics, prone to oral infection) and drug-seeking behaviors must be recognized. Contacting the dentist after hours is an example of drug-seeking behavior. Chronic chemical abusers are less inclined to maintain oral hygiene, to have regular examinations, and to keep appointments for follow-up care. Recognizing the previous signs of substance abuse is important in order for oral care providers to help patients get into medical care for addiction. The dentist was advised to request the patient to come to the office for consultation. At that appointment, concerns about the possibility of narcotic abuse should be shared, specifying the failure to keep the appointments for the tooth extraction, which would resolve the dental pain. Concerns should be expressed in a caring, nonjudgmental manner.

If the patient is receptive, the physician should be contacted and, with the client listening, a communication of the events that necessitated the call is made. The dentist can assist the client with making a medical appointment to seek help for abuse of prescription narcotics. Confidentiality laws prevent the dentist from discussing the situation with the client's family members, unless approved by the client. In the case of a minor, state laws related to confidentiality for adolescents should be investigated with an attorney in order to receive direction on the oral health professional's obligations to report (or prevent the reporting of) the suspicions to the parent or court-appointed guardian. The dental professional could offer assistance in finding community resources to help advance the welfare of the patient. This is in keeping with the ADA Code, Section 2.B, Consultation and Referral, which states, "Dentists shall be obligated to seek consultation, if possible, whenever the welfare of patients will be safeguarded or advanced by utilizing those who have special skills, knowledge, and experience."

In 2005, the ADA recognizing the increasing need for helping clients with substance abuse drafted the following guidelines[4]:

1. Dentists are urged to be aware of each patient's substance use history, and to take this into consideration when planning treatment and prescribing medications.
2. Dentists are encouraged to be knowledgeable about substance use disorders—both active and in remission in order to safely prescribe controlled substances and other medications to patients with these disorders.
3. Dentists should draw upon their professional judgment in advising patients who are heavy drinkers to cut back, or the users of illegal drugs to stop using.
4. Dentists may want to be familiar with their community's treatment resources for patients with substance use disorders and be able to make referrals when indicated.
5. Dentists are encouraged to seek consultation with the patient's physician when the patient has a history of alcoholism or other substance use disorder.
6. Dentists are urged to be current in their knowledge of pharmacology, including content related to drugs of abuse; recognition of contraindications to the delivery of epinephrine-containing local anesthetics; safe prescribing practices for patients with substance abuse disorders—both active and in remission—and management of patient emergencies that may result from unforeseen drug interactions.
7. Dentists are obliged to protect patient confidentiality of substance abuse treatment information, in accordance with applicable state and federal law.

Dental Management Considerations

Drug interactions with some abused drugs and drugs used in dentistry can occur. There is a significant interaction between cocaine and vasoconstrictors used in local anesthesia due to the cardiovascular effects of cocaine.[5] Cocaine increases myocardial oxygen demand by raising blood pressure, pulse rate, and myocardial contractility. Simultaneously, cocaine promotes vasoconstriction of the coronary arteries and promotes thrombosis by activating platelets and increasing levels of clotting factors in circulating blood making it a major cause of MI among young adults.[6] The effects of cocaine are greatest within the first several hours after cocaine use, but the risk remains elevated for several days. For this reason, cocaine users should be advised to refrain from "using" for at least 18 hours prior to a dental appointment in which a vasoconstrictor is planned.[6] An exploratory study also reported an increased risk for MI for marijuana users who have coronary heart disease.[7] Heavy marijuana users should be advised to discontinue use for at least 1 week before dental treatment due to cardiovascular effects of cannabis and increased CV effects with vasoconstrictors.[8]

Methamphetamine (meth) abuse is increasing in the United States and this drug has severe oral effects (meth mouth) and abrasions of the skin caused by the affected user picking away the skin after having the sensation of bugs crawling under their skin. Cardiac disease occurs in some meth users with signs including irregular heartbeats, tachycardia, and increased blood pressure.[9] Clinicians should be cautious when administering local anesthetics, sedatives, general anesthesia, or nitrous oxide and when prescribing narcotics because of potential drug interactions. The oral health professional should instruct the meth user to refrain from using for 24 hours prior to an appointment on which local anesthesia with a vasoconstrictor is planned. Meth users often consume large quantities of carbonated sugary soft drinks. When they are using meth, they may go for days without eating and are not concerned with toothbrushing. The caries in meth users is affected by long periods of xerostomia and the normal protective capacities of the saliva are lost. Meth use stimulates periods of excessive chewing, tooth grinding, and clenching, which compromise the dentition. The "red flags" for oral health professionals in identifying the meth user are listed in Box 7-1.[3]

Box 7-1

Red Flags for Dental Professionals

Oral healthcare professionals should watch for the following characteristics of meth use.

- Accelerated tooth decay in teenagers and young adults that is not accounted for by other factors.
- A distinctive pattern of decay on the buccal smooth surfaces of the teeth and the interproximal surfaces of the anterior teeth.
- Malnourished appearance due to appetite suppressant effects of meth and increased activity levels of meth use.
- Poor compliance with and poor response to preventive oral care, combined with a history of unreliability in keeping dental appointments.
- Excessive tooth wear and broken teeth because of excessive grinding and clenching.

(Adapted from Klasser GD, Epstein J. Methamphetamine and its impact on dental care. J Can Dent Assoc 2005;71:759–762.)

Oral Complications of Drug Abuse

Articles discussing oral effects of drug abuse identify chronic xerostomia and increased caries, especially at the gingival margin, severe periodontal attachment loss with gingival recession, *Candida* infection, and squamous cell carcinoma as major concerns.[1,10,11] Candidiasis is associated with chronic xerostomia and nutritionally deficient, immunocompromised conditions. Injection or intravenous (IV) drug users are at high risk for HIV and other bloodborne infections. IV drug injection users also have the highest rate of IE.[12]

Implications for Practice

The following issues should be considered when treating clients who abuse controlled substances (Box 7-2):

Box 7-2

Treatment Plan Implications for Substance Abuse

- Review medical history for CVD, IE, bloodborne infection, liver disease, and immunosuppression and make appropriate modifications related to providing oral care.
- Determine need for antibiotic prophylaxis prior to probing and therapy.
- Instruct client to avoid using controlled substances for 2 to 7 days if vasoconstrictor will be used during oral procedures.
- Monitor vital signs during each appointment and do not treat if blood pressure is ≥180/110. Use low concentrations of vasoconstrictor.
- Recommend non-narcotic analgesics for pain and a nonalcohol antimicrobial mouthrinse. Nitrous oxide can be used during therapy for analgesia.
- Monitor bleeding during treatment; use digital pressure to establish clotting.
- Use in-office fluoride therapy for caries control, plus a home fluoride program.

1. Medical consultation should be completed related to the presence of concurrent systemic disease, such as a history of MI, IE, or communicable diseases; reduced liver function; poor wound healing; and appropriate analgesics for oral pain. Standard precautions to avoid transmission of bloodborne diseases should be followed. Determination of functional capacity should be established prior to continuing with oral care when CVD is reported. Determination of need for antibiotic prophylaxis (prior history of IE) is appropriate. Vital signs should be monitored during each appointment.
2. The client should be instructed to refrain from using any drugs before the oral healthcare appointment. When cocaine use is discovered during the interview, and if local anesthesia containing a vasoconstrictor (such as epinephrine) is planned, the client must abstain from cocaine use for at least 18 hours prior to the appointment. The client must be advised to refrain from smoking marijuana for 1 week before an appointment when a local anesthetic containing a vasoconstrictor is planned. Blood pressure and pulse rate should be monitored prior to administration of the vasoconstrictor.

If blood pressure is ≥ 180/110 mm Hg, treatment should be delayed until vital signs are lower and the client referred for medical evaluation. In addition, if pulse rates are over 120 bpm treatment should be delayed. If the client is unable to control drug use and vital signs are acceptable, select a local anesthetic without a vasoconstrictor or use one with a low concentration of vasoconstrictor (1:200,000). Both of these practices can reduce the degree of effectiveness of the local anesthetic, however. Parenteral drug abusers may have a reduced response to local anesthetics, and larger amounts of the anesthetic may be required to provide pain-free therapy. In emergency situations and when the client has used drugs recently, a low concentration of vasoconstrictor (1:200,000) should be selected for emergency treatment. Nitrous oxide analgesia can be considered for added pain control.[5]

3. Postoperative pain medication should be in the non-narcotic category, unless other medical problems contraindicating their use exist.[1] Examples are aspirin, acetaminophen, or a nonsteroidal anti-inflammatory drug (NSAID) such as ibuprofen. NSAIDs have been reported to have equal analgesic relief for dental pain to that of codeine. These drugs may be contraindicated, however, if the client has gastrointestinal (GI) ulceration, significant liver dysfunction, or a blood marrow abnormality. Unrelieved pain can be a relapse trigger, and therefore, adequate pain control is a necessity in the recovering chemically dependent client. New modalities, such as **coanalgesia**, with low-dose ketamine in the opioid-addicted client have been shown to be effective.[13]
4. Monitor bleeding during treatment. While providing periodontal debridement, and if bleeding has not stopped within a few minutes, apply direct digital pressure (with fingers) to stimulate clot formation. Before rescheduling the client for additional treatment, refer for medical evaluation and blood laboratory studies related to clotting (international normalized ratio [INR]). Physician consultation with a recommendation for **hemostasis** is appropriate when bleeding is a problem. Refer to the medical section dealing with liver disease (see Chapter 9) in this self-study for laboratory values and criteria.
5. Increased dental caries can be managed with in-office and home fluoride therapy, restorative dentistry, and sealant application, when appropriate. Some drug abusers are young individuals, and sealants may be an appropriate consideration. Some drug abusers have severe oral disease and may require removal of teeth and placement of dentures (Fig. 7.1).

"Do you use tobacco (smoking, snuff, chew, bidis)? If so, how interested are you in stopping? Circle one: VERY, SOMEWHAT, NOT INTERESTED."

There is a strong correlation between use of tobacco and oral cancer. Tobacco is responsible for most of oropharyngeal cancers in the United States. Tobacco use is implicated in chronic obstructive pulmonary disease, ischemic heart disease, and atherosclerosis. Statistics reveal that more than 400,000 deaths in the United States each year can be attributed to cigarette smoking, making it the leading preventable cause of premature mortality. In addition, using tobacco products is associated with increased periodontal disease and a poor response to periodontal therapy. Vasoconstriction associated with the chemicals in tobacco decreases circulation in oral tissues and reduces healing of oral tissues. Extrinsic stains on teeth and halitosis are associated with use of tobacco.

A newer fad appealing to teenagers in the United States is the use of **bidis**. Bidis are filterless cigarettes imported from India and Southeastern Asia. They contain tobacco, but are wrapped in nonporous leaves and sold in a variety of flavors including vanilla, strawberry, chocolate, mango, cinnamon, cherry, and clove. According to the Centers for Disease Control and Prevention, approximately

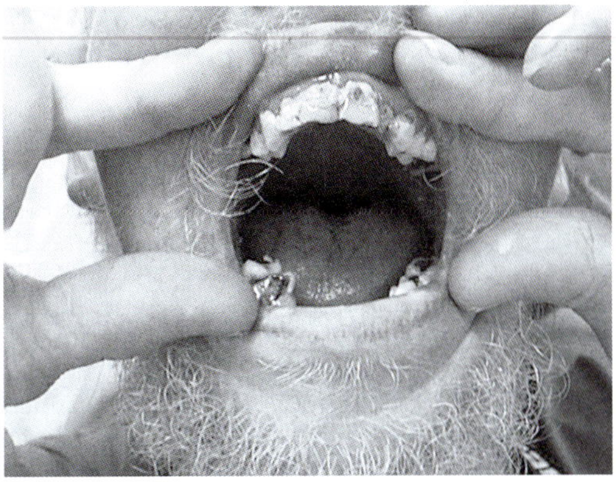

Figure 7.1 ■ Clinical photograph of a drug abuser with severe dental disease who reported taking multiple drugs (heroin, cocaine, phencyclidine, others).

2% of high school students and middle school students in the United States smoke bidis.[14] Bidis are being mistaken for healthy cigarettes because they look natural. Another appeal is that they cost less than conventional cigarettes. However, the leaves they are wrapped in are nonporous and do not burn easily, making the smoker inhale harder and more often to keep it lit. An average of 28 puffs is needed for a bidi compared to 9 puffs for a cigarette. In addition, bidis are both mutagenic and carcinogenic. Studies conducted in India revealed that bidi smoking is associated with an increased risk for oral cancer, lung cancer, and stomach and esophageal cancers.[15–17] Bidi smoking is associated with a greater than threefold increased risk for coronary heart disease and heart attack, as well as almost a fourfold increased risk for chronic bronchitis.[16,18]

The ADA and American Dental Hygienists' Association (ADHA) both recommend that members of the professions offer smoking cessation programs in their offices or have information on smoking cessation programs to provide to clients interested in quitting tobacco use. The ADHA program "Ask, Advise, and Refer" can be accessed online through the ADHA Web site (www.adha.org). It provides information for planning a smoking cessation program within the dental office. Specifically, the protocol recommended for a tobacco cessation intervention system in the dental office is to be brief, provide simple measures, and follow-up as needed. The emphasis on this program is to maintain the flow of the practice routine and not be too time consuming for either the dental care provider or the client.

This brief tobacco cessation intervention involves three steps: Ask, Advise, and Refer.[19] For those clients who indicate a history of smoking, Ask the following:

- Do you use tobacco? If no, have you ever used tobacco in the past?
- Determine if client is current, former, or never tobacco user.
- Determine the form, frequency, and duration of tobacco use.
- Document tobacco use status in the dental record.

Step 2, *Advise*, involves

- In a clear, strong, and personalized manner, urge every tobacco user to quit.
- Employ the "teachable moment": link oral findings with advice.
- Tobacco users who have not succeeded in previous attempts should be told that most people try repeatedly (on average 3 to 8 times) before permanent quitting is achieved.

Step 3, *Refer*, recommends the dental hygienist or dentist to

- Ask client if he or she is willing to make a quit attempt at this time. If unwilling to make a quit attempt, reassess his or her willingness at next visit.
- If client is willing to make a quit attempt, provide assistance by referring to the National Network of Tobacco Quitlines, 1-800-QUIT NOW.
- Use reactive referral—provide client with a 1-800-QUIT NOW wallet card and urge client to call the tobacco quitline.
- Use proactive referral (if available)—request written permission to fax contact information to tobacco quitline. Inform client that tobacco quitline staff will provide assistance.
- Schedule a follow-up telephone call.

This protocol provides personalized quit plan tearsheets, pharmacological product guides for FDA-approved medications, consumer guide, tobacco use stickers, tobacco cessation intervention cards follow-up record, and intervention action plan for the dental team. A new product "the electronic cigarette" is available but limited research regarding health benefits and risks of use has been completed.

Dental Management

Tobacco products influence the oral cavity by reducing blood flow necessary for healing of oral tissues and by reducing host immune responses. Both effects can result in poor healing. Vasoconstriction reduces the blood-supplied nutrients required for adequate healing. Host resistance is compromised through a diminished leukocyte protective function. These factors reduce the prognosis for responding to periodontal therapy in the client who uses tobacco products. The following issues should be considered when providing oral health care for the client who uses tobacco products:

1. The oral health education plan in the client who smokes should include the relationship of tobacco to CVD, lung cancer, oral cancer, periodontal disease, and a poor response to periodontal therapy.
2. The client should be asked whether there is interest in stopping the smoking habit, and if "yes," information on smoking cessation should be provided.

3. The oral cavity should be examined for other tobacco-related diseases (e.g., leukoplakia, nonhealing ulcerations, gingival recession, hairy tongue, and nicotine stomatitis) at each scheduled appointment.
4. For clients with periodontal infection, consider a more frequent continuing care schedule, for example, a 3-month schedule.
5. Vital signs should be monitored due to the strong association between smoking and atherosclerosis and coronary artery disease (Box 7-3).

Box 7-3

Management of the Tobacco Abuser

- Educate the client on the health effects and oral effects of tobacco use.
- Offer smoking cessation information.
- Perform oral cancer, head and neck examination at every appointment.
- Monitor periodontal tissue health; consider more frequent continuing care schedule when appropriate.
- Monitor vital signs.

Self-Study Review

1. Use of local anesthetics or gingival retraction cords with epinephrine in clients using cocaine may cause:
   a. tachycardia and a decrease in blood pressure.
   b. tachycardia and an increase in blood pressure.
   c. bradycardia and a decrease in blood pressure.
   d. bradycardia and an increase in blood pressure.
2. Intravenous drug users are at high risk for developing all of the following EXCEPT one. Which one is the EXCEPTION?
   a. Increased caries
   b. Infective endocarditis
   c. Severe periodontal disease
   d. Pulpal infection
3. Postoperative pain medication recommended for clients who abuse recreational drugs include:
   a. acetaminophen and ibuprofen.
   b. codeine and ibuprofen.
   c. aspirin and acetaminophen-oxycodone (Percocet).
   d. oxycodone and ibuprofen.
4. When cocaine use is identified and local anesthesia is planned, the client should be advised to refrain from drug use:
   a. 1 day before the appointment.
   b. 1 week before the appointment.
   c. 1 month before the appointment.
   d. refraining from drug use is not indicated in this case.
5. When marijuana use is identified and local anesthesia is planned, the client should be advised to refrain from drug use:
   a. 1 day before the appointment.
   b. 1 week before the appointment.
   c. 1 month before the appointment.
   d. Refraining from drug use is not indicated in this case.
6. Delaying treatment in clients who report using controlled substances is indicated in which of the following situations? Select all that apply.
   a. Blood pressure is ≥ 180/100 mm Hg.
   b. Temperature is elevated above 98.68°F.
   c. Pulse rate is over 120 bpm.
   d. Client has a history of cardiovascular disease.
   e. Client has reduced liver function.
7. The prognosis for responding to periodontal therapy in clients who use tobacco products is less than favorable as a result of all of the following EXCEPT one. Which one is the EXCEPTION?
   a. Vasoconstriction of vessels
   b. Reduced host immune response
   c. Inhibition of growth factors
   d. Diminished leukocyte protective function
8. From the following list, identify the oral diseases associated with using tobacco products.
   a. Caries
   b. Chronic obstructive pulmonary disease
   c. Nicotine stomatitis
   d. Hairy tongue
   e. Squamous cell carcinoma
   f. Cardiovascular disease

  g. Periodontal disease
  h. Halitosis

9. Bidis are a new fad used by teenagers in the United States. Although they contain nicotine, they are made from natural ingredients and are safer than cigarettes.
  a. Both statements are true.
  b. Both statements are false.
  c. The first statement is true, and the second statement is false.
  d. The first statement is false, and the second statement is true.

"Do you drink alcoholic beverages? If yes, how much alcohol did you drink in the last 24 hours? How much do you typically drink in a week? If yes, are you in recovery?"

These questions are intended to identify the alcohol abuser who may have alcohol-related liver disease and to determine whether the client is in a recovery program to stop drinking. Alcoholism is a chronic psychiatric illness affecting more than 17.6 million people in the United States. Those affected may lose control over their use and begin craving alcohol. Identifying alcohol-abusing clients is important because they are at an increased risk for developing oral cancer, periodontal disease, and dental caries.[20] The alcoholic client often develops disease of the liver. Functions of a healthy liver include

1. Removal of toxic substances from the blood.
2. Formation of several clotting factors.
3. Metabolism of drugs.
4. Storage of energy sources (glycogen, vitamins).
5. Removal of waste products from blood.

Abnormal liver function leads to buildup of toxic substances, bleeding problems, and increased adverse reactions from drugs, including drug–drug interactions. There are several issues related to providing treatment to clients in this category.

1. Depression of immune response: Alcohol abusers often are nutritionally deficient, making them more likely to have reduced immune function. Chronic alcohol consumption can also decrease lymphocyte production and white blood cell function, impairing host immune function. These factors lead to increased oral infection. They may also have a poor response to treatment and require longer healing times. Immune function is greatest in the morning, so morning appointments may be indicated. There is no recommendation for antibiotic prophylaxis in the client with alcohol liver disease although a state of immunosuppression may exist.
2. Coexisting medical problems: Long-term alcohol abusers are likely to have bleeding ulcers in the GI tract resulting from the effects of alcohol on the GI mucosa.[20] Older clients who have two or more drinks per day have an increased prevalence of hypertension and are at risk for CVD and cerebrovascular disease (stroke). They may have poor functional capacity (unable to meet the 4 metabolic equivalent [MET] level). Liver function may be reduced by chronic inflammation of the liver (hepatitis), and liver disease, such as fatty liver and cirrhosis. This makes selecting drugs for pain control, infection, and stress reduction difficult since the liver is the main organ that manages the elimination of drugs. Many alcoholics cannot take aspirin because of bleeding ulcers in the GI tract exacerbated by the acidic, irritating nature of aspirin. Some alcohol abusers also abuse narcotic drugs. If the dentist uses narcotic analgesics for pain control and the client is currently abusing other narcotic substances, increased depression of the central nervous system (CNS) can cause a potential medical emergency. Dentists should be cautious in, and try to avoid, prescribing narcotic medications when any form of substance abuse is suspected. Acetaminophen, up to 4 g/day, and lidocaine local anesthetic can be used for pain control.[21,22] Dentists should avoid using metronidazole, meperidine (Demerol), and diazepam (Valium®); aspirin-containing products should only be used when the client has abstained from alcohol for 2 to 3 weeks, otherwise, increased bleeding is likely.[21]
3. Increased oral disease: Long-term alcohol abusers are unlikely to have regular dental or periodontal care. Salivary function is often diminished. This may result in increased rates of dental caries, untreated oral infection, and advanced periodontal disease with attachment loss. Reduced salivation associated with nutritional deficiency makes the long-term alcohol abuser prone to dental decay at the cervical third of the teeth (Fig. 7.2). Oral signs and symptoms of alcohol-induced nutritional

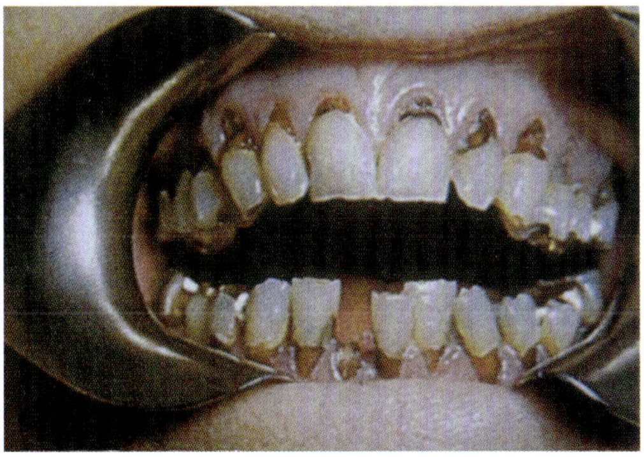

Figure 7.2 ■ Clinical photograph of dentition of chronic alcoholic.

deficiencies include glossitis, angular cheilitis, and gingivitis.[14] The alcohol abuser may frequently miss appointments for oral care and may be noncompliant with oral hygiene procedures.[20] All of these issues reduce the likelihood for having a successful outcome from periodontal care. The risk of developing oral cancer increases when more than two alcoholic drinks per day are consumed and the risk continues to rise with increasing levels of alcohol intake.[20] The floor of the mouth and lateral borders of the tongue are common sites for squamous cell carcinoma.

4. Liver dysfunction: Long-term alcohol abusers may have poor liver function, reducing the ability of the liver to metabolize medications normally. Drug doses may need to be lowered to accommodate for this potential problem. Dentists should be cautious in prescribing narcotic analgesics (or any CNS depressant drug) that can increase the CNS depressant effects of alcohol. Non-narcotic analgesics, such as acetaminophen, aspirin, or NSAIDs (ibuprofen), are the options to consider. Each has its own potential problems. Acetaminophen is metabolized to a great extent in the liver and may be poorly metabolized when liver dysfunction is present. Large doses of acetaminophen may result in formation of a toxic metabolite that can cause fatal liver injury. However, research reveals that acetaminophen, in low doses and with short-term use, may be the best choice for pain control in the alcohol abuser who also has GI bleeding problems.[20–22] More acidic drugs, such as aspirin or NSAIDs, can be considered for pain relief in the client who does not have GI bleeding problems or ulcers and who has not consumed alcohol for 3 weeks.[21] However, these acidic agents may provide additional irritation to the stomach and are contraindicated when the client has GI ulceration and bleeding. The dentist should consult with the client's physician before prescribing any potentially addicting drugs, such as opioid analgesics or mood-altering medications, in clients with alcohol-induced hepatitis or cirrhosis.[20,21]
5. Increased bleeding and liver disease: Blood clotting factors are synthesized in the liver. Any condition that depresses liver function and formation of clotting factors can result in increased bleeding. In the client who has chronic liver dysfunction, such as alcoholic cirrhosis or hepatitis, bleeding can result from platelet abnormalities.[20,21] Blood studies should be completed before surgery, including complete blood cell count, a coagulation profile (INR), and liver function studies.[20] Vitamin K injections may be needed a few days before any surgical dental procedure to increase the formation of vitamin K–dependent clotting factors. A physician consultation and appropriate laboratory tests are necessary to determine the risk of increased bleeding in alcoholic liver disease.
6. Behavior management: There may be behavior management problems in the client who presents for oral care under the influence of alcohol. It may be necessary to reschedule the appointment when the client is under the influence of alcohol. Certainly, communication and oral healthcare teaching opportunities would be diminished in that situation. However, not all alcoholics present management problems during treatment. The term "functional alcoholic" is applied to persons who drink alcohol at inappropriate times but who go to work and function in the workplace. The clinician must make the determination whether to reschedule the appointment on the basis of the patient's behavior.
7. Oral manifestations of alcohol abuse: Oral complications can include opportunistic infec tions (associated with having an immunocompromised condition), such as candidiasis; xerostomia leading to increased dental caries; predisposition to squamous cell carcinoma (oral cancer); chipped teeth or areas of erosion from frequent vomiting; and periodontal attachment loss as a result of poor host resistance and lack of regular oral care.[20] Alcohol consumption and smoking are considered to be primary causes of oral cancer.

8. Oral care product selection: Alcohol-containing mouthrinses are contraindicated in the alcohol abuser. Chlorhexidine antimicrobial rinse (Peridex) sometimes used to reduce periodontal inflammation contains a high concentration of alcohol. A nonalcohol-containing chlorhexidine is available and would be indicated as the most effective antimicrobial mouthrinse (Butler Oral Products). Other alcohol-containing rinses, such as the Listerine product, should not be recommended. Most of the fluoride mouthrinse products contain no alcohol, but the clinician should check the alcohol content before recommending any oral rinse product. For the client in recovery from former alcohol abuse, nonalcohol products are mandatory to reduce the chance of recovery failure.
9. Tobacco and alcohol use: Alcohol abusers frequently use tobacco products, and the combination of the two products predisposes them to develop squamous cell carcinoma. A thorough oral examination for clinical evidence of this condition, which represents the most common oral cancer, is recommended. Any nonpainful oral ulceration that has been present for more than 2 weeks should be referred for biopsy. The most common locations for oral cancer include the lateral border of the tongue and the floor of the mouth; however, any area of oral mucosa can be affected. Tobacco has been associated with an increased level of periodontal disease and a reduced ability of oral tissues to heal during periodontal care procedures.

Dental Management

Providing oral health care for clients with a history of alcohol use and alcoholic liver disease poses several challenges. For the dental hygienist potential bleeding problems must be considered. When planned procedures will involve significant bleeding, a physician consultation and request for a coagulation test (INR) is recommended. For the client who is currently drinking large amounts of alcohol, and bleeding is expected during oral procedures, the client should be advised to abstain from alcohol intake for at least 5 days for clotting factors to develop.[21] If oral procedures involve significant bleeding and digital pressure is inadequate to control bleeding, mouthrinses to initiate clotting (tranexamic acid, aminocaproic acid) can be considered.[21] Dental auxiliaries do not prescribe medications, but they may be asked to recommend over-the-counter analgesics. The best choice for the alcohol abuser with GI disease appears to be acetaminophen, but the client must be cautioned to take no more than 4 g/day and for no more than a few days.[21] Behavior-related problems may or may not pose a management problem. The client who comes to the appointment smelling of alcohol should be informed that oral care appointments require a sober client and that presenting for treatment under the influence of alcohol will not be tolerated. Maintenance appointments should be frequent (every 3 months) and should include a thorough head and neck examination for oral cancer and an oral examination of mucosa for suspicious lesions that do not heal within a normal time interval.[22] The client who is in an alcohol recovery program may be taking a drug called disulfiram (Antabuse). This drug causes the person to have severe GI distress, nausea, and vomiting if alcohol is ingested. The dental relevance for the client taking Antabuse is that alcohol-containing oral rinse products are contraindicated (Listerine, Peridex, etc.). Chlorhexidine rinses have been shown to reduce gingival inflammation. A nonalcohol-containing chlorhexidine rinse has been shown to be as effective as the alcohol-containing chlorhexidine in reducing gingival inflammation.[23] Table 7.1 includes management considerations for the alcohol-abusing dental client.

THE HEALTHCARE PROFESSIONAL WHO ABUSES SUBSTANCES

The journal of the ADA has published a section related to employees who are suspected of abusing substances.[24] The section is entitled "Ethical Moment." It describes a hypothetical situation in which a dental hygienist (RDH) has worked in a dental practice for a number of years and, within the previous 5 months, demonstrated erratic behavior resulting in complaints by the staff. The dentist confronted the RDH with these behaviors and seeming lack of cooperation with the dental team and received a response that she had been under personal stress. She said these problems were resolved recently and things would improve; however, the next week she missed work for three days due to "car trouble." On the fourth day, she arrived at work with noticeable bruises on her arms, bloodshot eyes, and alcohol was detected on her breath. The Ethical Moment column continued with advice to the dentist on handling the situation. It explained the serious consequences for the practice, the staff, and the patient care. It referred the

Table 7.1 Management of the Alcohol Abuser

Oral pain	Acetaminophen in low doses, up to 4 g/day
Oral examination	Oral cancer examination at every dental or dental hygiene appointment
Oral infection	Treat infections with appropriate anti-infective; physician consultation for drug selection in cirrhosis or alcoholic hepatitis client
Product recommendations	Avoid alcohol-containing products
Behavior management	Reschedule a client who comes to dental appointment under the influence of alcohol

dentist to the ADA Principles of Ethics and Code of Professional Conduct but advised the employer to gain information on employment law issues. For this information, consultation with an attorney was advised. According to the ADA Code Section 2.C, describing uses of auxiliary personnel within the principle of nonmalfeasance (or "do no harm") the dentist is obligated to protect the health of patients by only assigning to qualified auxiliaries those duties that can be legally delegated. Dentists are further obligated to supervise patient care provided by auxiliary personnel as they work under the direction of the dentist. The advice noted that the RDH may pose a harm to patient care if allowed to provide treatment while impaired, and the supervising dentist who, under law is obligated to ensure adequate care is provided to clients, is ethically obligated to safeguard the welfare of the patient. In Section 2.D of the code "Personal Impairment," employers with knowledge that a colleague is practicing dentistry when impaired must report this evidence to the professional assistance committee of a professional society. In this case, the person is an impaired staff member, but the dentist is ethically obligated to limit the activities of the RDH in the office that could endanger the patients or the staff. State law may require reporting suspected impairment to the appropriate licensing authorities. Most states have a professional assistance program for professionals who have addiction problems and can get help from the profession. The dentist was advised to establish an office policy that explicitly prohibits employees from being under the influence of alcohol or illegal drugs during working hours and that advises violators that they are subject to dismissal if they do not seek professional help for the addiction. The employer should provide encouragement to help the employee become free of the addiction and into a recovery program, be understanding of the personal problems but make it clear that coming to work in an impaired state will not be tolerated. The employee must realize that her welfare is important to the dentist and the staff and the welfare of the patients and office personnel is of utmost importance. These discussions should be documented in the employee file and the employee should sign that it is understood that excessive absenteeism may be a reason for dismissal.

Self-Study Review

10. Healthcare professionals who abuse substances should be treated in all of the following manners EXCEPT one. Which one is the EXCEPTION?

- a. Terminated from their job.
- b. Reported to the appropriate licensing authorities.
- c. Counseled to seek professional help.
- d. Limited to duties that will not jeopardize the health of the other clients.

11. Long-term alcohol abuse may result in poor liver function. If medications need to be prescribed after dental treatment:

- a. doses will need to be lower than usual.
- b. doses will not be affected.
- c. doses will need to be higher than usual.
- d. the practitioner should not prescribe medications for a client with alcohol abuse.

12. The combination of alcohol abuse and use of tobacco products places the client at risk for:

- a. candidal infections.
- b. opportunistic infections.
- c. squamous cell carcinoma.
- d. cervical root caries.

13. Bleeding problems can occur in the alcoholic client as a result of:
    a. abuse of other drugs.
    b. alcoholic hepatitis.
    c. reduction of platelet formation.
    d. suppression of bone marrow function.
14. An alcohol abuser who has gastrointestinal disease and dental pain may require analgesic medication. Which medication is the safest to use?
    a. Antabuse
    b. Acetaminophen
    c. Aspirin
    d. Ibuprofen
15. For how long should an alcohol abuse client refrain from using alcohol when undergoing periodontal therapy?
    a. 1 day
    b. 3 days
    c. 5 days
    d. 8 days
16. Clients who abuse alcohol and are taking Antabuse should be counseled to use oral mouthrinses such as Listerine or Peridex. These oral rinses will be well tolerated by the client.
    a. Both statements are true.
    b. Both statements are false.
    c. The first statement is true, and the second statement is false.
    d. The first statement is false, and the second statement is true.

Legal Implications for Addiction

Drug prescribers are counseled to write prescriptions for narcotics only on a short-term basis. The licensing boards in various states monitor prescription practices for over-prescribing, especially for people in health care who may be prescribing for themselves. Healthcare providers must be aware of the possibility of drug interactions between controlled substances and alcohol and agents used in dentistry. When an individual has signs or symptoms of being impaired by controlled substances or alcohol, a frank discussion should ensue that includes patient information related to the serious cardiovascular risks when a local anesthetic with a vasoconstrictor is needed. The dental record should always be documented properly with warnings provided to the client to protect the dental practice against a malpractice lawsuit. If a recommendation for referral for help with substance, alcohol, or tobacco addiction is made, this should be documented in the record. The dentist should work with the medical team or addiction counselor to coordinate oral care. The client will need to sign a medical release form so the dentist can obtain client medical information. For clients referred for medical help, future appointments for oral care should include follow-up of the referral if the client is in a recovery program and encouragement to continue in recovery programs. Appropriate documentation in the dental record of the conversation should be made.

CHAPTER SUMMARY

The identification and screening of dental clients with chemical dependency is becoming an important issue in client assessment. Oral care professionals should take an active role in screening for general overall health issues, and when related to abuse of controlled substances, alcohol, or tobacco, make appropriate referrals for the addiction. Preventive health care can not only save teeth, but may save a life. Oral care providers may be the source to make the connection between substance abuse and getting those affected into a recovery program.

Review

1. Describe four aspects that must be considered when treating an individual who abuses recreational drugs.
2. Describe management considerations and recommendations for support for the client who asks for assistance in quitting smoking.
3. List three issues that must be considered when rendering treatment to an individual with alcohol abuse.

Case Study

Case A

Mason Briggs, a 23-year-old client, presents to the office for restorative dental care involving a crown preparation. His medical history is significant for previous infective endocarditis (IE) and use of recreational drugs including marijuana and cocaine. The client states that he used marijuana last evening because he was anxious about having a crown preparation and wanted to be calm for this appointment. He has not used cocaine within the past week. The client reports that he took his prescription of amoxicillin 1 hour before the dental appointment. His vital signs are pulse 68 bpm, respiration 14 breaths/min, and blood pressure 110/70 mm Hg, right arm, sitting.

1. Why did the client take amoxicillin for the dental appointment? What dosage should the client have taken for this appointment?
2. What potential risks exist for the client during a crown preparation given that he has recently used marijuana?
3. Given the client's medical history, should the dentist proceed with treatment? Why or why not?
4. If the dentist decided to postpone treatment until next week, what recommendations should be made concerning preparation for treatment?

Case B

Joseph Morton, III, a 35-year-old client, presents for a routine prophylaxis. On entering the dental office, he appears somewhat disoriented, is staggering, and has alcohol on his breath. The dental hygienist inquires about his use of alcohol, and the client responds that he regularly drinks at least four or five vodka martinis at lunch and immediately after work, followed by several bottles of beer at home. The client reports that he had several martinis at lunch and just finished two beers before arriving for his evening appointment. His vital signs are pulse 80 bpm, respiration 18 breaths/min, and blood pressure 130/80 mm Hg, right arm, sitting. The dental hygienist proceeds to perform an oral examination.

1. What types of clinical findings should the hygienist be looking for as part of the oral examination?
2. During the course of the oral examination, the client repeatedly becomes argumentative and verbally abusive. What would you recommend concerning treatment for this client?
3. If the dental hygienist were to perform a debridement procedure and the client complained of posttreatment pain and requested pain medication, what type of analgesic medication would be appropriate?
4. If the client presented with alcohol abuse and a GI condition, which analgesic and maximum dosage should be recommended?

Chapter Eight

Women's Issues (Pregnancy, Lactation, Menopause) and Antibiotic Prophylaxis

Objectives

After completing the self-study chapter the reader will be able to:

- Describe the treatment plan considerations for the pregnant client and for the lactating client.
- Describe the treatment plan considerations for the client taking birth control pills or hormone replacement therapy.
- Describe treatment considerations when osteoporosis is reported on the health history.
- Identify circumstances in which antibiotic prophylaxis is indicated before providing oral healthcare and the regimen for prophylaxis.
- Discuss management of a client who requires antibiotic prophylaxis for multiple dental hygiene appointments.

Key Terms

Antibiotic prophylaxis: use of antibiotics to prevent infection in cardiac valves caused by bacteremia

Bacteremia: the presence of bacteria in the blood

Infective endocarditis: infection within tissues lining the heart or within valves of the heart, caused by bacteria within the circulating blood that infect these cardiac tissues

Parturition: the act or process of giving birth to a child

Periodontopathogen: bacteria responsible for periodontal disease, principally gram-negative anaerobic microorganisms, including *Actinobacillus actinomycetemcomitans*, *Prevotella* species, and *Porphyromonas* species

Teratogen: any drug capable of causing a birth defect in the fetus

Valvulopathy: a disorder of valve function causing a variety of cardiac disorders, such as arrhythmia, pulmonary hypertension, heart failure, and cardiogenic shock

MEDICAL CONDITION

INTRODUCTION

The next section on the American Dental Association (ADA) Health History Form involves women. The section entitled WOMEN ONLY contains questions on pregnancy, nursing, and medications used for birth control or hormone replacement.

This is followed by questions for both sexes related to indications for **antibiotic prophylaxis** to prevent **infective endocarditis** (IE) and to be administered prior to oral procedures.

"FOR WOMEN ONLY: Are you or could you be pregnant? Number of weeks:____"

It is necessary to identify the client who is pregnant because some medications used as a part of oral health care may be contraindicated in pregnancy. The first and third trimesters of pregnancy are associated with the greatest risk for medical emergencies or increased risk to the fetus from drugs or ionizing radiation. For these reasons, the safest time to provide oral health care during pregnancy is during the second trimester. Any drug being considered for use by the oral healthcare provider in a pregnant woman must be investigated in a drug reference for the pregnancy category assigned by the U.S. Food and Drug Administration, called the FDA pregnancy category (Table 8.1). Categories A and B are considered safe for use during pregnancy. Categories D and X are not recommended for use during pregnancy. Category C drugs should only be used if the benefit is considered to be greater than the potential risk involved. The category is assigned on the basis of the available animal or human studies with the drug.

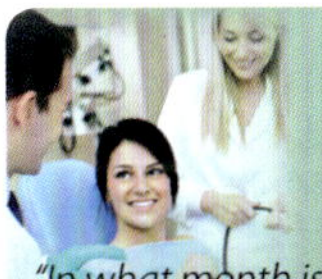

Follow-up Questions

Proper follow-up questions for a positive response would include

"In what month is your pregnancy? Have you had any problems with your pregnancy? Are you having morning sickness?"

These questions provide information on the trimester of pregnancy and alterations needed to deal with nausea or any other complication reported. During the first trimester, the organs of the fetus are forming. This is a critical time for teratogenicity caused by taking medications or receiving ionizing radiation. The client who is experiencing morning sickness would be appointed at a time when they are least likely to experience complications, such as in the afternoon.[1] Strategies for prevention of decay (when vomiting occurs frequently) should be recommended to the client, such as rinsing the mouth, but not toothbrushing, immediately after the vomiting episode. Toothbrushing immediately after regurgitation removes some of the

Table 8.1 FDA Pregnancy Categories

Category	Definition
A	Controlled studies have failed to demonstrate a risk to the fetus in any trimester.
B	No evidence of risk in humans. Either animal findings show risk, but human findings do not; or if no human studies have been done, animal findings are negative.
C	Risk cannot be ruled out. Human studies are lacking and animal studies are either positive for fetal risk or lacking. Potential benefits may justify potential risks.
D	Definite human fetal risks; may be given in spite of risks if needed in life-threatening conditions; benefits of taking drug may outweigh potential risks.
X	Absolute fetal abnormalities; not to be used any time during pregnancy because risks outweigh benefits.

(Adapted from Facts and Comparisons. Philadelphia, PA: Wolters Kluwer Health. A-4.)

fluoride-rich enamel surface. Sodium bicarbonate or magnesium hydroxide (milk of magnesia) rinses will neutralize acid in the mouth after vomiting.[1] Toothbrushing should be delayed until the pH in the mouth returns to normal.

Dental Drugs Acceptable for Use during Pregnancy

Only a few drugs used in dentistry are considered safe for use during the first trimester of pregnancy. Drugs prescribed during pregnancy are only used if the expected benefit to the mother is thought to be greater than the risk to the fetus. Drugs should be avoided during the first trimester, and if needed should be given in the lowest effective dose and for the shortest duration possible.[2,3] Lidocaine or prilocaine (Pregnancy Category B) can be used safely as a local anesthetic during pregnancy and epinephrine used in small doses (two cartridges 1:100,000) is acceptable.[2] Acceptable antibiotics include penicillins, clindamycin, and erythromycin (except the estolate form). All tetracyclines should be avoided during pregnancy. For oral pain, acetaminophen is considered to be safe. Nonsteroidal anti-inflammatory drugs (NSAIDs), such as ibuprofen, and aspirin should be avoided during pregnancy. The reasons are ibuprofen is related to embryonic implantation disturbances and during the third trimester, aspirin and NSAIDs can delay **parturition**, result in premature closure of the patent ductus arteriosus, complicate delivery, and increase the risk of maternal or fetal hemorrhage.[2,3] Codeine and other opioid analgesics should be avoided as they are associated with teratogenicity and neonatal respiratory depression.[2] Benzodiazepines and barbiturates, used by dentists for relief of anxiety, should be avoided during pregnancy due to an increased risk for an oral cleft (cleft lip, cleft palate).[3] A single exposure to nitrous oxide for no more than 35 minutes has not been associated with any fetal abnormalities nor low birth weight.[2]

Ionizing Radiation during Pregnancy

The developing fetus should be protected from ionizing radiation during the first trimester. This is a time of rapid cell division and organ development. These cells are especially sensitive to ionizing radiation, which leads to a concern regarding taking radiographs especially during the first trimester of pregnancy. However, the ADA has concluded that when radiation safety practices and a caries risk assessment are used, guidelines for taking radiographs during pregnancy need not be altered.[4] Placing a lead apron over the client's upper body (regardless of pregnancy status) is essential when taking radiographs. The lead apron should provide adequate safety for the developing fetus. Some authors suggest a second lead apron for the back of the body to ensure complete coverage of the fetal location.[1] Using fast-speed X-ray (F-speed) film reduces the exposure to ionizing radiation and is considered a safe practice.[4] Dental considerations related to exposing the pregnant client to ionizing radiation include:

1. X-ray exposures should be preceded by an oral examination and only taken if evidence of disease is noted that requires a dental X-ray. Radiographs should not be taken on a routine basis (i.e., every 6 to 12 months).
2. Full mid to upper body coverage with a lead apron that includes a thyroid collar (to protect the thyroid from radiation) is essential when exposing a client to radiation.
3. Take the minimum number of radiographs needed.
4. Determine whether X-rays can be delayed until after the delivery of the child.

This may reduce the anxiety of the pregnant woman regarding ionizing radiation's effect on the developing fetus. Radiographs should never be exposed unless the client understands the need for the radiographs and the dental practitioner has received the consent of the client.[5] Digital radiography imaging requires much less radiation than standard radiography images. The reduction is approximately 90% when compared with the dose from D-speed film and approximately 60% when compared with E-speed film.[4]

Treatment Plan Modifications and Appointment Planning

As stated earlier, the second trimester is recommended for elective oral healthcare procedures because this is the safest and most comfortable period of pregnancy. The blood pressure should be monitored because pregnancy-induced hypertension (preeclampsia) can occur.[6] This usually occurs after the 20th week of gestation. Hypertensive disorders are a leading cause of maternal mortality during pregnancy and are also associated with low birth-weight babies and perinatal mortality.[7] Pregnant clients with hypertension and abnormal weight gain should be referred for medical evaluation before receiving elective oral procedures, and appointments should be avoided that involve extended time periods.[2] Stress associated with dental infection or dental treatment may exacerbate the condition. Detection of a functional heart murmur is common during pregnancy, and the client may indicate a positive response to a health history question for "heart murmur." This heart murmur is temporary and occurs because of increased blood flow through the heart causing a systolic ejection murmur. Functional heart murmurs do not require antibiotic prophylaxis before dental procedures.

Oral health education should begin early in pregnancy. Oral problems are generally not directly attributable to pregnancy (one does not lose a tooth for every child), but pregnancy may exacerbate existing oral disease. For example, pregnancy gingivitis is a manifestation of biofilm-induced gingival inflammation. Nausea and vomiting are common during the first trimester of pregnancy, leading to enamel erosion. To prevent erosion, brushing should be avoided immediately after vomiting since the enamel is vulnerable to toothbrush abrasion following an acid insult. The client should be advised to rinse thoroughly with a sodium bicarbonate solution following each acid challenge. Fluoride products should be recommended and xylitol gum can be used to stimulate salivation and improve taste.

Safety considerations in the treatment plan for the pregnant client should include short appointments, monitoring of blood pressure and vital signs, a semisupine chair position, or if supine positioning is used to place a pillow to elevate the right hip and displace the weight of the uterus to the left and away from the vena cava, an afternoon appointment if the client is experiencing morning sickness or nausea, taking care not to cause gagging or induce the vomiting reflex, and following a protocol that reduces medical risks to the fetus (X-rays, drugs; Box 8-1).[1,5] Extensive dental procedures should be delayed until after parturition. Acute dental infection should be treated with incision and drainage to reduce the infection. If possible, tooth extraction should be delayed until after delivery.[6]

Box 8-1

Safety Considerations for the Pregnant Client

- Second trimester recommended for elective treatment
- Monitor blood pressure
- Short appointment, afternoon appointment if morning sickness occurs
- Semisupine chair position; if supine, place pillow under right hip (third trimester)
- Care to avoid stimulation of gag reflex
- Take X-rays only if necessary; complete coverage with lead apron
- Check FDA pregnancy categories to select safest drugs; consider risk/benefit before prescribing drugs
- Treat acute dental infection with incision and drainage; delay extensive dental treatment until after delivery of baby

Potential Emergency of Supine Hypotensive Pregnancy Syndrome (Syncope)

During the third trimester, there is a risk for syncope as a result of reduced blood flow to the heart and hypotension. This occurs when the client is placed in the supine position for treatment. The enlarged uterus compresses the vena cava, reducing the amount of blood returned to the heart. The reduced cardiac output that results (amount in = amount out) stimulates the heart to slow down and blood vessels to dilate. The result is low blood pressure and reduced oxygenated blood levels. The lack of adequate oxygenated blood can also result in fetal hypoxia. When the pregnant client is raised to an upright position, hypotension can develop, leading to unconsciousness.[6]

Prevention

One recommendation to prevent this potential emergency is to place a pillow under the pregnant client's right hip to displace the weight of the fetus to the left and away from the vena cava vein.[1,6] The client can bring the right knee up with the bottom of the foot resting on the dental chair to promote adjustment of the body to the left.

Management

If hypotensive supine pregnancy syndrome occurs, the client should be placed with the head at or below the level of the heart and with the abdomen rolled to the left. The right knee can be brought up to promote adjustment of the body to the left and a pillow placed under the right hip to stabilize the position. Provide supplemental oxygen by face mask (10 L/minute). If the heart rate falls below 60 bpm, call 911 because drugs to increase the heart rate may be needed.[6]

"Are you nursing?"

This question relates to appointment planning for follow-up care after the delivery of the baby and selection of drugs to use during oral healthcare procedures.

Application to Practice

Discuss with the client to determine a convenient time during her breast-feeding schedule to come for oral care. Let her schedule be the guide for appointment planning. The same considerations apply to drug use during lactation as apply during pregnancy. The clinician must check a drug reference to determine whether a precaution exists during lactation before using drugs in treatment. This information should be found in the section of the drug discussion entitled "Precautions." There is no safety risk to the infant from the mother having dental X-rays during lactation. To reduce the concentration of a drug in breast milk, a drug can be taken *after* breast-feeding and there should be at least 4 hours between taking a drug and breast-feeding (Box 8-2).[2] Box 8-2 includes clinical considerations during lactation.[3]

Box 8-2

Clinical Considerations for Patients Who Are Breast-Feeding

Advise to minimize infant exposure to drugs the mother is receiving, such as by timing feedings or pumping and discarding milk.

Teach mother to recognize drug effects in child.

Reduce drug dosage during lactation.

Ascertain the risk for drugs prescribed by DDS to reach breast milk.

(Adapted from Donaldson et al. JADA 2012.[3])

"Are you taking birth control pills or hormonal replacement?"

This question attempts to determine potential adverse drug effects that could impact the plan for oral procedures or identify conditions associated with taking hormones that could impact the oral care plan. The specific drug(s) taken for the reasons in the question above would be investigated for side effects, such as cardiovascular effects (hypertension is possible with some contraceptive medications). The Women's Health Initiative, a large study investigating adverse effects from hormone replacement therapy in postmenopausal women, determined that those women who took hormone replacement medication(s) were at an increased risk for cardiovascular events, and for those who took the estrogen/progesterone combination an increased risk for breast cancer was found. There is no specific follow-up question related to this item on the health history that relates to a medical emergency. When the blood pressure is taken, the values should be considered in terms of the normal limits of blood pressure, just as would be done with any drug that could increase blood pressure. When values are increased, and there are no concurrent medical factors that could be responsible, the values should be written and provided to the client with a suggestion to have a medical evaluation and discuss the role of the oral contraceptive in blood pressure elevation or hypertension.

There is a potential for a reduction in the efficacy of oral contraceptives when antibiotics are taken. The ADA Council on Scientific Affairs published recommendations to dentists regarding this issue.[8] The Council recommendations included:

1. Advising the client of a potential risk for reduced effectiveness of the oral contraceptive if antibiotics are taken concurrently with the oral contraceptive.
2. Recommending that the client use an additional nonhormonal form of birth control during exposure to antibiotics.
3. Advising the client to continue taking the oral contraceptive while using antibiotics.

In the discussion of the issue, the Council noted research reporting that the failure rate of oral contraceptives used during antibiotic therapy was similar to the failure rate when oral contraceptives were used alone, and discussed a literature review that questioned whether the antibiotic–oral contraceptive interaction actually occurs.[9] The Council also cited evidence that some antibiotics commonly used in dentistry, such as amoxicillin, ampicillin, metronidazole, and tetracycline, may reduce the effectiveness of oral contraceptives, although the mechanism for this interaction is unclear. For this reason, it has been recommended that the client should be told to use a nonhormonal backup contraceptive method throughout antibiotic therapy and for 1 full week after completion or early cessation of the antibiotic course.[8,10]

HORMONE REPLACEMENT THERAPY

Both birth control medications and medications for hormone replacement therapy to relieve symptoms of menopause have side effects relevant to provision of oral procedures. These include increased blood pressure, nausea, increased incidence of dry socket, and increased bleeding. When discussing the drug history with the client, determine whether any of the side effects have occurred in the past.

Treatment Plan Modifications

The treatment plan should include strategies to monitor the client for the possibility of these side effects, such as:

1. Measuring the blood pressure during assessment of vital signs.
2. Asking the client whether she experiences nausea and using a semisupine chair position if the client gives a positive response to this question.
3. Examining for increased bleeding during the periodontal examination and instrumentation.
4. If the client is scheduled for tooth extraction, warning the client to watch for the signs of a dry socket (excessive pain, foul odor) and to return to the office should these signs occur (Box 8-3).

Box 8-3

Treatment Considerations for Hormone Therapy

- Monitor blood pressure
- Use a semisupine chair position if nausea occurs
- Assess for increased bleeding during periodontal examination
- Warn about risk of dry socket if extraction is planned
- Oral contraceptive: recommend additional form of birth control if antibiotic is taken throughout antibiotic therapy and for 1 full week after completion of antibiotic course

It is not uncommon for the dental auxiliary to be given the responsibility of providing postoperative instructions to clients following dental procedures.

"Please (X) a response to indicate if you have or have not had any of the following diseases or problems: osteoporosis."

Osteoporosis is identified in the medical section of the ADA Health History as a condition that

Self-Study Review

1. Which trimesters of pregnancy are associated with the greatest risk for medical emergencies?
    a. First and second trimesters
    b. First and third trimesters
    c. Second and third trimesters
    d. First, second, and third trimesters
2. Which U.S. Food and Drug Administration categories of drugs are considered safe for use with pregnant clients?
    a. A and B
    b. A and D
    c. B and D
    d. C and D
3. Syncope is common in the third trimester of pregnancy as a result of
    a. increased blood flow to the heart.
    b. increased blood flow to the left atrium of the heart.
    c. the weight of the fetus depressing the vena cava vein.
    d. the weight of the fetus stimulating the vena cava vein.
4. For those clients who use oral contraceptives and require antibiotic therapy, advise them to use a backup contraceptive:
    a. during the course of antibiotic therapy and for 1 week after antibiotic therapy is completed.
    b. during the course of antibiotic therapy and for 2 weeks after antibiotic therapy is completed.
    c. during the course of antibiotic therapy and for 1 month after antibiotic therapy is completed.
    d. during the course of antibiotic therapy only.
5. All clients, whether pregnant or not, should receive dental X-rays on a regular basis. Use of a lead apron and thyroid collar provides adequate safety for the client and developing fetus.
    a. Both statements are true.
    b. Both statements are false.
    c. The first statement is true, and the second statement is false.
    d. The first statement is false, and the second statement is true.

should be investigated during the health history review. It is included in this chapter because it is a common disability that occurs during menopause. It can affect both women and men, but women are more commonly affected.

PATHOPHYSIOLOGY DISCUSSION

Osteoporosis is a relatively common disorder characterized by loss of calcium in bones, leaving them thin and susceptible to fracture. The causes of osteoporosis include inadequate calcium in the diet; estrogen deficiencies associated with menopause or surgical removal of ovaries; a side effect of medications, such as prednisone; hyperparathyroidism; and unknown factors. Osteoporosis develops over many years and is associated with aging; therefore, a long asymptomatic period of bone change occurs with no clinical symptoms.[1] Diagnosis is often delayed until a fracture occurs. Predisposing factors for women include Caucasian and Asian races, slender build, early menopause, and fair skin. People who are sedentary are also predisposed to osteoporosis. Symptoms can range from no symptoms in the early stage to pain in the lower back and fractures in the late stage.[1] Although not life-threatening, the condition leads to fractures that, in the elderly, can cause serious complications, including death. As the disease progresses, the person becomes shorter and develops a hump in the upper back, called a "Dowager hump." These changes result when the vertebrae deteriorate from the pressure of the body weight. Diagnosis is by X-ray or by a specialized machine that measures bone density.

Relationship to Bone in the Jaw

It has been proposed that osteoporosis may be a factor in periodontal attachment loss by making alveolar bone more susceptible to resorption. The understanding of the exact role low bone mineral density (BMD) plays is unclear, as studies report both associations between osteoporosis and clinical attachment loss and others report negative or equivocal findings. In addition, many of the studies were uncontrolled, were poorly designed, had small sample sizes, and were restricted to a population of postmenopausal women, factors that limit the validity of the study conclusions.[11] A recent, large study investigated the association between periodontal disease and BMD in 1,347 older men who were followed for an average of 2.7 years. Parameters evaluated in the study were clinical attachment loss, pocket depth, amount of calculus and plaque, and bleeding. BMD was determined at multiple areas of the body by dual-energy X-ray absorptiometry and by ultrasound (heel). After adjustment for age, smoking, race, education level, body mass index, and calculus, there was no association between the number of teeth, periodontitis, periodontal disease progression, and either BMD or annualized rate of BMD change. The study reported little evidence of an association between periodontitis and skeletal BMD among older men.[12] A study of 135 postmenopausal women who were in good oral health at the beginning of a 3-year study were followed and clinical attachment was compared from the baseline values taken at the beginning of the study to those at the end of the 3-year period. The authors concluded there was no association between clinical attachment level and BMD, or that systemic bone density is a minor factor influencing attachment loss and that both may be a reflection of general health.[13] A more recent study of 1,256 women recruited from the Buffalo Center of the Women's Health Initiative Observational Study evaluated the influence of oral infection and age on the associations between osteoporosis and oral bone loss. When the entire group of women in the study was analyzed and adjusted for factors associated with osteoporosis, the results of oral bone loss were non-significant; however, when the cohort of women less than age 70 years was examined, there was an association between bone loss (as determined by radiographs, not by probe depth readings and clinical attachment loss) and mean alveolar height.[14] In order to understand the true relationships between osteoporosis and alveolar bone, large prospective studies are needed to clarify the issue.

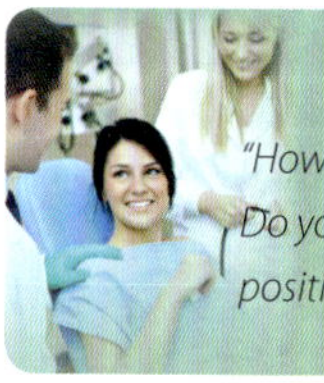

Follow-up Question

"How is your osteoporosis being treated? Do you have back pain that requires special positioning in the dental chair?"

Application to Practice

When osteoporosis is reported, client positioning should include supporting the back and the neck. Extensive neck manipulation should be avoided if osteoporosis is severe.[2] Some clients have no symptoms and do not require modification of the treatment plan. Osteoporosis may be a risk factor for periodontal bone loss, although this issue is unclear and more studies are needed to answer the clinical question.[14]

Self-Study Review

6. Periodontal disease progression is a feature associated with osteoporosis. Studies have shown that clinical attachment loss occurs with a decrease in bone mineral density.

a. Both statements are true.
b. Both statements are false.
c. The first statement is true, and the second statement is false.
d. The first statement is false, and the second statement is true.

7. Dental implications for the client diagnosed with osteoporosis include all of the following EXCEPT one. Which is the EXCEPTION?

a. Consider positioning in dental chair.
b. Protect the neck from excessive bending.
c. Prescribe calcium fluoride supplements.
d. Encourage plaque control and periodontal maintenance.
e. Recommend calcium and vitamin D supplements.

Osteoporosis is associated with causing ridge resorption in edentulous clients.[1] Treatment plan ning should address plaque control procedures to reduce periodontal attachment loss and encourage increased calcium plus vitamin D consumption to increase bone density. The most common drugs prescribed to treat osteoporosis are within the bisphosphonate class of drugs. For individuals who are taking bisphosphonate therapy follow recommendations included in Chapter 5.

"Please mark (X) your response to indicate if you have or have not had any of the following diseases or problems. Artificial (prosthetic) heart valve. Previous infective endocarditis. Damaged valves in transplanted heart. Congenital heart disease (CHD), including unrepaired, cyanotic CHD; repaired (completely) in last 6 months; repaired CHD with residual defects. Except for the conditions listed above, antibiotic prophylaxis is no longer recommended for any other form of CHD."

The American Heart Association's (AHA's) committees to develop guidelines for prevention of IE recently updated indications and timing for administration of antibiotics prior to oral procedures.[15] The medical conditions listed in the item above represent the 2007 indications for antibiotic prophylaxis prior to oral procedures in individuals who are at a *high risk for IE* due to **valvulopathy**. When bacteria enter the bloodstream, a condition termed **bacteremia** exists. The types of microorganisms within the bacteremia are relevant, in that some types of microorganisms are more likely to attach to and infect cardiac tissues than others. Bacteria that mainly inhabit the skin (*Staphylococcus aureus*), enterococci from the gastrointestinal tract, and microorganisms from the mouth and the pharynx (viridans group streptococci) are the three most common types of microorganisms to cause IE. However, this microorganism profile does not include subgingival gram-negative **periodontopathogens**. Periodontal bacteria are rarely a cause of IE. The number of worldwide cases of IE caused by periodontal pathogens is no more than 105 cases.[16]

The AHA has recommended prophylactic antibiotics prior to dental procedures since 1955, although no research showed that antibiotics could prevent the infection. Researchers thought that antibiotics might be helpful in preventing a serious cardiac infection that could result in death or extreme morbidity (need for a cardiac transplant). Amoxicillin is an antibiotic that can kill the three types of microorganisms that cause most cases of IE, so it is the drug of choice for prevention of IE. Second-line drugs are suggested when a penicillin allergy exists or when oral medications cannot be tolerated (Table 8.2). The effectiveness of these antibiotics is being compromised by development of antibiotic resistant bacteria. Most authorities report that the taking of antibiotics when they are not needed is the most likely cause of the increasing number of microorganisms developing resistance to penicillins and other antibiotics. Because there is no evidence that antibiotics prevented IE, and there are reports of IE developing even when prophylactic antibiotics were taken, plus the increasing antibiotic resistance problem worldwide, the AHA committee decided to reduce the conditions indicated for antibiotic prophylaxis and to only include cardiac conditions at the highest risk for mortality or morbidity if IE developed.[15]

Table 8.2 2007 AHA Regimen: Prophylactic Antibiotic Premedication to Prevent Infective Endocarditis
Indications: Prosthetic heart valve, previous IE, heart murmur or valvulopathy that develops in a transplanted heart, congenital heart disease: unrepaired congenital malformations, repaired congenital defects for 6 months following surgery, and repaired congenital defects with residual defects.
All oral antibiotics are recommended 30 minutes to 1 hour before appointment; no second dose is recommended. When antibiotic is inadvertently not taken, can be given up to 2 hours after appointment.
Dental procedures for which prophylaxis is recommended: All dental procedures that involve manipulation of gingival tissue or the periapical region of teeth, or perforation of the oral mucosa. Oral procedures that *do not need* prophylaxis: routine anesthetic injections through noninfected tissue, taking dental radiographs, placement of removable prosthodontic or orthodontic appliances, adjustment of orthodontic appliances, placement of orthodontic brackets, shedding of deciduous teeth, and bleeding from trauma to the lips or oral mucosa.
Regimen of antibiotics:
Amoxicillin—2 g adult, children 50 mg/kg; for patients unable to take oral medications: ampicillin 2 g IM or IV; child 50 mg/kg IM or IV or cefazolin or ceftriaxone 1 g IM or IV, child 50 mg/kg IM or IV.
If penicillin allergy exists:
Clindamycin—600 mg (child 20 mg/kg)
Clarithromycin or azithromycin—500 mg (child 15 mg/kg)
Cephalexin[a]—2 g oral tablet (child 50 mg/kg)
If penicillin allergy exists and cannot take oral medications: Cefazolin or ceftriaxone 1 g IM or IV; child 50 mg/kg IM or IV; clindamycin 600 mg IM or IV; child 20 mg/kg IM or IV.
Alteration to recommended regimen: If procedures cover several weeks, alternate between drug classes, or wait 10 days before next appointment if using same class of antimicrobial.

[a]Cephalosporins should not be used when allergic to cephalosporin or when anaphylaxis, angioedema, or urticaria with penicillins has occurred.

AHA, American Heart Association; IM, intramuscularly; IV, intravenously; mg, milligram; g, gram; kg, kilogram.

(Adapted from Wilson W, Taubert KA, Gewitz M, et al. AHA Guideline: prevention of infective endocarditis. Circulation 2007;116:1736–1754. DOI: 10.1161/CirculationAHA.106.183095.)

The antibiotic selected for antibiotic prophylaxis should be taken 30 minutes to 1 hour before the appointment, but only by those in the *high-risk group*. A pretreatment antimicrobial rinse is not recommended because there is no science that shows this practice prevents IE. In situations in which a client appears for an appointment and has inadvertently failed to take the prophylactic antibiotic, the new guidelines recommend that the antibiotic be given within 2 hours following the appointment. Ideally, however prophylactic antibiotics should be taken at least 30 minutes before initiating a bacteremia during treatment.[15] Taking any antibiotic, including AHA prophylaxis, can result in the formation of antibiotic-resistant microorganisms in the oral cavity. However, resistance is unlikely to persist 10 days after the antibiotic is terminated. For situations where the client is currently taking amoxicillin and has a cardiac condition that is indicated to receive antibiotic prophylaxis prior to the dental appointment, the clinician should prescribe one of the other antibiotics in the regimen. When multiple appointments prior to a 10-day interval are planned, the AHA recommends choosing an antibiotic from a different class on subsequent appointments to reduce the risk of antibiotic resistance. Another suggestion to reduce antibiotic resistance is to complete as much treatment as possible at one appointment, even if it will take 2 to 3 hours to complete treatment. Antibiotic resistance is less likely to occur if the client has two appointments and half the mouth is treated under antibiotic prophylaxis than if four appointments for separate quadrant debridement under antibiotic prophylaxis are planned. The practitioner should use as few antibiotic administrations as are necessary depending on the client's ability to endure the stress of a long appointment.[15] Some cardiac clients need short, stress-free dental appointments to reduce the risk of a medical emergency. For those clients who cannot tolerate long appointments, the following example for antibiotic prophylaxis is suggested.

Case Example

The client has advanced periodontal disease with heavy generalized subgingival calculus; has no penicillin allergy; has a history of IE; is awaiting a heart transplant and is unable to withstand long appointments; needs to complete treatment as quickly as possible; and requires five appointments for examination, radiographs, and subgingival debridement one quadrant per appointment. According to the American Heart Association the suggested regimen is to use amoxicillin (first-line antibiotic) on the initial periodontal examination appointment that includes periodontal probing. For the first of a four-quadrant debridement appointment schedule that occurs before a 10-day interval, select a different antibiotic, such as a macrolide (clarithromycin). For the second debridement appointment before a 10-day interval, select clindamycin. For the third debridement before a 10-day interval, cephalosporin can be prescribed, or wait for a 10-day interval and start over with amoxicillin. Rotate antibiotic classes according to this schedule until treatment is completed. This protocol follows the recommendation included in the AHA policy when multiple appointments in close proximity are needed (Box 8-4).[17] If treatment can be delayed for 10 days between appointments, then amoxicillin can be used at each appointment.

Box 8-4

Antibiotic Prophylaxis for Less Than a 10-Day Interval between Appointments

First drug of choice: amoxicillin

First debridement: macrolide

Second debridement: clindamycin

Third debridement: cephalosporin

Fourth debridement: amoxicillin

Penicillin Allergies

For the client who is allergic to penicillin, the protocol suggested in Table 8.2 can be modified to eliminate amoxicillin. Either one of the macrolide antibiotics (clarithromycin, azithromycin) or clindamycin can be selected. Eliminate amoxicillin in the rotational schedule, and possibly the cephalosporins (the chemical structure of penicillin and cephalosporin is similar and the client may also have an allergy to a cephalosporin). For the client with a penicillin allergy but who is not allergic to cephalosporins, then a cephalosporin can be used.

Efficacy of Antibiotic Prophylaxis in Dental Practice

The 2007 AHA guidelines for prevention of IE discussed four primary reasons for updating the IE guidelines. These included (a) that IE is much more likely to result from frequent exposure to random bacteremias associated with daily activities, such as brushing and flossing the teeth or chewing food, than from a dental appointment; (b) that administering prophylactic antibiotics before a dental procedure may prevent a very small number of cases of IE, and possibly no cases of IE would be prevented; (c) the risk of antibiotic-associated adverse events exceeds the benefit of prophylaxis; and (d) that maintaining oral health and good oral hygiene may reduce the incidence of bacteremia from daily activities, and is more important than prophylactic antibiotics before dental procedures to reduce the risk for IE.[14] The AHA committee noted that stents, coronary artery bypass grafts, and a heart transplant procedure are not indicated for antibiotic prophylaxis prior to oral procedures; however, when a transplanted heart subsequently develops valvulopathy, prophylactic antibiotics can be considered. There have been recommendations for antibiotic prophylaxis in other medical situations. A recent systematic review assessed the evidence of efficacy for this practice in eight medical conditions: cardiac-native heart valve disease; prosthetic heart valves and pacemakers; hip, knee, and shoulder prosthetic joints; renal dialysis shunts; cerebrospinal fluid shunts; vascular grafts; immunosuppression secondary to cancer and cancer chemotherapy; systemic lupus erythematosus; and insulin-dependent (type 1) diabetes mellitus.[18] The authors concluded that there is no scientific basis for the use of prophylactic antibiotics before dental procedures for these eight groups of patients. Communication with the lead author revealed that there is no scientific basis for using antibiotic prophylaxis in the client with a history of glomerulonephritis. Until a study is completed verifying that antibiotic prophylaxis prior to oral procedures prevents kidney infection, this practice is unfounded. The United Kingdom (NICE Guidelines) completely eliminated prescribing antibiotics to prevent IE and a follow-up study revealed no increase in the incidence of IE, thereby supporting the notion that antibiotics do not prevent IE. A similar study in the United States concluded the same thing—that antibiotic prophylaxis does not reduce the incidence of IE.[19]

Self-Study Review

8. Which of the following conditions requires prophylactic antibiotic coverage before dental treatment?
   a. Kidney stones leading to kidney infection
   b. Alcohol abuse
   c. Prosthetic heart valve
   d. Seizure disorder involving tonic contractions
9. Infective endocarditis (IE) can be caused by
   a. septicemia during oral treatment.
   b. anemia during oral treatment.
   c. bleeding during oral treatment.
   d. bacteremia produced during oral treatment.
10. Ideally when should prophylactic antibiotics be taken?
    a. 30 minutes before the appointment
    b. Within 2 hours of the appointment
    c. 30 minutes to 1 hour before the appointment
    d. 1 hour before the appointment and 3 hours after the appointment
11. The antibiotic of choice recommended for antibiotic prophylaxis to prevent IE is
    a. clarithromycin or azithromycin.
    b. clindamycin.
    c. amoxicillin.
    d. cephalexin.
12. Select from the following list, the three antibiotics that are recommended if a penicillin allergic client requires antibiotic prophylaxis.
    a. Clarithromycin
    b. Clindamycin
    c. Amoxicillin
    d. Azithromycin

CHAPTER SUMMARY

This chapter provides information concerning treatment considerations for the pregnant or lactating patient. It identifies considerations when the client is taking oral contraceptives or hormone replacement therapy. The chapter ends with a discussion of indications for antibiotic prophylaxis prior to oral procedures that involve tooth manipulation or the perforation of oral mucosa and identifies eight medical conditions that have no evidence base for antibiotic prophylaxis.

Review

1. Define the following terms: parturition, teratogen, and valvulopathy.
2. Identify four side effects of birth control and hormone replacement medications that are relevant for oral health care.
3. What procedure can be used during treatment to prevent syncope in the pregnant woman who is in her third trimester?
4. List the indications for which antibiotic prophylaxis is no longer indicated.

Case Study

Case A

Regina Bergen, a 28-year-old client, presents for an emergency appointment as a result of pain associated with tooth number 29. The client is 8 months pregnant and in good health. Oral examination reveals a large carious lesion on the occlusal surface of number 29. Restorative treatment is planned. Her vital signs are pulse 80 bpm, respiration 18 breaths/min, and blood pressure 110/60 mm Hg, right arm, sitting.

1. Which local anesthetic agent is considered safe for use during pregnancy?
2. Why would an NSAID be contraindicated for treatment of postoperative pain in this client?
3. Can radiographs be performed on this client?

The client returns 3 months later with facial swelling and continued pain associated with tooth number 29. She reports having delivered a healthy baby boy. Oral and radiographic examination of number 29 is performed, and the client is diagnosed with a periapical abscess. The dentist prescribes an oral antibiotic and refers the client to an endodontist for further evaluation. Medical history update reveals the client is taking an oral contraceptive. What specific recommendation would you make concerning antibiotic coverage and use of oral contraceptives?

Case B

Marjorie Logan, a 55-year-old woman, presents for a routine dental examination. She reports a history of hypertension and a pacemaker placed 3 years ago. She also reports a recent history of osteoporosis and hyperparathyroidism, for which she is being treated with calcium and prescription vitamin D. The client notes that she takes atenolol for her hypertension and feels well. She indicates that she exercises daily and can climb stairs without incident. Her vital signs include pulse 82 bpm, respiration 16 breath/min, and blood pressure 138/86 mm Hg, right arm.

1. What prophylactic antibiotic regimen is recommended for this client?
2. What are the initial signs of osteoporosis?

Chapter Nine

Blood-Related Abnormalities and Blood-borne Pathogenic Conditions

Objectives

After completing the self-study chapter the reader will be able to:

- Identify medical conditions associated with increased bleeding and determine when bleeding is likely to occur during oral health care.
- Describe prevention and management strategies for the various conditions that may result in increased bleeding.
- Describe treatment modifications associated with bloodborne diseases, including hepatitis, AIDS or HIV infection, and with sexually transmitted diseases.
- Identify postexposure prophylaxis (PEP) recommendations for bloodborne infections.
- Identify oral healthcare treatment modifications for bleeding disorders and anemia.
- Determine the risks of treating the client reporting a history of blood transfusion.

Key Terms

Blood dyscrasia: a pathologic condition in which any of the constituents of blood are abnormal or are present in abnormal quantities

Carrier: one who harbors disease organisms in the body, including the blood; capable of transmitting the disease to others

Ecchymosis: discoloration of the skin caused by blood within the local tissue; lesions are larger than pinpoint lesions

Hemostasis: the arrest or stopping of bleeding

Iatrogenic: any situation caused by the clinician or operator

Idiopathic: cause for condition is unknown

Petechiae: small, pinpoint collections of blood under the skin or mucous membrane

Platelet agglutination: clumping of platelets to cause a clot; involves adhesiveness or "stickiness" of platelet surface

Progeny: offspring or descendents, including cells produced by cell division

Seroconvert: the development of antibodies in response to vaccination

Sign: the objective evidence of a disease (e.g., observed by the healthcare professional)

Symptom: the subjective evidence of a disease (e.g., that reported by the client)

Thrombocytopenia: condition in which number of platelets is reduced, usually by destruction of red blood cell–forming tissue in bone marrow, associated with neoplastic diseases or an immune response to a drug

Thrombophlebitis: inflammation of a vein associated with clot formation within blood vessels

---

MEDICAL CONDITION

INTRODUCTION

This portion of the American Dental Association (ADA) Health History Form continues the assessment of the client's systemic health. The section is arranged to identify diagnosed disease conditions (YES answer), the absence of the disease condition (NO answer), or if the client does not know (DK) whether he or she has a specific disease condition. The "don't know" response may bring attention to situations where the client thinks he or she has **symptoms** of a disease or disorder but has not sought medical evaluation for it. It can also include situations where the client has been evaluated for a condition and the report was inconclusive. Any "don't know" responses require follow-up investigation related to why the client responded in this manner.

The chapters for the medical section will be organized to respond to each condition listed on the ADA Health History, generally in the order that it is listed on the form. However, when conditions with a strong relationship to each other are not grouped together on the form, they will be discussed together for this self-study reference (such as blood-related abnormalities and blood-borne diseases). The discussion for the medical section chapters includes

1. Pathophysiology of the medical condition
2. Appropriate follow-up questions related to determining disease control and risks to the client or clinician as a result of treatment
3. Treatment plan modifications and applications to practice
4. Potential emergencies that could occur because of the disorder and strategies to prevent the emergency from occurring
5. Management of the emergency, should one occur

This chapter will focus on blood-related abnormalities, such as abnormal bleeding, bloodborne diseases, sexually transmitted diseases, anemia, and blood transfusion.

"Please (X) a response to indicate if you have or have not had any of the following diseases or problems: abnormal bleeding, hemophilia, liver disease."

Abnormal bleeding problems can include a variety of conditions,[1] including:

1. **Blood dyscrasias** such as **thrombocytopenia**
2. Bleeding disorders such as von Willebrand disease (vWD) and hemophilia
3. Liver dysfunction associated with hepatitis or other liver disease complications (such as alcoholic cirrhosis)
4. Lack of clotting factor formation from disease or from drugs such as warfarin (Coumadin®)
5. Reduced **platelet agglutination** as a result of medications, such as aspirin (Box 9-1)

Box 9-1

Causes of Abnormal Bleeding

- Blood dyscrasia (thrombocytopenia)
- Bleeding disorders (vWD, hemophilia)
- Liver dysfunction (hepatitis, cirrhosis)
- Drug-induced clotting abnormalities (lack of platelet aggregation, lack of clotting factor formation)

The clinical implication of the bleeding disorders listed above is that each one has an increased risk for bleeding due to **iatrogenic** oral manipulation, such as instrumentation. It has been estimated that in a dental practice with 2,000 adults there will be 100 to 150 clients who may be at risk for increased bleeding during oral procedures.[2]

Signs and symptoms of these conditions are similar in that increased bleeding and collections of blood under the skin or mucous membranes, such as **ecchymosis** and petechiae, may occur. Laboratory blood tests to identify risks for uncontrolled bleeding include prothrombin time (PT), the international normalized ratio (INR), the number of platelets (Plt), the platelet function analyzer (PFA-100), and the activated partial prothrombin (aPTT).[1,2] The Ivy bleeding time test was formerly recommended to screen for disorders of platelet function and thrombocytopenia. Subsequent studies showed the test to be unreliable and it is no longer recommended.[2] Normal values and treatment indications for these tests are provided in Box 9-2.

PATHOPHYSIOLOGY OF THROMBOCYTOPENIA

Thrombocytopenia is a common cause of bleeding disorders. It occurs when there is a reduction in the formation of blood platelets or when mature platelets are injured. Clients with leukemia may have thrombocytopenia which results when the overgrowth of malignant cells takes the place of platelet precursor cells in the bone marrow. With fewer cells available to mature into platelets, blood levels of these cells fall. Another condition that can result in thrombocytopenia is liver disease. Liver dysfunction can cause overactivation of the spleen, and platelets are damaged in the process. Reductions in platelet levels or abnormalities in platelet function can result in excessive bleeding. Blood platelets are formed in the bone marrow and hematopoietic tissues, such as the spleen. Any situation that reduces the function of the bone marrow (drugs, disease) can result in low blood levels of platelets. For example, the toxic effects of cancer chemotherapy can reduce the synthesis of platelets by killing bone marrow cells. The function of platelets is to form clots. They do this by sticking together and clumping over an injured area of the body. This is analogous to the body's own "band-aid." Covering the injured area prevents further outward blood flow and allows healing to begin. The normal number of platelet formation is between 140,000 and 400,000 platelets per cubic millimeter of blood (expressed as mm^3).[2] Diagnosis of thrombocytopenia is determined by a laboratory platelet count. When the laboratory test reveals less than the normal number of platelets, but the cause cannot be determined, the condition is called "**idiopathic** thrombocytopenia."

Box 9-2

Laboratory Values and Clinical Implications

Test	Normal Range	Clinical Implication
Prothrombin time (PT)	11–15 s	Routine care can be performed when PT is <20 s
International normalized ratio (INR)	<2.5	Routine care can be performed when INR 2–3, MD consult when INR >3.5
Activated partial thromboplastin time (aPTT)	25–35 s	Routine care when aPTT is >1.5 normal, MD consult when >57 s
Platelet count	140,000–400,000/mm^3	Routine care 50,000/mm^3
Platelet function analyzer (PFA-100)	<175 s	Used when clopidogrel is taken and oral surgery planned

(Adapted from Tyler MT, et al. Clinician's guide to treatment of medically complex dental patients. AAOM. 2nd ed. 2001:4, 34; and Little JW, Falace DA, et al. Dental Management of the Medically Compromised Patient. 8th Ed. St. Louis, MO: Mosby, 2013:417–419.)

Management

Bleeding problems from thrombocytopenia generally occur at platelet levels less than 50,000/mm^3.[1,2] In the client with a history of a blood dyscrasia, appropriate laboratory tests should be ordered to determine the risk of providing oral health care. On the basis of the values of the laboratory test (Plt), the decision can be made whether to delay treatment or proceed with planned procedures that may involve bleeding. Most routine oral procedures can be provided when platelet levels are <50,000/mm^3. Infiltration and block local anesthetic injections can be provided when the platelet count is greater than 30,000/mm^3.[2] Aspirin, or aspirin-related products, should not be recommended to clients with thrombocytopenia because of the additive anticoagulant effect. When platelet levels are less than 50,000/mm^3, consult with the client's physician to determine whether a platelet infusion may be necessary before treatment and the time necessary between the infusion and appointing the client for treatment. The need for platelet transfusion can be reduced by using local hemostatic agents, such as tranexamic acid rinse.[2]

PATHOPHYSIOLOGY OF VWD

vWD is an inherited bleeding disorder that is caused by a deficiency or dysfunction of von Willebrand factor (vWF), a plasma protein that initiates the adhesion of platelets at sites of vascular injury and also binds and stabilizes blood clotting factor VIII in the circulation.[3] This condition is the most common *inherited* bleeding disorder. In vWD, the inherited defect can cause bleeding by poor platelet adhesion to tissue surfaces or a reduction in the concentration of factor VIII. The platelets do not stick to surfaces because vWF is missing. There are several variants of vWD. Type 1 is the most common form (70% to 80%) and is characterized by a partial deficiency of vWF and lower than normal levels of factor VIII. It is considered to be a mild form with the least risk of hemorrhage. The more severe forms of vWD are types 2 and 3. Generally, in type 1 vWD bleeding occurs only after surgery or trauma. There is no single ideal laboratory test to diagnose vWD. Initial tests for patients with excessive bleeding include a complete blood count, aPTT, and PT.[3] Extraoral signs of vWD may include **petechiae** of skin. Gastrointestinal (GI) bleeding and epistaxis (nosebleeds) are often reported in types 2 and 3 and they represent the greatest risk for increased bleeding during oral procedures.[2,3]

Management

Uncontrolled bleeding is associated with types 2 and 3, and follow-up questioning would be directed toward identifying the type of vWD and revealing problems with bleeding after minor injury or surgery, and if frequent nosebleeds occur. Clients with the milder type 1 form may not report a history of "at home" bleeding problems. There is a low risk for hemorrhage when the aPTT is below 50 seconds and increased bleeding can usually be controlled with local measures.[1,2] Consultation with the physician is recommended to order a laboratory test for aPTT and to determine necessary medical treatment before oral procedures involving bleeding. The current clinical practice guidelines recommend that minor bleeding associated with simple dental extractions can be controlled with the drug DDAVP administered by a physician prior to the dental appointment.[3] DDAVP stimulates the release of vWF from endothelial cells and is used to manage minor bleeding. Local hemostatic rinses, for example, aminocaproic acid and tranexamic acid, can be used to manage mild mucocutaneous bleeding in vWD.[3] Careful suturing of the extraction socket is also important. Aspirin and other nonsteroidal anti-inflammatory drugs (e.g., ibuprofen, naproxen) should be avoided.[3]

PATHOPHYSIOLOGY OF HEMOPHILIA

Hemophilia is an inherited disorder that results in lack of formation of clotting factors and has a wide range of severity. There are three main forms. Hemophilia A involves a deficiency of factor VIII and represents the most common inherited coagulation disorder.[2] It comprises approximately 80% of genetic coagulation disorders. Hemophilia B (also called Christmas disease, or factor IX deficiency) accounts for approximately a 13% prevalence. Lack of factor XI involves approximately 6% of those affected.[2]

Management

The client with a history of hemophilia is at risk for hemorrhage after oral healthcare procedures that involve bleeding. However, most clients do well with proper medical management involving the administration of drugs to decrease bleeding or the infusion of platelets or plasma-containing clotting factors. This requires consultation with the client's physician and the administration of the necessary agents before the dental appointment. Laboratory tests necessary before treatment that involves bleeding include the PT/INR and the aPTT. In each of the conditions affecting bleeding discussed earlier, the physician would supervise the administration of necessary blood transfusions and determine the timing between the medical management and the appointments for oral health care.

PATHOPHYSIOLOGY OF BLEEDING CAUSED BY LIVER DISEASE

Acquired coagulation disorder, such as liver disease, is the most common cause of prolonged bleeding.[2] The liver forms all of the protein coagulation factors needed for clot formation. In addition, liver disease often affects the spleen resulting in thrombocytopenia. The most common condition to result in liver dysfunction is hepatitis. Hepatitis is defined as inflammation of the liver. It occurs through a variety of causes, but a fairly common reason is viral infection in the liver. Alcoholic cirrhosis, discussed in Chapter 7, is a severe form of liver disease. Clients with liver disease can have a low platelet count secondary to effects on the spleen. The spleen normally removes platelets from the blood. The extraoral sign of this disturbance is bruising of the skin (called purpura or ecchymoses; Fig. 9.1). Petechiae may be found on the oral mucous membranes. This finding gives the clinician a clue that there is a risk for increased bleeding during treatment. Abnormal liver function resulting in increased bleeding occurs as a result of reduced formation of clotting factors and components necessary for the formation of fibrin. These are formed mainly in the liver. In addition, liver disease may cause portal hypertension that secondarily increases the function of the spleen to remove platelets. Abnormal bleeding associated with liver dysfunction or disease is the result of the following:

1. Reduced synthesis of blood-clotting factors
2. Abnormal fibrin function
3. Thrombocytopenia associated with platelet destruction by the spleen

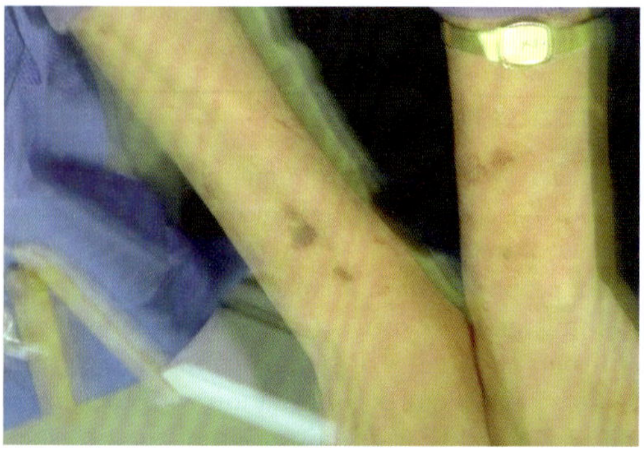

Figure 9.1 ■ Clinical photograph of ecchymoses on the arm of a client with liver damage as a result of hepatitis.

MEDICATION-RELATED CONDITIONS LEADING TO ABNORMAL BLEEDING

Most individuals who take medications that affect blood components which regulate bleeding do so because of a history of heart attack, stroke, or intravascular clotting (e.g., thrombophlebitis). Other medical conditions where these medications are used include following joint replacement surgery, cardiac valve replacements, and a variety of other less common medical conditions. Aspirin is used on a daily basis to prevent cardiovascular complications and to relieve chronic pain, such as in arthritis.

Antiplatelet Agglutination

Aspirin is the most commonly used medication that has an antiplatelet effect. This means that aspirin affects newly formed platelets in a way that makes platelets lose the ability to stick together. Blood remains fluid and clot formation is delayed. Prevention of clot formation is the reason for "taking a baby aspirin each day." It has been shown that low-dose aspirin can increase bleeding on probing (BOP) and impair diagnostic assessments.[4] In this study, patients with gingivitis were divided into three groups (group one took 81 mg aspirin, group two took 325 mg aspirin, group three was the placebo group that took no aspirin). There were significant increases in BOP in both aspirin groups and no changes from baseline in the placebo group. The effect of taking daily aspirin (100 mg tablet/day) was investigated, and it was determined that although the bleeding time was increased in aspirin therapy, this increased bleeding could be controlled by local digital pressure.[5] A recent study investigating the risks of aspirin and bleeding in dentistry concluded that removing the client from aspirin prophylaxis was more likely to result in death from intravascular clot formation than to create management problems related to excessive bleeding.[6] The authors felt that more information would be gained by questioning the client about excessive bleeding following injuries or trauma than from ordering laboratory tests to determine if the risk for bleeding was increased. The ADA agreed with this conclusion and recommended that aspirin and clopidogrel (Plavix®) therapy be continued (do not take patient off these drugs) for minor dental surgical procedures in patients who have coronary artery stents due to the significant thrombotic risks of discontinuing therapy.[7]

Lack of Clotting Factor Formation

The most common oral drug taken to reduce formation of blood clots within blood vessels is warfarin (Coumadin®). This drug is recommended for clients who have had a recent myocardial infarction (heart attack), cerebrovascular accident (stroke), or **thrombophlebitis**. Other conditions for which anticoagulant medications may be prescribed include having artificial heart valves and short-term therapy after total joint replacement surgery. The purpose of anticoagulation therapy is to reduce the risk of intravascular clot formation (thrombosis) while maintaining the lowest possible risk for bleeding. Warfarin accomplishes this effect by inhibiting the formation of vitamin K–related coagulation factors. The blood test to measure the level of anticoagulation (and to determine the risk of bleeding) when warfarin is taken is the PT or INR. The INR is a more accurate and standardized test and is widely accepted. If the INR is kept at levels of between 2 and 3, the bleeding risk is very low. If the INR is more than 5, the risk increases significantly.[8]

Clients on low-dose warfarin therapy (INR 2 to 3) to prevent formation of venous blood clots have a very low risk for hemorrhage (4.3% per year).[8] A recent systematic review on the intensity of anticoagulation therapy and outcomes concluded that INR levels greater than 3 but less than 5 had an absolute risk for combined thrombosis and bleeding of 7% per year.[8] It is likely that the absolute risk of thrombosis and bleeding at a ratio between 3 and 4 would be lower than 7%.[9] The bleeding risk is directly related to the drug's dose and level of anticoagulation and those clients on higher-dose therapy (INR greater than 5) have a greater risk for bleeding.[8] However, dental hygiene procedures involving periodontal instrumentation are considered safe at INR levels of 3.5 and bleeding can usually be controlled by digital pressure at the bleeding site.[2] A review of the literature reported on dangers of reducing the anticoagulation levels before oral surgery.[10] The author investigated more than 950 patients on warfarin therapy and found only 12 required more than local measures to control increased bleeding associated with dental surgery. In this study, five clients who had the dose of warfarin therapy reduced prior to oral surgery experienced serious embolism formation, and four clients died. The author concluded that dentists should continue the client on therapeutic levels of warfarin when oral surgery is planned and recommended a medical consultation to determine the client's level of anticoagulation before performing oral surgery.[10] If warfarin is being taken and the client has additional medical conditions leading to increased bleeding (such as liver disease, currently also taking aspirin, NSAIDs, or antibiotics), then the client must be managed on an individual basis with medical consultation.[2]

Application to Practice

The dental hygienist would question the client to determine what the INR number was at the last medical visit. Generally, the INR is monitored every 3 months. If the client cannot recall the number, the clinician should ask if the dosage of warfarin was changed at the last visit. If no dose reduction was made this is an indication that the levels were in the therapeutic range, and the risk for bleeding from periodontal procedures is low. Digital pressure should be successful to manage bleeding during periodontal procedures.

There are several effective protocols used to reduce bleeding during and after oral surgery in the client taking warfarin. These include rinsing with a hemostatic agent, such as tranexamic acid, taking aminocaproic acid (Amicar®), vitamin K injections, and the local application of an absorbable gelatin sponge (Gelfoam®) or other hemostatic agents.[11] When bleeding abnormalities are reported on the medical history, the clinician should consult with the client's physician or hematologist to determine the risk for uncontrolled bleeding during the oral procedure. Before surgery or procedures involving excessive bleeding are attempted, the client should be sent for hematologic laboratory tests to determine the INR level (Box 9-2). If hemostatic drugs or vitamin K injections are ordered by the physician for **hemostasis**, they must be taken before the appointment and according to the physician's recommendation.

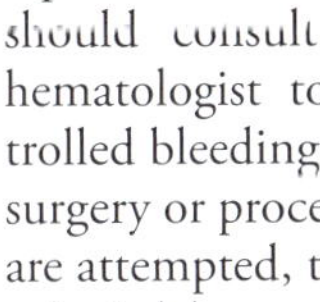

Follow-Up Questions

The appropriate follow-up questions would include

"What kind of bleeding problem do you have and do you know the cause? Do you have frequent nosebleeds? Have you had bleeding problems following dental or medical treatments, and if so, describe them? How do you control bleeding problems? Has your physician warned you about having dental treatment?"

These questions should identify the nature of the bleeding problem and the cause(s), previous problems associated with oral healthcare procedures, and strategies for controlling the bleeding episode. Frequent nosebleeds are a sign that bleeding problems may develop during oral procedures that involve bleeding. When treating a client, where very little is known about reasons for increased bleeding (frequently a client says increased bleeding after a cut has occurred but no medical evaluation was sought), the clinician can instrument one or two teeth and observe for clotting. If a clot does not form within a few minutes, digital pressure can be applied and treatment delayed until medical evaluation and blood tests have been completed. A physician consultation should be completed to determine the PT/INR in the client taking warfarin. When drugs are taken that have an antiplatelet effect, there is no reliable laboratory test to determine the risk of bleeding and bleeding should be controlled with digital pressure and local hemostatic agents, as needed. Low doses of aspirin have not been shown to cause clinical bleeding problems, so no modification of the treatment plan is necessary.

Potential Emergencies and Prevention

All of the above conditions pose a risk for hemorrhage or excessive bleeding. The most important information to discover when determining the risk for an uncontrolled bleeding emergency is whether the condition is controlled by current medical management. In most cases when conditions involving increased bleeding are known and measures are taken to reduce the risks of hemorrhage, a few problems occur. The greatest risk involves not knowing that the condition exists and proceeding with oral care that causes bleeding. In this situation, excessive bleeding is not expected. Excessive bleeding usually occurs within several hours after the oral procedure and the client calls the dental office to report the hemorrhage. For hemophilia and severe vWD, infusions of blood factors might be ordered by the physician before the appointment. The client can have an appointment for oral care the day after the infusion. Infusions of platelets may be ordered for the thrombocytopenia client. Verification of adequate platelet levels would be determined by the hematologist. Figure 9.2 reveals a client with idiopathic thrombocytopenia who was unaware of the condition until she had an oral prophylaxis.

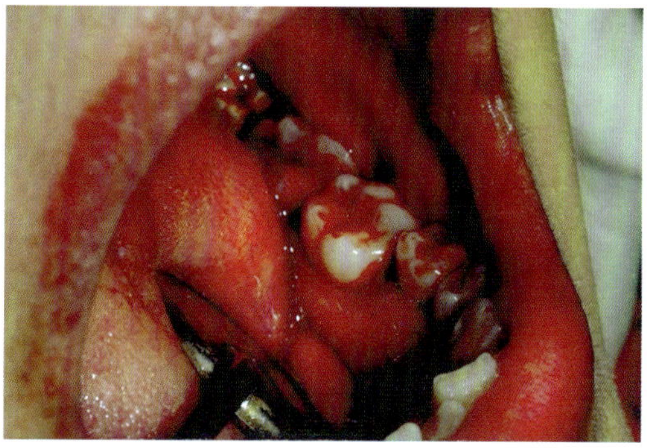

Figure 9.2 ■ Clinical photograph of uncontrolled bleeding after a dental hygiene oral prophylaxis appointment. Patient was later determined to have idiopathic thrombocytopenia.

She reported that during the night after her dental hygiene appointment she "spit out several blood clots the size of a 50-cent piece." The clinical photograph was taken approximately 16 hours after the appointment. Note that the gingivae are still bleeding freely.

Management

Antifibrinolytic medications or rinses (aminocaproic acid, tranexamic acid) have been used successfully to manage bleeding after tooth extraction in hemophilia clients and in clients taking warfarin. For most cases when the medical history indicates a potential for increased bleeding, the clinician will monitor the bleeding levels during treatment, and if clotting is prolonged, apply digital pressure to the soft tissue or gingivae. This may encourage clot formation. Clients with excessive bleeding should not be dismissed until bleeding is stopped or controlled. Postoperative instructions might include mild rinsing with cold water or applying a moistened tea bag to the area. The tannic acid in tea leaves has a coagulation effect.

"Please (X) a response to indicate if you have or have not had any of the following diseases or problems: hepatitis, jaundice."

Self-Study Review

1. An INR of 5 is contraindicated in a client who requires periodontal debridement because the client is at increased risk of hemorrhage.

a. Both the statement and reason are correct and related.
b. Both the statement and reason are correct, but NOT related.
c. The statement is correct, but the reason is NOT.
d. The statement is NOT correct, but the reason is correct.
e. NEITHER the statement NOR the reason is correct.

2. The most common inherited blood disorder is:
a. hemophilia.
b. von Willebrand disease (vWD).
c. factor IX deficiency.
d. thrombocytopenia.

3. Examples of inherited coagulation disorders include all of the following EXCEPT one. Which is the EXCEPTION?
a. Thrombocytopenia
b. Hemophilia A
c. Hemophilia B
d. Factor IX deficiency

4. The normal number of platelet formation is:
a. 100,000 to 150,000 mm^3.
b. 100,000 to 300,000 mm^3.
c. 150,000 to 400,000 mm^3.
d. 150,000 to 450,000 mm^3.

5. From the following list, identify which blood studies are prolonged in hemophilia?
a. Platelet count
b. Bleeding time
c. Activated partial thromboplastin time
d. Prothrombin time
e. INR
f. PFA-100

6. The form of vWD with the least risk of hemorrhage is type:
a. 1.
b. 2.
c. 3.
d. 4.

7. Minor bleeding associated with simple dental extractions in those with vWD is best controlled by:
a. NSAIDs.
b. DDAVP.
c. Sutures.
d. Tranexamic acid.

Six forms of hepatitis have been reported in the medical literature.[2] These include hepatitis A (HAV), hepatitis B (HBV), hepatitis C (HCV), hepatitis D (HDV), hepatitis E (HEV), and non-A–E hepatitis. Hepatitis forms transmitted by the fecal–oral route (transmitted by food or fluid contaminated with feces) include hepatitis A (HAV) and hepatitis E (HEV). These forms of hepatitis do not result in a **carrier** state, so carry no risk for bloodborne transmission to the oral healthcare worker (HCW) during treatment. Bloodborne hepatitis forms include HBV, HCV, HDV, and possibly non-A–E hepatitis. This last group includes hepatitis that appears to have a viral origin but that cannot be attributed to a specific virus, the etiology is unknown.[2] HCWs are considered to be at high risk for contracting bloodborne infections, such as hepatitis and HIV, from occupational transmission when they come into direct contact with infected blood. There is little to no risk of contracting HAV, HEV, and non-A–E hepatitis.[2] The two most significant bloodborne hepatitis infections are HBV and HCV. Both are capable of developing into a carrier state.

Approximately 10% to 15% of those infected with HBV become persistently infected as carriers, and more than 85% of those infected with HCV become carriers. It appears, however, that HBV is more likely to occur than HCV.[2] HBV causes approximately 300,000 acute infections annually in the United States. Estimates of approximately one million carriers of HBV and four million carriers of HCV have been reported.[17] Chronic infection leads to liver failure and malignancy. Specific blood tests have been developed to detect both viruses in the blood-bank system, and transmission via blood transfusion is rare. A sign of hepatitis or liver damage is jaundice. This self-study will supplement information found in clinical textbooks and focus on identifying treatment modifications for oral care. This includes identifying risks for emergency situations involving uncontrolled bleeding, as well as management procedures to prevent the transmission of bloodborne disease to the patient or the clinician.

TRANSMISSION OF HEPATITIS B IN THE DENTAL OFFICE

In the past 10 years, there have been 91 cases of HCW-to-patient transmission of HBV in settings where no breaches in infection control practices could be identified and 38 cases of HCW-to-patient transmission of HCV transmission.[13]

Prevention of bloodborne disease in healthcare settings is accomplished by strict adherence to standard infection control practices. Apparently such practices were inadequate in blocking the transmission of HBV from one patient to another patient following oral surgery.[14] In 2001, a patient-to-patient transmission of HBV in a dental setting was reported. The 60-year-old patient who was not sexually active and had no risk factors for HBV was diagnosed with HBV infection. She had never received the vaccine for HBV. Her case was reported to the state health department, which follows the protocol recommended by the Centers for Disease Control and Prevention. The state health department's epidemiologic investigation found that the patient had none of the traditional risk factors for HBV, but had recently had oral surgery. An investigation of the oral surgery practice where the patient received treatment revealed that another surgical patient seen earlier on the same day was on the state's reportable disease registry for HBV. Molecular epidemiologic techniques indicated the same genetic profile between the two patients. The office followed standard infection control practices, and all staff had been vaccinated and were negative for HBV. The investigators could only speculate that a lapse in cleanup procedures occurred after treating the source patient. Perhaps contaminated blood was left on an instrument(s) despite following standard procedures. Another possibility is some areas on equipment could have been missed during cleanup, with subsequent cross-contamination. This case should raise awareness to the importance of strict compliance with standard bloodborne pathogen precautions and to the real possibility that bloodborne infection can be transmitted during oral procedures.[14]

PATHOPHYSIOLOGY OF HEPATITIS B

HBV is transmitted through injection drug use or from becoming contaminated with the body fluids of an infected person. This discussion focuses on methods of transmission that may occur in the dental office. In dentistry, this can include instrument cut injuries or needlestick injuries to the operator during treatment of an HBV carrier. Other occupational injuries capable of transmitting HBV include splashes of infected blood onto mucous membranes or broken skin. There are reports prior to 1987 of HBV being transmitted to patients from an infected HCW because of inadequate infection control procedures, such as not wearing gloves.[13] When the viral particles enter the body they deposit in the liver and begin the destruction of the hepatic cells. Signs of acute HBV infection can include fever, flulike symptoms, malaise, and fatigue. As the disease progresses and liver cells are destroyed, jaundice or yellow skin may be seen, called the "icteric stage." The majority of clients have no symptoms, a situation described as "a subclinical infection." These clients develop antibodies (anti-HBVs) that provide permanent immunity from reinfection with HBV, and the disease resolves. The presence of anti-HBVs in the serum is a marker for immunity. It occurs in clients who have had the infection resolved by the immune system, or in the client who has had the HBV vaccine series and **seroconverted**. If the infection is not cleared by the immune system, the HBV incubation period is 2 to 6 months.[15] The infected person develops serum markers that relate to the degree of infectiousness. The presence of serum HBV surface antigen (HBsAg) and hepatitis B e antigen (HBeAg) indicates the person is infectious to others.[15]

Management of Hepatitis B

The major issue related to preventing occupational transmission of hepatitis involves having the HBV vaccine series followed by serology testing to verify formation of protective antibodies. Because vaccination for HBV is strongly recommended for those involved in dentistry, it is not as significant an issue as are those bloodborne diseases that have no immunization. However, some dental HCWs who took the vaccine series did not seroconvert and developed no immunity to HBV. Some were unable to take the vaccine series for various reasons. Those HCWs are at risk for becoming infected with HBV as they have no immunity. To reduce the risk of exposing the clinician or others to the virus, recommendations include wearing personal protective equipment, following standard precautions, and ensuring the clinician does not injure himself or herself during oral healthcare procedures. If the HCW with low antibody levels (or those nonvaccinated) is exposed to blood from a client who is a carrier of HBV, there is an injectable immunoglobulin that may protect the HCW from being infected, called HBIG (hepatitis B immunoglobulin). This must be taken within a few days of exposure to HBV to provide maximum protection. The postexposure prophylaxis (PEP) for exposure to hepatitis in an HCW who did not seroconvert or who could not take the vaccine for medical reasons is included in the HIV/AIDS discussion in this chapter. Postexposure guidelines were updated December 20, 2013 and no changes were made that affect oral healthcare workers (Box 9-3).

PATHOPHYSIOLOGY OF HEPATITIS C

This form of hepatitis frequently results in the development of a carrier state. The HCW treating a carrier is at risk for HCV transmission if a needlestick or instrument injury occurs during treatment, often referred to as a percutaneous exposure. The onset of chronic HCV infection is often unnoticed as it is characterized by an absence of symptoms. Some people who develop a persistent infection carry the virus for 10 to 20 years before symptoms manifest. It is estimated that 85% of HCV infections develop a carrier state. Few people develop an acute infection. When symptoms develop, they can include abdominal discomfort, nausea, vomiting, and jaundice.[15]

Management of Hepatitis C

There is no vaccine for HCV, nor is there an immunoglobulin that confers protection if occupational exposure to the virus occurs. The PEP for exposure to HCV in the HCW is included in the HIV/AIDS discussion in this chapter.

PATHOPHYSIOLOGY OF HEPATITIS D

This form is referred to as delta hepatitis. It cannot occur unless the person is coinfected with HBV. Delta hepatitis depends on components of the HBV to be able to replicate. In the United States, most HDV infections occur in injection drug users and hemophiliacs. It can progress so that the person infected becomes a chronic carrier of both viruses. Chronic HDV infection often progresses to cirrhosis. Immunity through the HBV vaccine confers immunity to HDV.

PATHOPHYSIOLOGY OF NON-A–E HEPATITIS

The non-A–E group is a catch-all group for all the hepatitis virus conditions not in any of the other categories. It may not be attributable to a viral etiology and may be an autoimmune response. No etiology has been identified.[2]

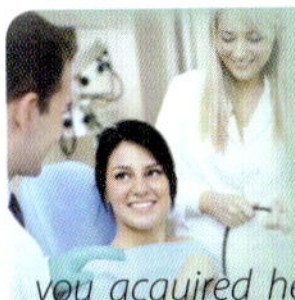

Follow-Up Questions

"What type of hepatitis did (do) you have? If unknown, do you know how you acquired hepatitis? What type of treatment did you receive and was it successful to resolve the viral infection? Have you been tested to determine if you are a carrier for any hepatitis virus? Do you have liver damage and bleeding problems? What medications do you use for pain?"

Identifying potential carriers of bloodborne infections is important in the case of an accidental exposure to the clients' blood allowing a portal of entry into the body, such as a splash or needlestick. All clients are treated as if they are infectious, but if an injury occurs and the carrier status of the client is known, time can be saved in testing for the presence of infection in the client's blood. When a history of increased bleeding as a result of liver disease is reported, the clinician must evaluate the level of risk for uncontrolled bleeding during treatments involving bleeding. The liver is the main organ responsible for drug metabolism. To prevent a drug interaction or adverse effect, it is helpful to know what medications the client has taken with success. This reduces the risk of recommending a product that may result in further damage to the compromised liver.

Self-Study Review

8. Identify the types of hepatitis that do not carry a risk to the oral healthcare clinician during treatment.
   a. HAV
   b. HBV
   c. HCV
   d. HDV
   e. HEV
9. The hepatitis virus that is dependent on HBV to replicate is:
   a. HCV.
   b. HDV.
   c. HAV.
   d. non-A–E.
10. Which of the following forms of hepatitis pose the greatest risk for occupational exposure?

a. HCV
b. HAV
c. HEV
d. HDV

11. Jaundice is a sign of which stage of hepatitis?
    a. Subclinical
    b. Acute
    c. Icteric
    d. Chronic

12. The presence of which serum markers indicates a person is infectious?
    a. HBsAg and HBcAg
    b. HBsAg and HBeAg
    c. HBbAg and HBcAg
    d. HBbAg and HBeAg

Box 9-3

Resources for Bloodborne Pathogen Standards

CDC: CDC Guidance for Evaluating Health-Care Personnel for Hepatitis B Virus Protection and Postexposure Management 2013. MMWR 62 (RR10).

OSHA: www.osha.gov/SLTC/dentistry?control.html OSHA: www.osha.gov?OshDoc/toc_fact.html HIVDENT: www.hivdent.org

National Clinician's Postexposure Prophylaxis

Hotline: http://www.nccc.ucsf.edu/about_nccc/pepline

"Please (X) a response to indicate if you have or have not had any of the following diseases or problems: AIDS or HIV infection."

According to the newest estimates new HIV infections in the United States reached 56,300 in 2006, about 40% more than the previous estimate of 40,000 annual infections.[16] More than one million individuals aged 13 years and over are living with HIV/AIDS in the United States, with the largest number of HIV/AIDS cases occurring among men who have sex with men (53%) and black individuals (45%).[16]

The disease has affected the practice of dentistry more than any other single infectious disease. Although there is no cure for the viral infection, many new drugs have been developed that suppress the viral replication and improve life expectancy for those infected.[17]

In an attempt to reduce transmission in the dental office, the U.S. Centers for Disease Control and Prevention (CDC) introduced the concept of standard precautions. Standard precautions mean that all clients are treated as if they were infected with a bloodborne disease. The Occupational Safety and Health Administration (OSHA) is the governmental agency that regulates all healthcare facilities to ensure employee safety. It administers the OSHA Bloodborne Pathogen Standard and requires employers to enforce safe work-related practices and to provide personal protective equipment and vaccines. The development of serology tests to identify antibodies to HIV has produced a relatively safe national blood supply system of donated blood. Web-based resources for bloodborne pathogen standards are given in Box 9-3.

PATHOPHYSIOLOGY DISCUSSION OF AIDS AND HIV INFECTION

HIV (also referred to as HIV-1 virus)[15] is transmitted through body fluids, such as blood products. Routes of transmission that are possible in the dental office include puncture wounds with contaminated needles and contact with infected blood products from splashes or spatter onto mucous membranes. When the virus enters the blood, it infects specific cells, such as monocytes, macrophages, and T-helper lymphocytes with CD4 receptors.[15] HIV uses the DNA and RNA in the lymphocyte to reproduce itself. Once the viral DNA enters the host nucleus, infection is established and **progeny** of the host cell are HIV-1 infected. At some point, the viral copies break out of the lymphocyte and infect other cells. Eventually the virus reduces the numbers of protective lymphocytes, resulting in immune suppression. When specific immune-related disease conditions occur, the HIV infection status enters a stage called acquired immune deficiency syndrome (AIDS). An AIDS diagnosis is made when the person develops life-threatening malignancies and opportunistic infections, and CD4 levels are less than 200 cells/mm^3.[15]

Early symptoms include a flulike illness, but some infected persons have no early symptoms.

After several weeks to months, the infected person develops antibodies to the virus and is described as being HIV positive or having HIV disease (HIVD). Laboratory tests to diagnose HIV infection include a screening test (enzyme-linked immunosorbent assay [ELISA]) and, if this test is positive, a verification test, called the Western blot. The infected person can transmit the virus to others exposed to his or her body fluids. In dentistry, this can occur from spatters or splashes of infected blood to the eyes, nose, or mouth and through needlestick or other percutaneous injuries.

Oral Manifestations of AIDS and HIV Infection

Oral manifestations of HIVD are key indicators of disease progression and are associated with CD4 counts less than 200 cells/mm^3 and a viral load greater than 3,000 copies/mL.[18] There are a variety of potential oral conditions associated with an HIV status. These include candidiasis, hairy leukoplakia, a rapidly progressive form of periodontal disease, linear gingival erythema, necrotizing ulcerative periodontitis, aphthous ulcerations, wart-like lesions, and a malignancy of blood vessels, called Kaposi sarcoma. When the immune system is significantly suppressed, some clients develop a widespread form of candidiasis, called oropharyngeal candidiasis (Fig. 9.3). Symptoms include burning mucosa, taste disturbances, pain, and difficulty in eating. Candidiasis is treated with antifungal medications. Antiviral medications can provide temporary regression of the lesions associated with HIVD. These opportunistic infections and malignancies are rarely seen in the client with a healthy immune system.

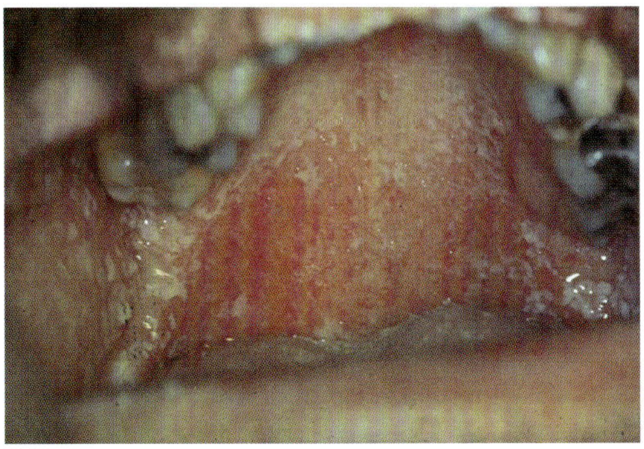

Figure 9.3 ■ Clinical photograph of oropharyngeal candidiasis.

Clinical Implications of AIDS and HIV Infection

The main oral care consideration for a client with a medical history of AIDS or HIV status (other than occupational transmission from infected blood) is to prevent infection in the oral cavity. These clients are at high risk for having postoperative oral infection after oral surgery or periodontal scaling. Clinicians should prescribe antibiotic prophylaxis for clients with HIVD who are severely neutropenic (500 polymorphonuclear neutrophils/mm^3), and elective dental procedures are contraindicated in those with a neutrophil count of less than 500 cells/mm^3.[12] However, prophylactic antibiotics are not recommended unless severe neutropenia exists. A recent study investigating oral complications following various oral procedures (both surgery and nonsurgical procedures) in the HIV-positive individual found a low complication rate, although the presence of oral lesions, smoking habit, or HIV stage B status may be predictive factors of oral complications in HIVD.[18]

Clients with HIV infection are treated no differently than clients without HIV in the dental office and personal protective equipment (mask, gloves, protective glasses) is used as a part of standard procedures.[19] Home care instruction should include the role of bacterial plaque in periodontal infection and nontraumatic plaque removal techniques. An antimicrobial mouthrinse can be recommended for daily use.

Medication Effects

The client with a history of AIDS or HIVD may be taking as many as six or seven different drugs (or more) on a regular basis. These drugs are used to manage the HIV infection, the opportunistic infections seen as part of the syndrome, and the effects of the disease (nausea, wasting syndrome). The current multiple-drug combination therapy can cause adverse side effects and drug interactions. Topical medications for candidiasis (such as nystatin) often contain sugar to disguise the unpleasant taste and must be used several times a day. This can lead to development of caries in the caries-prone individual, suggesting a need to use home fluoride products daily. Drugs used in dentistry that interact with antiviral HIV therapy include sedative agents (midazolam [Versed®], triazolam [Halcion®]) and analgesics (meperidine [Demerol®] and propoxyphene [Darvon®]).[12] Side effects that can require modification of the treatment plan include

GI symptoms (nausea, vomiting) and hyperglycemia. GI symptoms may require using a semisupine chair position. Blood sugar levels greater than 200 mg/dL may result in poor response to treatment and increased infection after therapy.[12] Medications taken may cause blood dyscrasias, resulting in bleeding and increased infection. Other toxicities involve the cardiovascular system, so vital signs should be monitored at each appointment.[12] HIV infection cannot be cured and is managed with antiviral drugs for the life of the client. All medications reported should be investigated in a suitable drug reference before any oral health care is provided.

Barrier Protection

Standard precautions require that all equipment used as part of oral healthcare delivery is covered with disposable barriers and disinfected with a tuberculocidal-quality disinfectant solution as part of normal delivery of services. The HCW must wear a mask, gloves, and protective glasses to provide a barrier against infectious bloodborne microorganisms. All nondisposable instruments are sterilized, and the sterilizing equipment is monitored for biologic effectiveness on a regular basis. Blood-soaked gauze must be placed in a red biohazard bag and disposed of in a designated area separate from regular waste products. If local anesthesia is used, the needle should not be recapped by hand and must be disposed of in a red sharps container. There is a risk of occupational exposure to the virus through needlesticks or percutaneous injuries. Settings where dental treatment is provided are now required to have a designated infection control officer. This person directs the procedure to follow when mercury spills occur in the office or if the HCW is exposed to percutaneous injuries or splashes.

An exposure that might place the HCW at risk for HIV infection is defined as a percutaneous injury (e.g., a needlestick or cut with a sharp object) or contact of mucous membrane or nonintact skin (e.g., exposed skin that is chapped, abraded, or afflicted with dermatitis) with blood, tissue, or other body fluids that are potentially infectious.[19] Saliva and sputum are not considered potentially infectious unless they are visibly bloody and the risk for HIV transmission from these fluids is low.[19]

For human bites, clinical evaluation must include the possibility that both the person bitten and the person who inflicted the bite were exposed to bloodborne pathogens, although transmission by this route has been reported rarely and no occupational exposures have been reported.

Occupational Exposure Recommendations

The U.S. Public Health Service guidelines for management of occupational exposures to HIV and recommendations for PEP were updated in 2013.[19] The principles of exposure management were not changed from the earlier 2005 guidelines, but recommendations regarding HIV PEP were updated to include additional pharmacologic therapies. It was emphasized for HCW (including those involved in dental care) to adhere to HIV PEP when it is indicated for an exposure, to consult with a medical expert regarding management of exposures (or to determine if an exposure has actually occurred), to follow-up exposed workers regarding adherence to PEP, and to monitor adverse events, including seroconversion. Timely postexposure management and initiation of HIV PEP should be considered as urgent medical concerns. If occupational exposure to blood occurs and the source exposure client has reported an infection with any infectious bloodborne microorganism (HIV, HBV, HCV, etc.), or subsequent testing reveals the source client has an infectious bloodborne infection, the occupational blood exposure should include the following[20]:

- Provide immediate care to the exposure site by washing the wound and skin with soap and water.
- Determine the risk associated with the exposure by considering the type of fluid involved (blood, bloody fluid, other potentially infectious fluid containing concentrated viral particles) and type of exposure (percutaneous injury, bite resulting in blood exposure, splash or spatter to mucous membranes).
- Evaluate exposure source by medical history or by blood testing for bloodborne pathogens (HIV antibody, HBV, HCV) using a rapid HIV antibody testing method. A new test was recently approved by the FDA (OraQuick Advance HIV1-2 Antibody Test) for use with oral fluids and preliminary HIV results can now be obtained in 20 minutes.
- Initiate PEP as soon as possible (within hours) and do not delay while determining the infection status of the source. The severity of the wound should be considered (superficial injury is less severe and injury with a large-bore hollow needle or deep puncture wound with visible

blood is most severe). PEP should include 3 or more antiretroviral drugs. The drug regimen should be taken for 4 weeks. The HCW should be monitored for drug toxicity at baseline and after 2 weeks of starting PEP. There are reports of HCWs with needlestick injuries who developed HIV infection after a needlestick injury while treating an HIV-infected client, and who took combination drug therapy as described earlier.[20]

- Perform follow-up testing and provide counseling within 72 hours to include advising exposed HCW to seek medical evaluation for any acute illness occurring during follow-up. This should be done regardless of whether the exposed HCW received PEP.[19]
- Perform HIV-antibody testing for at least 4 months after exposure (e.g., at baseline, 6 weeks, and 4 months), and if illness that is compatible with an acute retroviral syndrome occurs, initiate antiretroviral drug therapy. For HCW who are infected with HCV after exposure to a source coinfected with HIV and HCV follow-up is extended to 12 months.[19]
- Advise exposed persons to use precautions to prevent secondary transmission during the follow-up period.
- Evaluate exposed persons taking PEP within 72 hours after exposure; monitor for adverse reactions from drug regimen for at least 2 weeks.[19,21]

Although recommendations for follow-up testing, monitoring, and counseling of exposed HCW are unchanged from those published previously,[22] greater emphasis is needed on improving follow-up care provided to exposed HCW to increase adherence to HIV PEP regimens and to provide alternate therapy when adverse effects are untolerable.

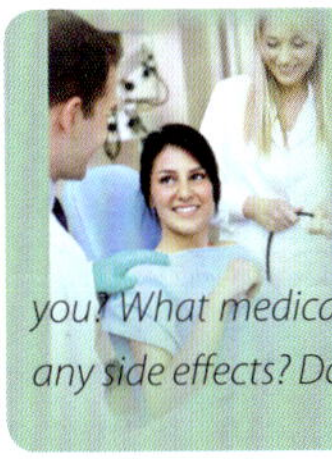

Follow-Up Questions

"When was your last complete blood count and do you have the results with you? What medications are you taking and have you had any side effects? Do you bleed a long time following a cut?"

A systematic review of risks for complications for HIV-positive patients undergoing invasive dental procedures concluded that no studies involving periodontal therapy, oral prophylaxis, or scaling and root planning were found. It was determined that the risk for complications from these procedures was low in the client with HIVD.[21] With the exception of bleeding disorders, no special precautions are necessary. For the client with HIVD who has an absolute neutrophil count of less than 500 cell/mm^3, antibiotic prophylaxis is recommended.[12] Current drug therapy can bring the viral load to very low levels. Viral load is monitored to determine the effectiveness of the drug therapy and to detect development of resistance to antiviral agents. For the investigation of drugs taken for HIV therapy, each side effect experienced is managed according to the problem caused. Blood dyscrasias can occur, and bleeding must be monitored during treatment. For medications with sugar that are administered to be swished in the mouth several times daily, recommend a home-based daily fluoride regimen. The client must be told to contact the dental office if increased pain, poor healing, or development of acute dental infection occurs following oral care.

Application to Practice

The USPHS recommendations for PEP described earlier should be followed. Clinicians must use standard precautions and personal protective equipment to reduce exposure to bloodborne pathogens. The risk for transmission is reduced when percutaneous injuries involve only small amounts of blood.

The use of the source person's viral load as a measure of viral titer for assessing transmission risk has not been established. Although a lower viral load (or one that is below the limits of detection) probably indicates a lower titer exposure, it does not rule out the possibility of transmission. If an HCW is exposed to contaminated blood as a result of a break in gloves or a needlestick or instrument injury, the incident must be recorded in an occupational exposure report (Box 9-4).

POTENTIAL EMERGENCIES

The most relevant emergency to discuss is one related to protection of oral HCWs from transmission of bloodborne pathogens. The HCW in the dental facility who gets a needlestick or who gets cut with a blood-contaminated instrument is at risk for occupational exposure to bloodborne pathogens.

- Prevention: Standard precautions and the wearing of personal protective equipment is a method to protect the oral HCW from occupational exposure to disease during treatment. Methods of protection during equipment

Box 9-4

The Occupational Exposure Report

- Date and time of exposure
- Details of procedure being performed, where and how the exposure occurred, and when in the course of handling the device the exposure occurred
- Details of the exposure, including the type and amount of fluid or blood and the severity of the exposure (for a needlestick: depth of injury, whether fluid was injected; for instrument cut: the estimated volume of blood contacting the skin and the condition of the skin [intact, chapped, abraded])
- Details about the exposure source (HIV-infected: stage of disease, history of antiretroviral therapy, viral load, antiretroviral resistance information)
- Details about the exposed HCW (e.g., HBV vaccine series and postvaccine response status)
- Details about counseling, postexposure management, and follow-up

(Adapted from Kuhar DT, Henderson DK, Struble KA et al. Updated U.S. Public Health Service guidelines for the management of occupational exposures to human immunodeficiency virus and recommendations for postexposure prophylaxis. Infect Control Hosp Epidemiol 2013;34(9):875-892.)

cleaning and disinfection include wearing thick utility gloves, placing instruments in covered trays to prevent sharp points from causing operator injury, and cleaning instruments within trays in an ultrasonic cleaner. The operator should consciously avoid inflicting personal injury from puncture wounds during oral healthcare procedures.

- Management: It is well known that clients with one bloodborne disease are at an increased risk for other bloodborne infections. It is important to know the serology status of the client in terms of what infections were identified in the completed blood tests. A physician consultation is recommended to obtain accurate information. PEP should be instituted quickly (within hours) and not delayed until after determination of serology testing of the source patient.

Self-Study Review

13. Identify which of the following exposures places the HCW at risk for HIV infection.
    a. Needlesticks
    b. Contact of mucous membrane with blood
    c. Bloody saliva
    d. Mercury spills
14. Of the following list, which medications used in dentistry interact with antiviral HIV therapy?
    a. Sedative agents
    b. Antidepressants
    c. Muscle relaxants
    d. Analgesics
15. The governmental agency that regulates all healthcare facilities to ensure employee safety is:
    a. OSAP.
    b. OSHA.
    c. CDC.
    d. CDCP.
16. Antibiotic prophylaxis is recommended for the client with HIVD who has an absolute neutrophil count of:
    a. <500 cells/mm^3.
    b. <750 cells/mm^3.
    c. $<1,000$ cells/mm^3.
    d. $<2,000$ cells/mm^3.
17. Postexposure HIV antibody testing should occur for:
    a. 6 weeks.
    b. 3 months.
    c. 4 months.
    d. 1 year.

"Please (X) a response to indicate if you have or have not had any of the following diseases or problems: sexually transmitted diseases."

Sexually transmitted diseases (STDs) and sexually transmitted infections (STIs) can include a wide variety of diseases, both bacterial (syphilis, gonorrhea) and viral (genital herpes). STIs are differentiated from STDs in that an STD is an infection that can be transmitted during symptomatic periods whereas an STI is an infection that can be transmitted when there are no symptoms.[23] The infections listed are transmitted in the general population through direct sexual contact and are not bloodborne diseases. The discussion of STDs is included in this chapter because other bloodborne disease conditions have a relationship to sexual transmission. This discussion will focus on the clinical relevance regarding HCW protection for clients who respond positively with this item on the health history. A key principal to remember is that an individual is just as likely to acquire an STI from someone with no presenting symptoms, as from someone with symptoms. Standard precautions greatly minimize this risk during oral care.

PATHOPHYSIOLOGY OF SEXUALLY TRANSMITTED DISEASES

Pathophysiology of the specific STD is specific to the infecting microorganism. STD lesions may contain the contagious microorganism. Transmission occurs if the operator's glove barrier becomes compromised or infectious fluids are splashed onto the operator's mucous membranes (eyes, nose, mouth). Locations of infectious lesions from STDs can include the oral or genital mucosa. Oral manifestations appear clinically different depending on the infecting microorganism, ranging from ulcerations to papillary growths.

Syphilis is caused by direct contact with the spirochete, *Treponema pallidum.*[24] Following a low incidence of syphilis in the United States for the last two decades, rates are now increasing, primarily in men.[25] In this report, the increase was attributed primarily in men who have sex with men accounting for more than 60% of new cases and are often associated with HIV coinfection and high-risk sexual behavior. Unlike other sexually transmitted diseases (e.g., HIVD) the spirochete that causes syphilis is readily transmissible by oral sex, kissing at or near an infectious lesion, and vaginal or anal intercourse, with the primary lesion described as a *chancre.*[24] The majority of extragenital chancres occur in the mouth (40% to 79%). The second most common mode of transmission is *in utero* or at delivery if the newborn comes into contact with a contagious lesion. Nonsexual cutaneous transmission has been reported among HCWs and laboratory personnel whose unprotected hands have contacted the infectious agent.[26] Once acquired, syphilis can pass through four distinct stages of disease: primary syphilis, secondary syphilis, latent syphilis, and tertiary syphilis, with each stage characterized by different symptoms and levels of infectivity.[24] Only the tertiary stage of syphilis is considered to be noninfectious. Diagnosis is made primarily by serologic assays (e.g., venereal disease research laboratory [VDRL] and the rapid plasma reagin assay). Penicillin, administered by injection, is the treatment of choice. For individuals with a penicillin allergy, the drug of choice is oral doxycycline.[27] Tests are available to evaluate serological response and the results should be obtained prior to intraoral procedures. The same barrier personal protection practices are recommended (mask, gloves, and glasses) to reduce the risk of disease transmission, although aerosolized microorganisms are possible when an infectious chancre is present.

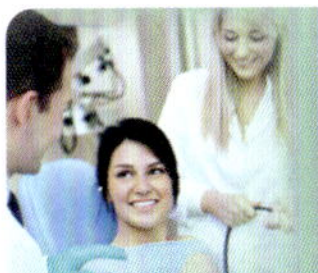

Follow-Up Questions

"What type of STD did you have? How long ago were you diagnosed? Have you been treated and has the infection been resolved? Do you have ulcers or lesions in your mouth?"

Application to Practice

Treatment decisions in the client who reports a history of sexually transmitted disease is to determine whether the infection has been cured, is not infectious, and is not capable of transmitting the disease to the HCW. If medical treatment resolved the disease, serology tests indicate noninfectivity, and no infectious oral lesions are present, there is no risk for disease transmission. Oral ulcerations that represent signs of the disease can include microorganisms that are infectious. For clients with oral lesions who are currently receiving medical treatment, the appointment should be rescheduled until successful treatment has eliminated the microorganism and the lesions have resolved. Medical consultation should be completed before rescheduling for oral health care to verify that the disease was resolved with treatment.

"Please (X) a response to indicate if you have or have not had any of the following diseases or problems: anemia."

Another disease involving blood components is a disease of the red blood cell (RBC) or a reduction of essential components in the RBC. There are different types of anemia, and the specific type must be identified to determine the treatment recommendations. In general, symptoms of anemia include fatigue, palpitations, shortness of breath, abdominal pain, bone pain, tingling of fingers, and muscle weakness.[2]

Signs include jaundice, pallor, splitting of the fingernails, liver and spleen enlargement, lymphadenopathy, and blood in the stool.[2] Oral signs include a smooth, painful red tongue.

PATHOPHYSIOLOGY DISCUSSION OF ANEMIA

Anemia is defined as a blood disorder characterized by a decrease in hemoglobin or hemoglobin function. This generally results from a decrease in the number of RBCs that carry hemoglobin to body tissues, although there are other conditions that can result in anemia. Hemoglobin carries oxygen to cells and is necessary for wound healing. Therefore, poor oxygenation of the wound results in reduced healing of body tissues. Reduced healing after oral healthcare procedures that produce a wound is the main factor that affects oral healthcare considerations. There are several types of anemia. Among these are

1. Iron-deficiency anemia
2. Pernicious anemia
3. Inherited anemias (such as sickle cell anemia or thalassemia)
4. Secondary anemia from blood loss (bleeding ulcers, leukemia, excessive menstruation)
5. Conditions requiring increased metabolic need for iron, such as pregnancy and lactation

All are caused by different factors, but they result in the same clinical consideration of reduced healing. Not all anemias will be discussed; however, the more common anemia-related conditions and the indications for dental management will be included. The reader is encouraged to refer to more comprehensive texts for anemias not included in this discussion.

Iron-Deficiency Anemia

This condition results from increased blood loss, usually from heavy menstrual flow or from GI bleeding as a result of ulceration. Another etiologic factor for iron-deficiency anemia is reduced absorption of iron from the diet because of a malabsorption problem. Iron-deficiency anemia is reported to occur during pregnancy and lactation as a result of increased dietary iron requirements. Laboratory tests reveal a hypochromic, microcytic type of RBC.

Pernicious Anemia

This form of anemia results when there is a lack of intrinsic factor in the stomach. Intrinsic factor is required for vitamin B_{12} absorption. This nutrient is needed for the maturation of RBCs in bone marrow. Pernicious anemia occurs more commonly in people aged 40 to 70 years. Early symptoms that might be detected as part of oral healthcare treatment include weakness, tingling in the fingers (paresthesia), and muscular weakness leading to ineffective use of a toothbrush and other oral physiotherapy devices. Medical treatment includes regular injections of vitamin B_{12}.

Sickle Cell Anemia

This condition is an inherited defect of the sickle cell trait causing the RBC to be deformed. This leads to a defect in the hemoglobin within the cell. It is described as an autosomal recessive trait disorder having a mild form with no symptoms (sickle cell trait) and affecting about 10% of carriers and a more severe form (sickle cell disease) affecting up to 98% of carriers.[28] African-Americans or Negroid populations are mainly affected. The RBC becomes sickle-shaped when low blood oxygen levels occur, if dehydration occurs, or when the pH of blood is reduced.[2] The result is stagnation of blood within blood vessels, increased blood viscosity, hypoxia, and intravascular occlusion leading to organ failure and stroke. The clinical signs of sickle cell disease are caused by hemolysis of the RBC producing a variety of symptoms, such as facial pallor, musculoskeletal pain, and jaundice. Infection is common, and prophylactic penicillin is often prescribed for children with the condition.[2] It is unlikely that a client experiencing a sickle cell crisis will come for oral healthcare treatment as this condition has severe symptoms (pain, infection, fever) that would preclude a visit to a dental facility.

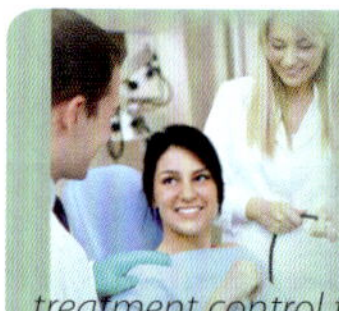

Follow-Up Questions

"What type of anemia do you have? Are you being treated and does the treatment control the condition? Has your physician given you any warnings regarding medical or dental treatment, or drugs to avoid? Do you have slow healing problems?"

The decision to proceed with oral healthcare procedures in the client with anemia involves determining whether the disease is controlled. When medications control the signs and symptoms of the disease, treatment is not contraindicated. Those clients with severe forms of anemia will be under current medical care to maintain life. Physician referral to assess disease control is required. Physician warnings to the client must be considered and followed up with medical consultation if the HCW has questions about medical warnings. Healing must be monitored after treatment procedures that produce a wound.

Application to Practice

Dental management of the client with anemia might include frequent, short appointments to identify infection or poor healing responses early and to reduce stress. Effective plaque control may prevent oral infection. Use of low concentrations of epinephrine in local anesthetics (LA; 1:100,000) or using an LA without vasoconstrictor will reduce blood stagnation. Acetaminophen (APAP) or opioid/APAP combinations for oral pain are recommended. If sedation is needed, it can be accomplished with diazepam or nitrous oxide with oxygen levels greater than 50% using a high flow rate.[2] Clients with unstable anemia must have a medical consultation before surgery or extensive dental treatment. The medical consultation should include blood counts and platelet counts. Low platelet counts may require management to reduce the risk of increased bleeding episodes. Blood transfusion may be necessary before surgery. Oral infection must be treated early and aggressively with antibiotics.

Sickle Cell Management

There are special dental management considerations for sickle cell anemia (SCA). Oral health care should be completed in a noncrisis period of the disease with attention to avoiding long appointments because of the risk of intravascular stagnation of blood. Oral infection can precipitate a crisis, so prevention of oral disease is essential. Local anesthetics that contain low doses of vasoconstrictors are recommended to avoid intravascular occlusion of RBCs.

POTENTIAL EMERGENCIES

These are variable depending on the cause of anemia. In the client with SCA, the greatest emergency is related to an exacerbation of sickle cell crisis during treatment.

Prevention

Prevention relies on assessing the degree of disease control that exists. For those clients with SCA, a physician consultation to determine disease control is recommended. For other anemias, the client should be questioned about problems related to infection, healing, and disease effects. The clinician would examine the client for extraoral signs of uncontrolled anemia, such as facial pallor, fatigue, muscle weakness, and shortness of breath. Short appointments and a stress reduction protocol may be considered in anxious clients.

Management

Because infection and poor wound healing may result after oral treatment in the anemic client, management procedures involve using nontraumatic instrumentation methods. Oral infections should be treated early and aggressively with antibiotics. Medical consultation to guide treatment of oral infection may be required in poorly controlled disease.

"Please (X) a response to indicate if you have or have not had any of the following diseases or problems: Blood transfusion (date)."

A question on blood transfusion with the transfusion date could relate to a client having bleeding disorders, experiencing an injury resulting in excessive blood loss, or other reasons, such as transfusion during hospitalization. Blood transfusion was formerly a risk factor for transmitting bloodborne diseases. Many hemophiliacs acquired HIV infection as a result of receiving infected blood products before the identification of the screening blood test for HIV. The date gives the clinician an idea of the time interval since the transfusion. If the client requires frequent blood transfusions this indicates an increased risk for bleeding during oral health care. If a client reports a single blood transfusion several years in the past, with no complications and no development of bloodborne disease, there generally is no need for follow-up. The main concerns with a blood transfusion, therefore, relate to determining the cause for the transfusion, the risk for an increased bleeding tendency during treatment, and the issue related to contracting a potentially transmissible bloodborne disease with an occupational risk to the clinician should a percutaneous injury or splash accident occur.

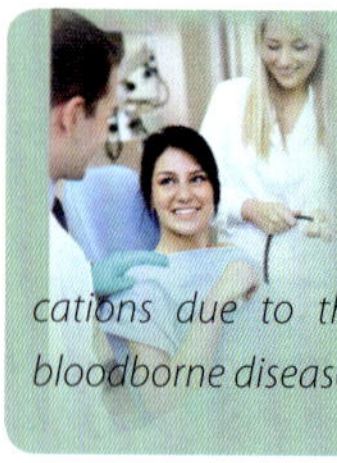

Follow-Up Questions

"Why did you need to have a blood transfusion? Have you had any complications due to the transfusion? Were you tested for bloodborne disease following the transfusion?"

The clinical protocol would be determined on the basis of the response to the follow-up questions and will relate to any complication reported. For example, if the transfusions are necessary to control a blood disease, the risk for bleeding must be determined. Another consideration is in cases in which bloodborne hepatitis has occurred, the reader should refer to the discussion of hepatitis; if HIV transmission has occurred, the reader is referred to that section.

Application to Practice

The clinician should focus on the reason for the blood transfusion for guidance on planning care. Bleeding disorders can result in excessive bleeding and are discussed at the beginning of this chapter.

Self-Study Review

18. Oral ulcerations associated with STD are infectious. Dental hygiene treatment can be performed as long as barrier personal protection is used.
- a. Both statements are true.
- b. Both statements are false.
- c. The first statement is true, and the second statement is false.
- d. The first statement is false, and the second statement is true.

19. What anemia represents an inherited defect of red blood cell anatomy and a defect in the hemoglobin within the cell?
- a. Iron-deficiency anemia
- b. Sickle cell anemia
- c. Pernicious anemia
- d. Thalassemia

20. The decision to proceed with oral healthcare procedures in a client with anemia involves:
- a. determining whether the disease is controlled.
- b. prescribing prophylactic antibiotics.
- c. using stress reduction strategies.
- d. providing education about plaque control to prevent oral infection.

21. All of the following represent a primary concern relative to a client who presents with a history of blood transfusion EXCEPT one. Which one is the EXCEPTION?
- a. The cause of the transfusion
- b. The risk for increased bleeding during treatment
- c. Potential for contracting a transmissible bloodborne disease
- d. The risk of poor wound healing

CHAPTER SUMMARY

This chapter provided a review of conditions that can be associated with abnormal bleeding during and after dental and dental hygiene procedures. Diseases associated with risks for occupational exposure and prevention strategies were discussed. Understanding the significance of follow-up questions related to specific systemic diseases is important to effectively prevent and manage emergency situations during oral health care.

Review

1. Define the following terms: idiopathic, petechiae, ecchymosis, and seroconvert.
2. List the four major causes of abnormal bleeding.
3. Identify the major components of an occupational exposure report.
4. List the follow-up questions that should be asked of the client with a history of a blood transfusion.

Case Study

Case A

Alfred Bridgewater presents with a history of thrombophlebitis that occurred 6 months ago. He reports using Coumadin daily, and a recent Doppler study was negative for recurring deep vein thrombosis. His vital signs are pulse 70 bpm, respiration 14 breaths/min, blood pressure 130/70 mm Hg, left arm, sitting.

1. What is the function of Coumadin?
2. List three other conditions for which Coumadin is prescribed.
3. Which blood tests are used to measure anticoagulation in clients taking Coumadin?
4. If the client required a tooth extraction, what preventive measures should be taken to avoid a medical emergency?
5. After extraction, the client appears to have excessive bleeding. What strategies can be used to manage this event?

Case B

Krystal Jordan, a 19-year-old African-American client, presents for an oral prophylaxis. She reports a history of SCA. The client has been under the care of her family practitioner and states that her condition is stable. Her vital signs are pulse 65 bpm, respiration 15 breaths/min, blood pressure 100/60 mm Hg, right arm, sitting.

1. What type of preliminary questions would you ask this client before offering treatment?
2. What symptoms would you expect to see in this client if she had uncontrolled anemia?
3. List four strategies that the clinician should use in treating this client.

Chapter Ten

Medical Conditions Involving Immunosuppression

Objectives

After completing the self-study chapter the reader will be able to:

- Identify treatment modifications for providing oral health care to clients undergoing cancer, chemotherapy, or radiation treatments.
- Specify disease conditions or drug therapies that predispose the client to immunosuppression and list treatment modifications for this situation.
- Describe the signs of uncontrolled diabetes and the treatment plan modifications for the client with diabetes.
- Describe the treatment modifications for the client with inflammatory autoimmune diseases, including systemic lupus erythematosus (SLE) and rheumatoid arthritis (RA).
- Identify disease conditions that involve persistent swollen glands, unexpected weight loss, and oral ulcerative disease and describe treatment modifications for these situations.

Key Terms

Benign: noncancerous, will not move from local area of the body

Hyperglycemia: abnormally high levels of glucose in the blood

Hypoglycemia: abnormally low levels of glucose in the blood, usually caused by taking too much insulin

Insulin resistance: the condition in which insulin receptors will not bind with insulin and hyperglycemia results because blood glucose cannot enter the cells

Ketoacidosis: high acidic pH of tissues accompanied by increased ketones in body resulting from inappropriate protein metabolism

Malignant: abnormal cells capable of invading tissue and causing death

Mucositis: inflammation of a mucous membrane, often manifesting as an ulceration

Osteoradionecrosis: the destruction and death of bone tissue from radiation therapy

Palliative: therapy designed to soothe or relieve uncomfortable symptoms, not a cure

Pathology: the study of disease

Stomatotoxic: chemotherapy that causes injury to oral mucosal cells

Trismus: a prolonged spasm of muscles of the jaw area

Xerostomia: loss of salivation, dry mouth

MEDICAL CONDITION

INTRODUCTION

The conditions grouped in this section deal with diseases that affect the host immune system. These include drug-induced or radiation-induced immunosuppression and conditions that cause depression of immune activity (diabetes, SLE). Clinical signs of problems when immunologically related conditions are present include enlarged lymph nodes and oral ulcerations, so they are included in the chapter. Weight loss can occur as a result of effects of the disease and can also reduce the function of the host response. These conditions will be discussed according to the most common causes of the immune system response.

"Please (X) a response to indicate if you have or have not had any of the following diseases or problems: cancer/chemotherapy/radiation treatment, drug, or radiation-induced immunosuppression."

PATHOPHYSIOLOGY OF MALIGNANCY

Cancer research has revealed that the majority of malignancies develop as a result of genetic cellular mutations that lead to abnormal activation of cell growth and mitosis. A variety of chemical, physical, or biologic factors increase the probability of mutation. These contributing factors include:

1. Ionizing radiation, such as diagnostic X-rays or ultraviolet light.
2. Chemical substances, such as those found in cigarette smoke.
3. Chronic physical irritants.
4. Hereditary tendency, such as inheriting the *HER2* gene for breast cancer.
5. Viruses, such as Epstein-Barr (lymphoma) and human papilloma virus (cervical cancer, oral cancer).

The main difference between the normal cell and a **malignant** cell of the same tissue is that the cancer cell continues to grow and does not have a natural cycle leading to death. Furthermore, most malignant cells do not remain in the local tissue area but travel to other body sites, a process called metastasis. A **benign** tumor commonly grows within a local area and does not invade surrounding tissue or spread through the body. Malignant cells travel through both the lymphatic and circulatory systems. Some cancers have the ability to cause new blood vessels to grow into the tumor and supply the nutrition needed for cellular growth. Because cancer cells proliferate indefinitely, they compete with normal cells for nutrients. In addition, they often replace cells responsible for normal function, causing normal body functions to cease. A good example is a malignancy of breast tissue that metastasizes to the liver, replaces normally functioning liver cells, and causes liver function to be impaired or to stop completely. Risk factors for developing malignancies include:

1. Hereditary predisposition.
2. Advancing age.
3. Environmental factors, such as occupations that require an increased amount of skin exposure to sun or ultraviolet light.
4. Working in an industry that includes carcinogenic substances such as asbestos.
5. Frequent exposure to contributing factors for malignancy, such as tobacco smoke, alcohol, and pesticides.

CANCER TREATMENTS

The use of drugs to kill or suppress cancer cells is called chemotherapy. Other common treatments include surgical removal of the malignant tissue, immunotherapy to stimulate the host immune response, and radiation to kill malignant cells.

Chemotherapy

Chemotherapeutic drugs work within different areas of the cell cycle to kill the malignant cells. Rapidly dividing cells are most sensitive to these drugs.

They often affect both normal cells and malignant cells. It is not uncommon for rapidly dividing *normal* cells of the gastrointestinal (GI) tract and oral mucosa to be affected, resulting in painful ulcerations, called **mucositis**. Other side effects from cancer chemotherapy drugs include fungal infections (candidiasis) and bacterial infection in the oral cavity, exacerbation of herpetic viral lesions, a transient loss of taste, **xerostomia**, and nausea and vomiting. Fungal and viral infections add to the oral discomfort. The mouth can become so painful that it is difficult to eat. These factors can adversely affect basic nutrition requirements. **Palliative** agents intended to relieve discomfort include products to coat the ulcerations and oral rinse mixtures that must be mixed by a pharmacist. These may include over-the-counter (OTC) agents, compounded oral solutions containing one teaspoon each of Maalox®, alcohol-free Benadryl® elixir, and viscous lidocaine (Miracle Mix, prescription required for this product which is compounded by the pharmacist), and frequent use of warm baking soda and salt water rinses (1/2 teaspoon of baking soda, 1/2 teaspoon of salt in one cup of warm water). Antifungal agents, such as nystatin or posaconazole (Noxafil®) suspension, may be used as a rinse, Mycelex® troches (lozenge that slowly dissolves in the mouth), or oral systemic antifungal medications are used to manage fungal infections. There are a wide variety of chemotherapeutic drugs, and each drug has side effects. These occur as a result of suppression of bone marrow activity and include leukopenia, thrombocytopenia, and other blood dyscrasias.

Radiation Therapy

Radiation is used after surgical removal of a tumor or when surgery is not an option to remove a malignancy. Radiation destroys the ability of cells to divide. Certain cancer cells are susceptible to radiation; however, normal cells are also affected. Radiation therapy is delivered to a planned treatment field at each appointment, with treatments given at various times, for example, daily or weekly up to 7 weeks. Cancer cells are more susceptible to radiation than normal cells, although not all malignant cells respond to radiation. Like surgery, radiation therapy is usually localized or directed at a specific area. Oral cancer is often treated with surgery, followed by head and neck radiation to destroy any remaining cancer cells. Radiation treatment may involve implanting radioactive seeds directly into the tumor to kill from within the tumor mass. Chemotherapy can be administered concurrently with radiation for some head and neck cancers. Oral side effects from head and neck radiation often include xerostomia, skin erythema, mucositis, candidiasis, and loss of taste. Some malignancies (Hodgkin disease and breast cancer) are treated with irradiation to the chest. Therapeutic irradiation of the chest can affect the heart sac, causing scarring. This may result in inflexibility of the heart muscle. Inflammation of the heart sac with fluid collection is also possible. When this is a possibility, clients are counseled by the radiation oncologist and informed consents are signed before treatment. Radiation in the chest area may result in damage to cardiac tissues. During the subsequent 10 to 20 years the clients may undergo pathologic changes of heart valves, predisposing them to infective endocarditis, and may exhibit atherosclerosis of coronary vessels increasing their risk for myocardial infarction.[1,2]

MUCOSITIS

Mucositis occurs as a painful ulceration of mucous membranes in the gastrointestinal tract. The discomfort from the ulceration can affect the ability to eat and decrease quality of life significantly. The Mucositis Study Group of the Multinational Association of Supportive Care in Cancer (MASCC) and the International Society of Oral Oncology (ISOO) completed a systematic review of issues involving oral mucositis (OM) to update the 2007 guidelines for the prevention and treatment of OM in cancer patients.[3,4] The recommendations made are discussed below.

Hematopoietic Stem Cell Transplantation, Radiation Therapy, Chemotherapy

One of the most problematic oral side effects of these therapies is OM, an ulcerated area on the mucosa of the oral cavity. The outcomes based on this 2013 systematic review included a recommendation, a suggestion, and no guideline.

The recommendation involves use of a low-level laser for the prevention of oral mucositis in adult patients receiving hematopoietic stem cell transplantation conditioned with high-dose chemotherapy, with or without total body irradiation. A new suggestion was made for low-level laser for the prevention of oral mucositis in patients undergoing radiotherapy for head and neck cancer, without concomitant chemotherapy. No guideline was possible in other populations and for other light sources due to insufficient evidence.[3] Low-level laser therapy and phototherapy (light therapy) interact with cells without increasing heat in the tissues. Authors added that additional well-designed research is needed to evaluate the efficacy of laser and other light therapies in various cancer treatment settings.

Laser therapy is begun at the beginning of chemotherapy and would be provided in the oncology center.[3]

Cryotherapy

Cryotherapy is a treatment where ice is held in the mouth during intravenous (IV) infusion of chemotherapy for various time periods. A systematic review analyzed the strength of the literature and defined clinical practice guidelines for the use of oral cryotherapy for the prevention and/or treatment of oral mucositis caused by cancer therapy.[4] Oral mucositis occurs as a painful ulceration of mucous membranes in the GI tract and can affect the ability to eat and decrease quality of life. It occurs in individuals receiving radiotherapy, stem cell transplant, and chemotherapy. Guidelines for treatment of this condition are available based on systematic review of clinical research.[3,4] Currently, research supports the use of cryotherapy and laser therapy to prevent this condition. Laser therapy is also being investigated as a potential option for treatment of OM, but additional studies are needed.

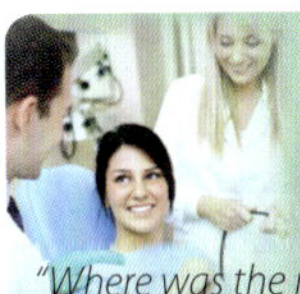

Follow-up Questions

For the client treated for cancer in the past:

"Where was the malignancy? What type of treatment did you receive? Was the treatment successful? Do you have any residual effects from the treatment? Are you still under care of your oncologist? How often are your follow-up appointments?"

In most cases when cancer treatment cures or moves the client to the remission phase, there is a return to normal body function and the client can be treated as a healthy person. Malignancies of the head and neck may result in significant oral dysfunction. In those cases in which treatment has resulted in a permanent disability, such as permanent loss of salivary flow resulting in chronic xerostomia, management is directed at the specific oral problem. Clients with a history of therapeutic chest irradiation for the malignancy should be questioned to determine whether cardiac valvular disease has induced endocarditis in the past. Follow-up care with the oncologist is very important to monitor for recurrence of the tumor or cancer.

Current Cancer Therapy

When the client reports recent or current cancer therapy, the following questions should be asked:

"Does your oncologist know you are here today? Did you have lab work done before this appointment? What type of cancer do you have and what area of your body is affected? May I have permission to contact your oncologist about your treatment? When did (or will) your treatment start? What type of treatments are you receiving? Has your physician given you any instructions related to having oral health treatment?"

APPLICATION TO PRACTICE

Initial Diagnosis

For the client who has been referred by the oncologist for oral care before initiating cancer treatment, it is essential to initiate an oral examination and complete the indicated treatment immediately. The examination should include a thorough examination of hard and soft tissues, as well as radiographs to detect **oral pathology** not evident by clinical examination. Any type of inflammation or disease must be resolved before cancer treatment (head and neck radiation and most chemotherapeutic regimens) to reduce oral complications. If periapical pathology or periodontal disease is not resolved before immunosuppression that results from head and neck oncologic therapy, there is an increased risk for **osteoradionecrosis** and increased infection in the mouth. When possible, oral health care should begin at least 14 days before initial cancer therapy. Before cancer treatment begins, the dentist and dental hygienist should take the following steps:

- Identify and treat existing infections, problem teeth, and tissue injury or trauma.
- Stabilize or eliminate potential sites of infection.
- Remove orthodontic bands if highly **stomatotoxic** chemotherapy is planned, or if the bands will be in the radiation field.
- Evaluate dentures and appliances for comfort and fit.
- In adults receiving head and neck radiation, extract teeth that may pose a future problem to prevent extraction-induced osteoradionecrosis.
- In children, extract loose primary teeth and teeth that are expected to loosen during treatment.

- Instruct patients on oral hygiene methods, use of fluoride gel, nutrition, and the need to avoid tobacco and alcohol.

If oral surgery, such as tooth extraction, is necessary, it should be completed no sooner than 7 to 10 days before the time the client will become myelosuppressed.[4] By adding oral care to the cancer pretreatment regimen, one can:

- Reduce the risk and severity of oral complications.
- Improve the likelihood that the client will tolerate optimal doses of treatment.
- Prevent oral infections that could lead to potentially fatal systemic infections.
- Prevent or minimize complications that can compromise nutrition.
- Prevent, eliminate, or control oral pain.
- Prevent or reduce incidence of bone necrosis in radiation patients.
- Preserve or improve oral health.
- Improve quality of life.[4]

Current Treatment

For clients who request oral health care and are currently in cancer treatment, there are specific recommendations for the treatment plan. Determine that the client's oncologist is aware of any dental and dental hygiene appointments. These appointments should be scheduled when blood counts are at safe levels (Box 10-1). Laboratory blood work should be done 24 hours before oral health treatment to determine whether the client's platelet count, clotting factors, and neutrophil counts are sufficient to prevent hemorrhage and infection. Postpone oral healthcare procedures when the platelet count is less than 50,000 platelets/mm^3, clotting factor levels are more than 5 international normalized ratio (INR), and the neutrophil count is less than 1,000 cells/mm.[3] When an implanted central venous catheter or port is in place, consult with the oncologist to determine whether or not antibiotic prophylaxis is recommended to prevent infection within the catheter or port. The American Heart Association (AHA) no longer recommends antibiotic prophylaxis for catheters and ports, but the oncologist may want the client to be prophylaxed for other reasons. If oral surgery is required, it should be completed at least 7 to 10 days before the next round of immunosuppressive chemotherapy. When radiation therapy is administered to the facial muscle area, fibrosis and **trismus** may develop. Advise the client that frequent practice of stretching exercises (such as opening the mouth widely and then closing it) are necessary to keep the muscles functioning properly. Some suggestions to help the client manage xerostomia include:

- Encourage frequent sips of water.
- Suggest using liquids to soften or thin foods.
- Recommend using sugarless gum or sugar-free hard candies to help stimulate salivation.
- Suggest using a commercial oral lubricant (saliva substitute).
- Use non–petroleum-based lip balm products (cocoa butter, lanolin).[5]
- Consider prescribing salivary stimulant drugs, such as pilocarpine[4] or cevimeline (after consultation with radiation oncologist, as it is contraindicated in some patients).

Box 10-1

Minimal Blood Laboratory Values

- Have blood work completed 24 hours before oral surgery or invasive procedures.
- Postpone oral treatment when platelet count is less than 50,000 platelets/mm^3 or abnormal clotting factors are present.
- Postpone treatment when neutrophil count is less than 1,000 cells/mm^3.

These strategies will reduce the discomfort of xerostomia. The non–petroleum-based lip moisturizers allow the lip tissue to retain moisture.

Mucositis is a debilitating condition that can result from cancer therapy. For clients who seek help with painful oral tissues, the following strategies are recommended:

- Detect, culture, and treat oral infections early.
- Suggest OTC agents, bicarbonate/soda mouthrinses, and prescribe topical anesthetics, as discussed earlier.
- Prescribe systemic analgesics (after consultation with oncologist).
- Encourage clients to avoid eating irritating or rough-textured foods.[4]

The National Cancer Institute CancerNet PDQ and the Cancer Information Center[7] has information on oral care to guide the client receiving chemotherapy or head and neck radiation. This can be requested by asking for the publication "Oral Complications of Chemotherapy and Head/Neck Radiation" at 1-800-4CANCER.

The body temperature should be monitored for fever as it may relate to oral infection. After chemotherapy has been completed and the client's immune system has returned to normal levels, the continuing care schedule can be instituted. This schedule is determined according to the client's oral health status similar to that determined in the normal dental client. Some groups in the past recommended that individuals being treated for cancer be cautioned not to use alcohol-containing mouthrinses. The basis for that recommendation came from concerns that alcohol-containing mouthrinses (such as Listerine) might cause oral cancer and also may promote xerostomia. Studies do not support those fears. A literature review of alcohol-containing mouthrinses and oral cancer found six studies reporting negative effects (no oral cancer) and three studies with positive effects.[8]

A follow-up of one case–control study showed negative results. One other positive study was reanalyzed and authors concluded the study's positive finding resulted from recall bias. The authors concluded that it is unlikely that use of mouthwashes containing alcohol increases the risk of developing oral cancer.

The Oncology Nursing Society has published guidelines for managing mucositis.[9] Traditional practices such as recommending the following were considered but NOT recommended: Chlorhexidine, antimicrobial lozenges, acyclovir and its analogs, pentoxifylline, and granulocyte-macrophage–colony stimulating factor mouthwashes, sucralfate, and combined rinses (Miracle Mix) were NOT found to be effective in the prevention and treatment of OM. Although some oral health professionals continue to recommend these products, there is no evidence to support these practices.

Bone Marrow or Stem Cell Transplantation Patients

These clients will be unlikely to seek elective dental care because of the pronounced immunosuppression that accompanies the treatment. Although these problems begin to resolve when hematologic status improves, immunosuppression may last for up to a year after the transplant, extending the time that oral complications can occur. After bone marrow transplantation and when the oncologist releases the client for oral treatment, the oral healthcare provider should:

- Examine the tongue and oral mucosa for infection, such as *Herpes simplex* viral and *Candida albicans* fungal infections.
- Monitor the oral health for dry mouth, plaque control, tooth demineralization, dental caries, and infection.
- Consult the oncologist before any oral health procedure, including oral prophylaxis.
- Delay elective oral procedures for 1 year.
- Follow client for long-term oral complications and manage, as needed.
- Follow client carefully for second malignancies in oral regions.[5]

Long-Term Problems after Head and Neck Radiation Treatment

When radiation is administered to the head and neck area as part of cancer treatment, some complications can remain for years after treatment has ended. The client may no longer be under the care of an oncologist, and it is the oral healthcare provider's responsibility to monitor oral complications that remain. Often the information provided during treatment about oral health will affect how a client deals with subsequent complications. Oral healthcare programs for the client receiving head and neck radiation treatment should address the following risks:

- High-dose radiation treatment carries a lifelong risk of osteoradionecrosis.
- Because of the risk of osteoradionecrosis, people who have received radiation should avoid invasive surgical procedures (including extractions) that involve irradiated bone.
- Radiation to the head and neck may permanently reduce the quantity and quality of normal saliva, so ongoing oral care is crucial to oral health. Daily fluoride application, good nutrition, and oral hygiene are especially important.
- Radiation may alter oral tissues, so dentures may need to be reconstructed. Some people can never again wear dentures because of friable tissues and xerostomia.
- A dentist should closely monitor children who have received radiation to craniofacial and dental structures for abnormal growth and development.[8]

Supplemental Fluoride Program

Fluoride rinses are inadequate to prevent tooth demineralization. A daily 5-minute application of a 1.1% neutral pH sodium fluoride gel or a 0.4% stannous fluoride unflavored gel in custom-made trays is required to deliver a high concentration of fluoride to the dentition. The trays should be fabricated so that all tooth structure is covered and should extend at least 3 mm beyond the gingival margins. Several days before radiation therapy clients should start a daily 5-minute application of a 1.1% neutral pH sodium fluoride gel or a 0.4%

stannous fluoride unflavored gel. Patients with porcelain crowns should use a neutral pH fluoride. The trays should be fabricated so that all tooth structure is covered without irritating the gingival or mucosal tissues. Clients with radiation-induced salivary gland dysfunction must continue lifelong daily fluoride applications.[9,10] The trays should be checked periodically, and new trays constructed as needed. According to the National Institute for Dental and Craniofacial Research (NIDCR), if the client prefers not to use the custom tray, the fluoride gel can be brushed onto the teeth. High-concentration fluoride products are available by prescription for home use (5,000 ppm fluoride) and may be preferred by the patient over a custom tray.

Oral Health Information

The NIDCR and the National Cancer Institute have designed materials to assist oral healthcare providers in management of clients being treated for cancer (Box 10-2). All materials are provided at no charge. They report that nearly one-third of cancer patients undergoing radiation and chemotherapy treatment or bone marrow transplantation are susceptible to oral complications that can compromise or even result in a need to stop the treatment. Some oral care considerations[7,9] for the client undergoing treatment for cancer include:

1. After meals, the oral cavity should be rinsed and/or wiped, as wiping is frequently necessary when excessive xerostomia has developed.
2. In addition to rinsing, mechanical plaque removal is necessary, even for those who are edentulous. If xerostomia is present, plaque is thick and will not rinse away. Mechanical plaque removal includes use of gauze, toothettes, toothbrush, and interdental aids such as floss, proxabrush, or wooden wedge.
3. Toothettes may not thoroughly cleanse the dentition, although they are effective for cleaning surgical areas and for cleaning the alveolar ridges of edentulous areas, the palate, prominent palatal tori, and the tongue. A sensitive or super-soft toothbrush may be more tolerable for plaque removal.
4. A denture brush is used on dentures. Dentures must be cleaned often and should be brushed, then rinsed, after meals.
5. Oral care products should be selected carefully and products that are irritating or injure the mucosa should not be used. It is unclear if the nonalcohol chlorhexidine is helpful to prevent infection. Flavoring agents in toothpaste can irritate and burn gingivae and mucosa, so a mild toothpaste, such as one for children, should be considered.
6. Lip care is important to prevent drying and cracking. A moisturizer should be suggested for the lip area.

Box 10-2

Materials for Oral Healthcare Providers from NIDCR

Material for professionals:

- Oral Complications of Cancer Treatment: What the Oral Health Team Can Do (OCCT-1)
- Oral Complications of Cancer Treatment: What the Oncology Team Can Do (OCCT-2)
- Oral Care Provider's Reference Guide for Oncology Patients (OCCT-3)
- Oncology Reference Guide to Oral Health (OCCT-4)
- Sample kit for the oral health professional (OCCT-9)

Materials for clients:

- Head and Neck Radiation Treatment and Your Mouth (OCCT-5)
- Chemotherapy and Your Mouth (OCCT-6)
- Who's on My Cancer Care Team? (OCCT-7)
- Three Good Reasons to See a Dentist (OCCT-8)
- Free materials from National Cancer Institute available at http://www.cancer.gov/cancertopics

Materials available at: http://www.nidcr.nih.gov/OralHealth/Topics/CancerTreatment/OralComplicationsCancerOverview.htm

POTENTIAL EMERGENCIES

Emergency situations of uncontrolled bleeding and increased infection are possible.

Prevention

Questions to ask the medical oncologist to prevent adverse events include:

- What is the client's complete blood count, including absolute neutrophil and platelet counts?
- If an invasive oral health procedure needs to be done (tooth extraction, deep scaling), are adequate clotting factors present to prevent excessive bleeding?
- Has the client been advised to receive antibiotic prophylaxis before oral healthcare procedures?

- What is the scheduled sequence of cancer treatments so that safe oral health treatment can be planned?[5]

Questions to ask the radiation oncologist include:

- What parts of the mandible or maxilla and salivary glands are in the direct path of radiation?
- What is the total dose and impact of radiation the client will receive to these areas?
- Has the vascularity of the alveolar bone been previously compromised by surgery?
- How quickly does the client need to start radiation treatment?
- Will there be concurrent chemotherapy with the radiation treatment?[5]

Oral health examination before cancer treatment should include:

- Establish a schedule for dental and dental hygiene treatment to begin at least 14 days before cancer treatment begins, when possible.
- Postpone elective oral surgical procedures until cancer treatment is completed and blood counts have returned to normal limits.
- Identify and treat sites of low-grade and acute oral infections, such as caries, periodontal disease, endodontic disease, and mucosal lesions.
- Identify and eliminate sources of oral trauma and irritation such as ill-fitting dentures, orthodontic bands, broken teeth, and other dental appliances.
- Before radiation treatment, identify and treat potential oral problems within the proposed field of radiation.
- Instruct clients about oral hygiene (Fig. 10.1).
- Educate clients on preventing demineralization and dental caries (fluoride).[5]

Management

Because there are a variety of emergency situations that are possible, ranging from increased bleeding to increased infection, the management would relate to the particular problem. Refer to the section on uncontrolled bleeding (Chapter 9) for management of this problem. For problems with infection, the oncologist must be consulted to establish a complete blood count. Antibiotics must be selected after culture and sensitivity tests are completed. The oral flora changes during chemotherapy (especially in leukemia clients), and antibiotics normally used for oral infection may not be effective.[11]

When the white blood cell count is adequate and the client is covered with adequate antibiotic blood levels, the area must be debrided of infectious and necrotic tissue to establish an environment for healing. Because the client with

Self-Study Review

1. For individuals undergoing initial cancer therapy, oral health care should be performed:
   a. at least 14 days before cancer therapy when possible.
   b. at least 14 days after initial cancer therapy.
   c. between cancer therapy sessions.
   d. oral health care should not be performed until cancer therapy is completed.
2. For clients who require oral health care during cancer therapy, laboratory blood studies should be performed to:
   a. determine baseline values.
   b. determine whether antibiotics are needed.
   c. prevent hemorrhage and infection.
   d. prevent immunosuppression.
3. From the following list, identify the conditions for which oral health procedures should be postponed.
   a. Platelet count is less than 50,000 mm^3.
   b. INR is >5.
   c. Neutrophil count is <1,000 cells/mm^3.
   d. A central venous catheter is being used.
   e. Xerostomia is present.
4. Individuals with a history of bone marrow or stem cell transplants should delay elective oral procedures for:
   a. 1 month.
   b. 6 months.
   c. 9 months.
   d. 1 year.
5. Radiation treatment carries a lifelong risk of all of the following EXCEPT one. Which one is the EXCEPTION?
   a. Osteoradionecrosis
   b. Xerostomia
   c. Friable oral tissues
   d. Gingivitis
6. Radiation therapy clients with salivary gland dysfunction should use daily fluoride applications:
   a. during cancer therapy.
   b. lifelong.
   c. 6 months after cancer therapy.
   d. 1 year after cancer therapy.

Three Good Reasons To See a Dentist BEFORE Cancer Treatment

Feel better Your cancer treatment may be easier if you work with your dentist and hygienist. Make sure you have a pretreatment dental checkup.

Save teeth and bones A dentist will help protect your mouth, teeth, and jaw bones from damage caused by radiation and chemotherapy. Children also need special protection for their growing teeth and facial bones.

Fight cancer Doctors may have to delay or stop your cancer treatment because of problems in your mouth. To fight cancer best, your cancer care team should include a dentist.

Protect Your Mouth During Cancer Treatment

Brush gently, brush often

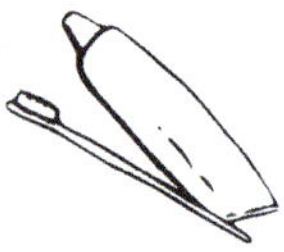

- Brush your teeth—and your tongue—gently with an extra-soft toothbrush.
- If your mouth is very sore, soften the bristles in warm water.
- Brush after every meal and at bedtime.

Floss gently—do it daily

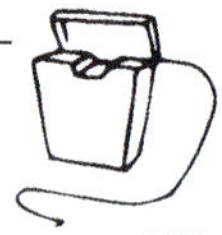

- Floss once a day to remove plaque.
- If your gums bleed and hurt, avoid the areas that are bleeding or sore, but keep flossing your other teeth.

Keep your mouth moist

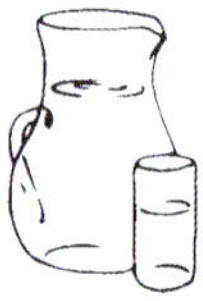

- Rinse often with water.
- Don't use mouthwashes with alcohol in them.
- Use a saliva substitute to help moisten your mouth.

Eat and drink with care

- Choose soft, easy-to-chew foods.
- Protect your mouth from spicy, sour, or crunchy foods.
- Choose lukewarm foods and drinks instead of hot or icy-cold.
- Avoid alcoholic drinks.

Keep trying (Quit Using Tobacco)

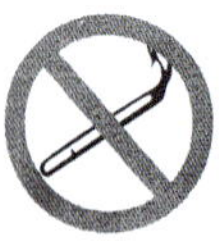

- Ask your cancer care team to help you stop smoking or chewing tobacco.
- People who quit smoking or chewing tobacco have fewer mouth problems.

Oral Health, Cancer Care, and You
Fitting the Pieces Together

A Service of the National Institute of Dental and Craniofacial Research, National Institutes of Health
Toll-free 1-877-216-1019

Figure 10.1 ■ U.S. Department of Health and Human Services: Three good reasons to see a dentist before cancer treatment begins. (Reprinted with permission from Oral Health, Cancer Care, and You: Fitting the Pieces Together information packet. Bethesda, MD: US Department of Health and Human Services, National Institutes of Health, National Institute of Dental and Craniofacial Research, 2002.)[5,6]

a history of oral cancer is at risk for additional oral malignancies, each maintenance treatment should include a thorough oral examination for other primary carcinomas in the oral cavity.

"Please (X) a response to indicate if you have or have not had any of the following diseases or problems: diabetes, if yes, specify below: type 1 or type 2? Excessive urination? Recurrent infections, if yes, indicate type of infection."

The Centers for Disease Control and Prevention estimates that nearly 26 million people in the United States have diabetes mellitus (DM). More than one-quarter of these cases are undiagnosed, and the individuals are unaware they have the disease. The prevalence of prediabetes exceeds 73 million in the United States and an even larger number are estimated to have prediabetes that has not yet been diagnosed.[12] This means an oral healthcare professional may be treating some clients with diabetes who report a negative reply to the DM question. For this reason, symptomatic questions to identify undiagnosed DM are included on the American Dental Association (ADA) Health History form, such as "Do you have excessive urination? Do you have frequent infections or heal slowly?" Although the former questions are included in the health history to identify individuals who need medical evaluation to determine if they have DM, individuals with diabetes may also be asymptomatic. Uncontrolled DM (defined by the American Diabetes Association as three consecutive nonfasting blood glucose readings 200 mg/dL or higher[13]) results in a variety of serious complications, resulting in cardiovascular disease, kidney disease, blindness, and limb amputation. DM is the number one reason for nontraumatic amputation. It is the most common reason for kidney transplantation, and it is the leading cause of blindness in individuals between 20 and 74 years of age. The most common cause of death in DM is cardiovascular disease. Hypertension is common in those affected with DM.

PATHOPHYSIOLOGY OF DIABETES

DM is a group of metabolic diseases characterized by increased levels of blood sugar or blood glucose (**hyperglycemia**) that results from defects in insulin secretion or how insulin is used in the body. In normal situations after carbohydrates are eaten and absorbed from the GI tract, the blood glucose levels rise. In response to this event, beta cells in islets of Langerhans of the pancreas secrete insulin into the bloodstream. Insulin binds to tissue cell receptors, allowing blood glucose to move from the circulation into the cell and be used for cellular metabolism. Levels of blood glucose return to normal after this normal physiologic event. The defect in carbohydrate metabolism in DM results in either inadequate levels of insulin secretion or an inability for the insulin secreted to bind to insulin receptors and enhance the movement of blood glucose into cells. This latter condition is called **insulin resistance** and is found, almost exclusively, in type 2 DM.

Type 1 DM often develops during youth, whereas type 2 DM is associated with onset during adulthood. Type 2 DM prevalence has recently been reported to be increasing in younger individuals. The reasons for this are unclear, but are thought to be related to obesity and lack of physical exercise.

Cardinal symptoms of type 1 DM include polydipsia (increased thirst), polyphagia (increased hunger), polyuria (increased urination), weight loss, weakness, infections, bed wetting, malaise, and dry mouth.[12] Symptoms of type 2 DM are less likely to include the "polys," develop slowly, and often go unnoticed by the client. Type 2 symptoms include weight loss or weight gain, frequent urination during the night (more than three times), vision abnormalities, loss of sensation, increased infections (urinary, skin, respiratory, periodontal), and weakness.[1] Oral signs of uncontrolled DM include granulomatous polyps (Fig. 10.2), periodontal abscesses (Fig. 10.3), candidiasis, taste impairment, cervical caries, xerostomia, parotid gland enlargement, and increased gingivitis and periodontal attachment loss.[14,15] Complications of uncontrolled DM, leading to disease in major organs of the body, are caused by atherosclerosis in capillaries and blood vessels. This results in impaired circulation to major organs and highly vascular tissues. DM also results in defects in polymorphonuclear leukocytes (neutrophils), causing poor healing and inability to fight infections. Warning signs of undiagnosed DM include frequent infections (skin, periodontal tissues, vagina, urinary tract), blurred vision, tingling or numbness in the hands or feet, and slow healing of cuts.

Classification of DM

There are three main forms of DM. These include type 1, type 2, and gestational DM. In type 1 DM, beta cells are destroyed and no insulin is secreted.

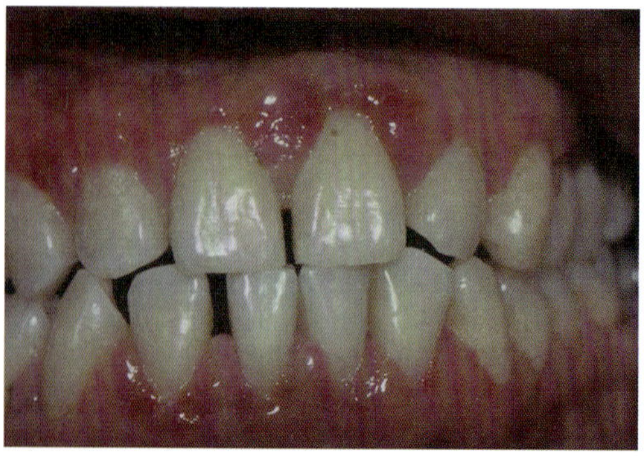

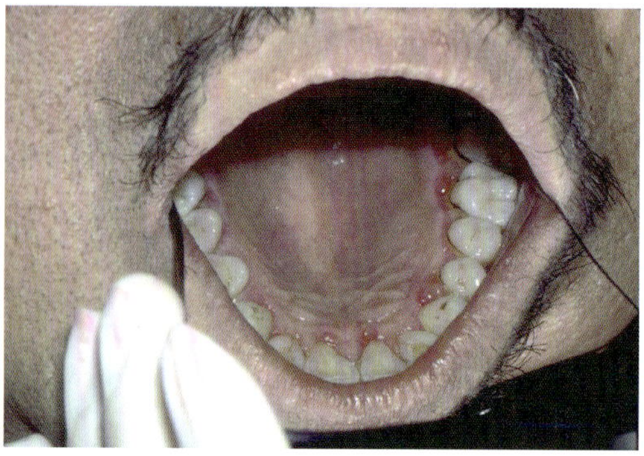

Figure 10.2 ■ Clinical photographs of granulomatous lesions in uncontrolled diabetes.

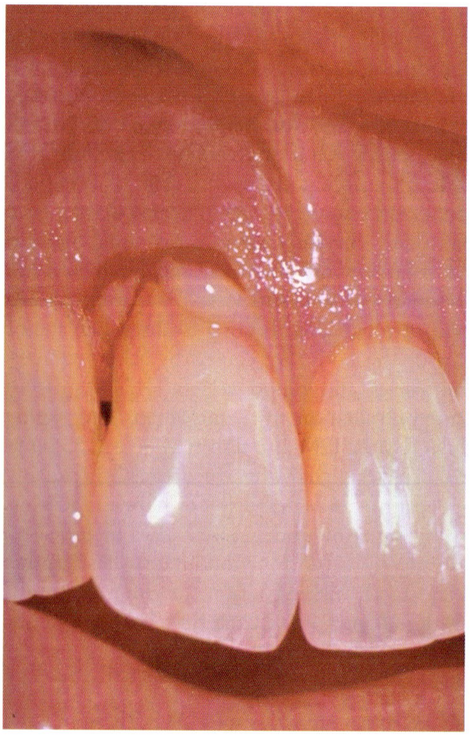

Figure 10.3 ■ Clinical photograph of periodontal abscess in uncontrolled diabetes.

In type 2 DM, beta cells remain, but secrete low amounts of insulin or the insulin secreted cannot interact with insulin receptors, resulting in insulin resistance. Gestational DM occurs during pregnancy, causing hyperglycemia that lasts until delivery of the baby.[1] Women with gestational diabetes and their infants are at an increased risk for developing type 2 DM in the future. Former names for type 1 DM include juvenile diabetes and insulin-dependent diabetes. Type 2 DM has been called adult-onset diabetes and non–insulin-dependent diabetes.

Etiology

Type 1 DM

Approximately 5% to 10% of cases of DM are type 1. Causes include hereditary predisposition, as well as autoimmune destruction of pancreatic beta cells. Some cases are idiopathic. The peak incidence occurs during puberty, but it can develop at any age. With an absolute deficiency of insulin preventing carbohydrates from being used for energy needs, protein and fat are metabolized to provide energy for body function. Ketone bodies result from metabolism of protein, leading to **ketoacidosis** of blood and diabetic coma. This is the most severe development of uncontrolled type 1 DM.

Type 2 DM

Approximately 90% to 95% of cases are type 2. Causes include hereditary predisposition, obesity, and sedentary lifestyle. Hereditary predisposition has a much greater influence than the genetic component in the etiology of type 1 DM.[1] High-risk ethnic groups include African-Americans, Hispanics, Native Americans, and Asian Pacific Islanders. In the past, it was thought that most cases occurred in people older than 45 years, but recently it is reported that increased numbers of younger individuals are diagnosed with DM. These diagnoses in younger people are related to an overweight condition and lack of adequate exercise. In fact, increased exercise helps move blood glucose into muscle cells and helps reduce hyperglycemia.

Long-standing DM presents a greater risk for organ dysfunction and complications from DM. In former guidelines systolic blood pressure (BP) was recommended to be <130 mm Hg as it was thought this level would reduce the risk for death. A review of research reported that this was not evidence-based and the risk for hypotension

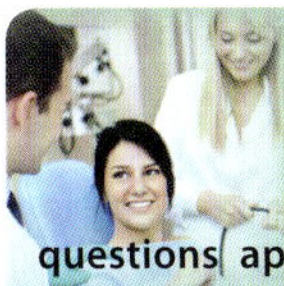

Follow-up Questions

When the client responds affirmatively to this question, follow-up questions apply regard less of the type of DM. Rather than asking "Is the diabetes controlled?" formulate questions related to evidence of control, such as A1C test results. These questions include:

"When were you first diagnosed? What have your recent blood sugar levels been? How often do you check your blood glucose levels? How often does your healthcare provider check your blood glucose levels? What is your most current A1C level? Do you heal slowly or have frequent infections? When was your last meal? Did you take your medication today? Have you experienced hypoglycemia recently? How many episodes of hypoglycemia have you had this week? Have you had any problems during dental treatment?"

was increased when BP was aggressively treated. Levels were revised in 2013 American Diabetes Association (ADA) guidelines to be maintained at <140/80 mm Hg.[13] The degree of disease control is determined from the results of daily blood sugar tests done at home by the client and semiannual or quarterly laboratory tests completed in the medical facility during medical evaluation. According to the ADA normal blood glucose is between 70 and 100 mg/dL. Normoglycemia is also defined as a fasting plasma glucose (FPG) test result of <100 mg/dL and a glucose tolerance test (GTT) of less than 140 mg/dL at 2 hours. In some individuals, these intermediate levels of glucose (FPG of 100 to 125 mg/L or a 2-hour GTT of 140 to 199 mg/dL) may lead to overt type 2 diabetes, cardiovascular disease, and microvascular complications. An FPG level of 100 to 125 mg/dL or an impaired glucose tolerance (IGT) of 140 to 199 mg/dL is in the prediabetes stage (Box 10-3). Clients with DM are counseled to keep FPG levels below 130 mg/dL so clinician questioning should be directed at those measurement values on waking in the morning. The client with prediabetes should have the same target BP as those with DM (<140/80 mm Hg).[13] Clients attempt to maintain blood sugar levels within this range each day through a combination of diet, exercise, and medications. Some clients with diabetes are able to control the from therapy and lifestyle habits alone. Clients with DM taking insulin are instructed to test blood sugar levels at various times during the day (before meals) and on waking in the morning by pricking the finger and placing the blood on a test strip.[13] The strip is then placed into a device called a glucometer. This digital device processes the blood on the test strip and reveals a number that corresponds with the blood sugar level. Clients with type 1 diabetes determine the dose level of insulin on the basis of the numbers revealed. This information allows the client to determine the level of disease control from therapy and lifestyle habits. Medical evaluation should occur quarterly. At that time a different laboratory test, called glycated hemoglobin or A1C test, reveals the control during the past 3 months. An A1C level of <7% is the goal according to the American Diabetes Association Guidelines (2013).[13] Therapy is designed on the basis of the results of the A1C test. When blood tests reveal frequent high blood sugar levels, the client is likely to have healing problems and increased infections.[10] The most common adverse effect from taking antidiabetic medications is **hypoglycemia**. This most often occurs as a result of taking antidiabetic medication and failing to eat the scheduled meal.

Medications Causing Hypoglycemia

The most common medications associated with causing low blood sugar levels include insulin and oral sulfonylureas (e.g., Glucotrol, Glynase, Micronase, and others). Hypoglycemia is the most

Box 10-3

Diagnostic Criteria for Prediabetes and Diabetes

	Fasting Plasma Glucose Test (FPG)	Two-Hour Oral Glucose Tolerance Test (OGTT)
Normal	Below 100 mg/dL	Below 140 mg/dL
Prediabetes	100–125 mg/dL (IFG)	140–199 mg/dL (IGT)
Diabetes	126 mg/dL or above	200 mg/dL or above

common medical emergency to occur in DM. It generally occurs when the client takes one of these medications but fails to eat food or a meal. The dose of the medication is calculated on the basis of the expectation that the client will consume food. Therefore, when food (which would increase blood sugar levels) is not eaten, the dose of the hypoglycemic drug becomes an overdose, resulting in hypoglycemia. A less common reason for hypoglycemia, unlikely to occur in a dental appointment, is excessive exercise.

Application to Practice

Because hypoglycemia is the most likely medical emergency to occur when treating a client with DM, the clinician must be able to recognize signs of hypoglycemia and behaviors that influence the condition. For those clients who report taking a hypoglycemic drug and who have not eaten, it is important to have a sugar source in the operatory, in case signs of hypoglycemia are observed. Signs of hypoglycemia include perspiration, confusion, diminished cerebral function and inability to respond to questioning in a rational manner, mood changes (argumentative, anxious, lethargy), hunger and nausea, and vital sign changes of low BP and tachycardia (Box 10-4). In addition, clients with mild hypoglycemia may experience no overt symptoms. Diminished salivary flow and increased glucose concentrations in cervicular fluid may alter plaque microflora and contribute to development of periodontal disease, caries, and oral candidiasis.[14] Oral burning sensation and taste disturbances are also associated with DM. Clients with DM and periodontal disease require more frequent (1 to 3 months) maintenance intervals to prevent excessive attachment loss depending upon their clinical presentation, host response to disease states, and adherence to home care instructions. Periodontal infection results in the need for higher doses of medication to control blood sugar levels. However, it is unclear if periodontal treatment plays a significant role in reducing antidiabetic medication dose requirements. Some studies showed treatment resulted in study subjects being able to reduce dose levels of antidiabetic drugs while others did not report any effect on medication dose. It is well known that smoking decreases the response to periodontal treatment; therefore, tobacco cessation counseling should be offered to the DM client as part of the oral healthcare treatment plan. Because hypertension is frequently found in the client with diabetes, BP should be monitored as part of the initial physical assessment.[12] The 2013 ADA recommendation raises the target for systolic BP from below 130 mm Hg to below 140 mm Hg on the basis of evidence that there is not a great deal of additional value, but there is an increase in risk in pushing systolic pressure much lower than 140 mm Hg.[13]

If targets are not achieved, drug therapy should be added.

Box 10-4

Common Signs of Hypoglycemia

- Perspiration
- Confusion, anxiety
- Mood changes (argumentative, agitated, anxious, lethargic)
- Diminished cerebral function, unable to respond to questions
- Tachycardia
- Hunger, nausea

Adverse events can lead to hypotension, unconsciousness, seizure, and hypothermia. (Adapted from American Diabetes Association Clinical Practice Guidelines. Diabetes Care 2013;36:S3.)

POTENTIAL EMERGENCIES

The most common emergency situation in diagnosed DM clients represents an overdose of medication, resulting in insulin shock or hypoglycemia. The individual with undiagnosed diabetes will exhibit severe hyperglycemia, leading to diabetic coma. Diabetic coma is unlikely to develop during a dental appointment as the symptoms preceding it develop slowly and cause the client to feel very ill and unlikely to come to a dental appointment. Signs of hypoglycemia develop quickly, causing hypoglycemia to be the most likely emergency in the dental patient with diabetes. Signs of ketoacidosis and diabetic coma include dry, warm skin; fruity breath odor; rapid, weak pulse; deep, slow or fast respirations to reverse respiratory alkalosis (called Kussmaul respirations); normal to low BP; and altered consciousness.[15] Signs of hypoglycemia include intense perspiration, weakness, normal to slow respirations, inability to think clearly, uncooperative attitude, hypertension initially, followed by hypotension in the late stage, and an altered level of consciousness. Inasmuch as glucose is essential for the function of brain cells, the inability to make rational decisions or the demonstration of irrational behavior often seen in the client experiencing hypoglycemia is understandable. However, it may make management of the situation difficult. The client may refuse to ingest the sugar to reverse the condition. According to the American Diabetes Association, blood glucose values less than 70 mg/dL defines hypoglycemia.

Prevention

The goal of medical management for DM is to keep blood sugar levels at a controlled level. Therapy involves diabetic education along with diet, exercise, and the possibility of antidiabetic drug therapy. Clients are advised to monitor blood sugar levels regularly to detect levels greater than 126 mg/dL (which represent uncontrolled disease) or to detect levels less than 70 mg/dL (which indicate hypoglycemia). The best way to prevent a medical emergency involving hypoglycemia during oral health care is to ensure the client has eaten a meal after taking hypoglycemic medication (insulin, sulfonylureas) and to observe the client for signs of hypoglycemia during the appointment. Offer glucose to reverse these symptoms.

Scheduling Healthcare Visits

For the client taking insulin, questioning should determine when the peak effect of the specific insulin preparation being used will occur. This is the time when hypoglycemia is most likely to develop. Avoid scheduling the appointment around this time. Ask the client to tell you the best time for the appointment to avoid hypoglycemia, depending on the type of insulin being used. Avoid lengthy appointments that extend into the DM client's meal pattern or snack time. Morning appointments are usually preferable.[14] If significant oral infection is present, the dentist may prescribe prophylactic antibiotics before periodontal therapy. Acetaminophen is the most appropriate analgesic for pain because aspirin and nonsteroidal anti-inflammatory drugs (NSAIDs) may interact with antidiabetic medications.

When signs of hyperglycemia are noticed in the client with diabetes (or signs indicating hyperglycemia in an undiagnosed client), oral health care should be delayed and the client should be sent for medical evaluation. Surgical procedures and invasive periodontal nonsurgical therapy can be provided when uncontrolled diabetes occurs but antibiotics should be considered to assist in the healing phase.[14]

Management

For the client with dangerously elevated blood sugar levels demonstrating signs of diabetic coma during oral healthcare procedures, the client should be managed by providing basic life support, calling the 911 emergency medical system (EMS), and allowing the EMS personnel to give necessary medication by IV route. Most dental offices do not have IV catheter equipment nor IV administered medications needed to reverse diabetic coma. This discussion will focus on the more common emergency to occur, which is hypoglycemia or insulin shock.

For the client with a recent history of hypoglycemia or when an invasive oral procedure (such as tooth extraction) is planned, it is a good practice to have the client bring their glucometer to the appointment to check their blood glucose levels prior to treatment.[14]

When blood glucose levels are <70 mm/dL, the risk for a hypoglycemic emergency is high. Hypoglycemia is managed according to the consciousness level of the client. Should the conscious client with diabetes show signs of hypoglycemia, provide a sugar source, such as candy, 4 oz of fruit juice, or a glucose tablet (administer three or four, one at a time) from the emergency kit. The unconscious client or the client who is unable to swallow would be managed by applying a sugar source to the vestibular mucosa. A recommendation is to have an OTC glucose gel or a tube of cake icing in the emergency kit as it is easy to squeeze into the vestibule. Ingestion of sugar will usually reverse signs of hypoglycemia within 15 minutes. If the client is uncooperative or loses consciousness, summon the 911 EMS and provide basic life support (open airway, monitor breathing and circulation, monitor vitals every 5 minutes). For dental offices that have equipment and knowledge on inserting an IV catheter, the dentist can administer 50% dextrose or intramuscular glucagon (1 mg) to reverse hypoglycemia.[14]

Self-Study Review

7. From the following list, identify the complications associated with DM.
   a. Blindness
   b. Cardiovascular disease
   c. Kidney disease
   d. Weight gain
   e. Loss of sensation
   f. Periodontal disease
   g. Liver dysfunction
8. The majority of DM cases are:
   a. type 1.
   b. type 2.
   c. gestational diabetes.
   d. secondary diabetes.
9. The most common medical emergency to occur in individuals with DM is:
   a. hypoglycemia.
   b. hyperglycemia.
   c. low BP.
   d. syncope.
10. A sugar source is needed to effectively treat hypoglycemia. Clients should use their glucometer device to check their blood sugar level prior to starting oral health procedures.
   a. Both statements are true.
   b. Both statements are false.
   c. The first statement is true, and the second statement is false.
   d. The first statement is false, and the second statement is true.

"Please (X) a response to indicate if you have or have not had any of the following diseases or problems: systemic lupus erythematosus."

SLE is discussed in this chapter because the drugs used to suppress the inflammation associated with the disease depress the immune inflammatory response. This leaves the client with a depressed host resistance. Ninety percent of cases are in young to middle-aged women.

PATHOPHYSIOLOGY OF SYSTEMIC LUPUS ERYTHEMATOSUS

SLE is one of a group of autoimmune diseases. Autoimmune diseases are disorders in which the body's immune system reacts against some of its own tissue and produces antibodies to it. In SLE, the immune system attacks multiple organs, such as the heart and the kidneys, as well as skin, joints, and muscles. The inflammatory disorder occurs in a variety of forms such as SLE, a blister-producing form (bullous), a neonatal form, and a chronic or a subacute cutaneous form (a less severe form affecting skin). Diagnosis is made by the presence of antinuclear antibodies (ANAs) in the blood. Skin lesions appear as pigmented, erythematous patches. When the face is affected, a characteristic butterfly pattern of rash occurs over the bridge of the nose, flaring on the cheeks (Fig. 10.4). Symptoms include severe pain in joints, severe fatigue, and bouts of fever. Oral ulcerations (Fig. 10.4) are sometimes reported. Inflammation can result in severe and irreversible damage to blood vessels and to kidney cells. Most deaths in SLE are as a result of kidney failure. Clients may be on hemodialysis or have a kidney transplant. There is no cure for SLE, but inflammation that occurs as part of the disease process is treated with immunosuppressive drugs, such as prednisone, hydrocortisone, and other drugs that suppress inflammation. Aspirin and other analgesics are used to reduce pain. The condition may regress to an arrested state of remission

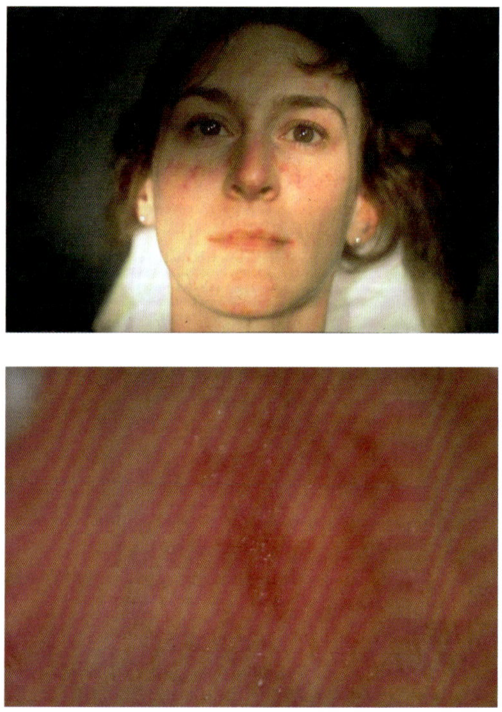

Figure 10.4 ■ Clinical photographs of SLE. Butterfly rash (top) and oral ulcerations (bottom) in the same client.

or progress to death. Autoimmune diseases often occur together, so that the person with SLE might have another autoimmune condition, such as Hashimoto thyroiditis or RA. SLE has been implicated as causing vegetative lesions on heart valves, inferring a risk for infective endocarditis. Other risks include increased bleeding, infection, adrenal insufficiency, and mucocutaneous ulcerations.[15,16,17]

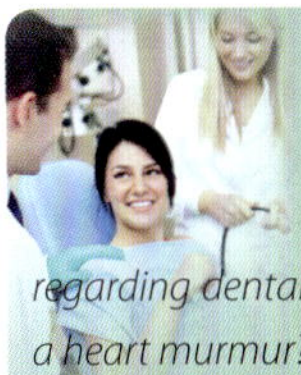

Follow-up Questions

"How long have you had SLE? Has your physician given you any warning regarding dental treatment? Have you been evaluated for a heart murmur? What drugs do you take to manage your symptoms?"

Questions should be related to determining the severity of the disease and the organ systems that have been adversely affected. Kidney failure is the most common reason for death in the client with a history of SLE. SLE is also associated with the presence of a heart murmur, but according to the most recent guidelines from the AHA for the prevention of endocarditis following oral procedures, heart murmur is no longer indicated for antibiotic prophylaxis prior to oral procedures (see Chapter 8). Drugs to suppress the inflammatory response, such as steroids (prednisone) are commonly used. Medication side effects should be investigated in a drug reference and determination made regarding the impact on oral health recommendations or the treatment plan. In the past, it was thought that clients on long term glucocorticoid steroid therapy should receive supplementary steroids for stressful oral procedures. The theoretical basis for this practice was that exogenous steroids suppress the function of the adrenal gland to an extent that insufficient levels of cortisol are possible during a stress response. This may increase the risk of acute adrenal crisis with hypotension, cardiovascular collapse, and shock. It is now considered that the risk for significant adrenal insufficiency, even following major surgical procedures, is very low and supplemental steroids are not recommended for routine oral procedures.[18]

Heart Valve Damage

Chronic SLE is associated with a risk for formation of vegetative lesions on cardiac valves. Autopsies after death as a result of SLE have revealed a high prevalence of these growths, leading researchers to question whether the client with SLE might require antibiotic prophylaxis to prevent infective endocarditis. There are no official guidelines advising antibiotic prophylaxis in these individuals prior to oral procedures.

Glomerulonephritis

Localization of immune complexes in the kidney can lead to the development of a rapidly progressive glomerulonephritis. In the past, it was suggested that glomerulonephritis may require antibiotic prophylaxis before oral health care, although no studies have been reported showing a benefit from antibiotics and there are no official guidelines advising antibiotic prophylaxis for glomerulonephritis. Chronic kidney disease predisposes an individual to hypertension. A physician consultation is indicated to determine the degree of damage to the kidney from SLE and medical recommendations prior to oral procedures.

Hematologic Disease

Anemia, leukopenia, and thrombocytopenia can occur as a result of both the disease process and drug therapy used to manage symptoms of SLE. Consequently, individuals are at risk for increased infection and increased bleeding episodes after oral trauma, such as that incurred in extensive periodontal scaling and in oral surgery.[17]

Application to Practice

The following treatment modifications are recommended for the oral care treatment plan[16]:

Before dental care:

- Consult with the patient's physician or rheumatologist to determine the degree of kidney damage and the management (dialysis, antibiotic prophylaxis, and so forth).
- Monitor vital signs and compare against limits of normal.
- Request complete blood count, platelet count, and prothrombin times before per-forming extensive surgical or periodontal scaling procedures.
- Postpone elective care during acute lupus flares or during high-dose steroid therapy.
- Assess potential for adrenal suppression, use replacement therapy as recommended by the physician.
- Use stress-reducing measures when appropriate, including sedative premedication and short, morning appointments.

During dental care:

- Assess oral mucosal disease and temporomandibular joint (TMJ) involvement.
- Use adjunctive hemostatic aids as needed when bleeding is a problem.
- Use stress reduction measures when appropriate, such as nitrous oxide and profound local anesthesia.

After dental care:

- Follow recommendations of rheumatologist if client has renal insufficiency or is on dialysis, regarding precautions in recommending NSAIDs or aspirin.
- Consult with physician regarding postoperative antibiotic use for patients receiving high-dose immunosuppressive therapy.

The potential for adrenal crisis may relate to presence of infection and pain, along with unstable adrenal function. Physician consult should include determination of adrenal stability.[18]

POTENTIAL EMERGENCIES

The most likely emergency situation is uncontrolled bleeding if the platelet count is very low. Treatment plan modifications may include a medical consultation to determine potential complications related to kidney dysfunction.

The client on long-term glucocorticoid (hydrocortisone, prednisone, others) therapy is classified as an American Society of Anesthesiologists (ASA) II or III risk. Stress reduction strategies should be used. Although very unlikely to develop signs of acute adrenal insufficiency, it includes feelings of extreme fatigue, weakness, skeletal muscle paralysis secondary to hyperkalemia, mental confusion, pain in the abdomen, back, or legs, hypotension, and hypoglycemia.[17,18] Hypoglycemia signs and symptoms include tachycardia, perspiration, nausea, weakness, headache, and convulsions leading to coma if sugar is not provided.

Prevention

A physician consultation should be completed prior to initiation of treatment to:

1. Determine the complete blood count and platelet levels and recommendations related to the proposed oral health care planned.
2. Request assessment of cardiac health and usual BP values.

A stress reduction protocol should be planned to reduce stress during oral healthcare procedures.

Management

When appropriate medical consultations are completed and medical advice followed, the SLE client should be able to receive oral health care with no complications. If signs of adrenal crisis occur (hypoglycemia, profuse sweating, mental confusion, weakness, nausea, hypotension),[18] activate the 911 EMS, place the client in the supine position with feet elevated, monitor vital signs, provide a sugar source, and provide basic life support measures until the emergency team arrives.

Self-Study Review

11. Individuals with SLE taking long-term corticosteroid therapy are at risk for acute adrenal insufficiency. They should be placed on supplemental steroids for oral procedures.
    a. Both statements are true.
    b. Both statements are false.
    c. The first statement is true, and the second statement is false.
    d. The first statement is false, and the second statement is true.
12. Antibiotic prophylaxis may be indicated for individuals with SLE who have all of the following EXCEPT one. Which one is the EXCEPTION?
    a. Have cardiac valve damage.
    b. Take immunosuppressive drug therapy.
    c. Have hypertension.
    d. Have signs of endocarditis.
13. A physician consult should be performed in clients with SLE to avoid potential problems such as hemorrhage and infection.
    a. Both the statement and reason are correct and related.
    b. Both the statement and reason are correct, but NOT related.
    c. The statement is correct, but the reason is NOT.
    d. The statement is NOT correct, but the reason is correct.
    e. NEITHER the statement NOR the reason is correct.

"Please (X) a response to indicate if you have or have not had any of the following diseases or problems: arthritis or rheumatoid arthritis."

RA is another autoimmune disease treated with immunosuppressive drug therapy. The same considerations discussed with SLE apply to the client with RA as corticosteroid drug therapies may be similar. It has been proposed that there is an association between periodontal attachment loss and RA.

While this relationship is unlikely to be causal, it is clear that individuals with advanced RA are more likely to experience more significant periodontal problems compared with their non-RA counterparts.[19] The two diseases could be very closely related through common underlying dysfunction of fundamental inflammatory mechanisms.

The nature of such dysfunction is still unknown; however, the clinical implications of the current data dictate that patients with RA should be carefully screened for periodontal disease.[19]

The other form of arthritis, osteoarthritis, is less severe and treated with mild analgesics. If it affects the TMJ, it can cause difficulties during oral healthcare procedures.

PATHOPHYSIOLOGY DISCUSSION OF ARTHRITIS

The condition referred to as "arthritis" relates to osteoarthritis, the most common form of arthritis. It is associated with aging and long-term "wear and tear" of the joint. In the TMJ, the disk between the mandibular condyle and the joint capsule of the maxilla degenerates, causing the bone of the condyle to contact the maxillary bone. The cause of the condition is not associated with inflammation. Extraoral examination of the TMJ may reveal crepitation as a sign of osteoarthritis in the joint. Pain may or may not be reported. When pain occurs, it is generally unilateral, whereas in RA the pain is bilateral.[1]

RA is a more serious condition. It is an autoimmune disease of unknown origin that results in inflammation in joints. Inflammation in joint spaces results in degeneration of joint tissue (cartilage and bone), redness, and swelling. The client has pain and stiffness when moving joints (bending knee, grasping, walking). As the disease progresses, joints become immobile and deform. When the fingers or wrists are affected, the ability to perform oral hygiene procedures may be impaired. Total joint replacement (TJR) might be necessary for severely affected joints. Women are more likely to have RA than men. Many individuals with RA have other autoimmune diseases. Sjögren syndrome (SS), an autoimmune disease characterized by the destruction of serous salivary cells in salivary glands, may also affect individuals with RA. A prime clinical feature of SS is xerostomia, a condition that can result in extensive caries and oral conditions associated with chronic xerostomia.

Treatment for RA requires disease-modifying drug therapy that results in immunosuppression. Bisphosphonate medication (e.g., Fosamax®) is often prescribed to improve bone health. All of the arthritic conditions require an investigation into the drugs used to manage symptoms of the condition, determination of alterations in dental chair position for client comfort, evaluation of malocclusion, a periodontal assessment, examination for osteonecrosis of the jaw, and assessment of the client's oral hygiene abilities and determining the need for modified oral physiotherapy (OPT) aids.

Drug Therapy

Many clients take daily anti-inflammatory agents to reduce the pain associated with arthritis. These may include aspirin, NSAIDs such as ibuprofen or naproxen, acetaminophen, or drugs with immunosuppression effects, such as prednisone, methotrexate, and newer, disease-modifying antirheumatic drugs (e.g., Enbrel®). As with any drug therapy, a drug reference must be consulted and attention paid to the dose taken, side effects, warnings, and dental considerations for each drug. Enbrel has a warning against taking the drug when infection is present. For the client taking this type of drug, any oral infection must be treated and resolved, similar to the client recommendation before initiation of cancer chemotherapy.

OPT Aids

Some clients with arthritis have malformed digits and joints between the fingers and are unable to grasp a toothbrush or to manipulate dental floss effectively. They may require powered toothbrushes with thick handles or flossaids with built-up handles to achieve good plaque control.

Follow-up Questions

Questions might be formulated to identify modifications needed during oral health care, such as:

"Are you having symptoms today? What position is most comfortable for you in the dental chair? Does your drug therapy control the symptoms of the disease? What areas of your body are affected? Do you have a problem grasping a toothbrush or using dental floss? Can you keep your mouth open for long periods of time? Does your medication cause bleeding problems?"

Application to Practice

Based on the client's responses, the clinician will determine whether modifications need to be made for positioning of the dental chair. Some clients may bring pillows to support the back or legs. During the oral and periodontal examination, attention will be paid to the effectiveness of current oral hygiene techniques and modifications made as needed. A quarterly maintenance schedule should be recommended when periodontal attachment loss is present. For the adolescent client with RA or other arthropathies, an assessment of occlusion is indicated. If the disease has damaged the mandibular condyles and malocclusion has resulted, referral for orthodontic treatment is indicated. Depending on the particular medications being taken on a chronic basis, side effects can include increased bleeding, oral ulcerations, dry mouth and lips, and reduced host response with increased risk for infection (Fig. 10.5). When drugs associated with immunosuppression (Enbrel) or blood dyscrasia (methotrexate) are taken, the client must be counseled regarding the need for strict plaque control to reduce oral infection. When the client is taking immunosuppressive drugs, the risk for spreading of infection is increased. The clinician must examine the oral cavity for evidence of infection and inform the client of the condition. Side effects for the specific medications being taken must be investigated in a drug reference. While it has been reported that individuals with RA may have an increased incidence of periodontal attachment loss, it does not appear that inadequate oral hygiene resulting from functional impairment is a primary factor in periodontal disease in this condition.[20] For individuals with chronic xerostomia, both professionally applied fluoride at maintenance appointments and daily home fluoride therapy are recommended. A final consideration relates to antibiotic prophylaxis in immunocompromised individuals with a TJR. The orthopedist following the care for the client with RA who has had a TJR would generally make this decision.

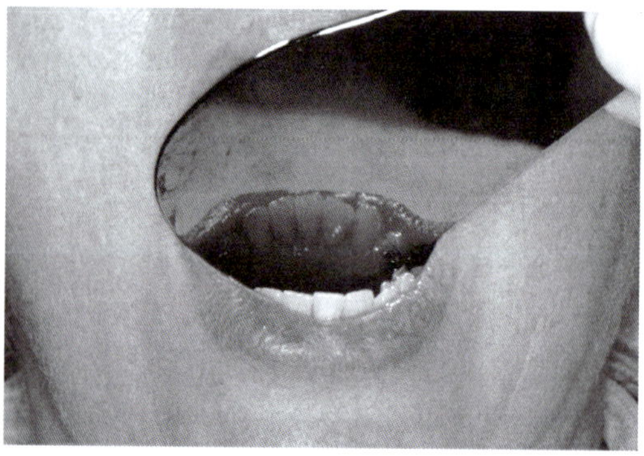

Figure 10.5 ■ Clinical photograph of dry lips in client taking methotrexate.

"Please (X) a response to indicate if you have or have not had any of the following problems: persistent swollen glands, rapid weight loss, night sweats, or sores or ulcers in the mouth."

These are signs of undiagnosed disease and are included on the ADA Health History Form to detect situations in which the client should be referred for a complete medical evaluation before proceeding with oral health care.

PATHOPHYSIOLOGY DISCUSSION

These signs could relate to a variety of problems, such as metastatic malignancies, disease in lymphatic tissues, metabolic disorders (such as diabetes), and any number of conditions that manifest as night sweats or oral ulcerations. These symptomatic questions are intended to identify the client who should be sent for medical evaluation to determine the cause for the particular symptom.

Follow-up Questions

"Do you know what is causing the symptom? Have you seen a physician regarding the symptom? If so, what was the outcome of the medical visit?"

Based on the responses to these questions, the clinician will determine whether referral for medical evaluation is necessary.

Application to Practice

Depending on the situation, the clinician may decide to delay elective oral health care until medical evaluation has been completed. Treatment that requires a good host response for healing should not be completed. Any lymph node that is fixed (nonmovable) and nonpainful should be referred for medical evaluation before elective procedures. These are two signs of metastatic disease in lymph nodes. Another example is when swelling of cervical lymph nodes causes the clinician to suspect Hodgkin lymphoma. The client would be referred for medical evaluation and elective oral health care delayed until the physician releases the client for treatment. A medical referral form and request for information should be sent to the client's physician.

"Please (X) a response to indicate if you have or have not had any of the following diseases or problems: organ transplant."

It is becoming more common to have a client with an organ transplant and this history can present in the child as well as the adult. Transplanted organs include hearts, lungs, livers, kidneys, and the pancreas. In addition, many clients are awaiting transplantation and have poorly or nonfunctioning organs. The dental management of these clients involves a variety of factors, including immuno suppression from immunosuppressive drug therapy and factors related to medically complex client care, such as the client receiving dialysis.

Pretransplanted Situation

In April 2011, the National Institute of Dental and Craniofacial Research updated guidance for dental management of the client awaiting organ transplant.[21] The following dental considerations are summarized from that document and are based on the effect of general health due to lack of organ function and the problems from dialysis.

Before treating a prospective transplant recipient, the patient's medical and dental histories should be reviewed and a noninvasive initial oral examination (without periodontal probing). After the examination, the current status of general health and effects on the immune system is considered. A physician consult may be needed. Decisions about the timing of treatment (AM or PM best?), the need for antibiotic prophylaxis, and precautions to prevent excessive bleeding should be considered during the discussion. Whether a patient can tolerate dental treatment is another crucial concern. When organ transplant is in the near future, it may be safer for patients to undergo dental treatment after transplant as the new organ improves the health.

Management

Several factors should be considered before starting oral procedures:

- ***Antibiotic Prophylaxis:*** Ask the patient's physician whether antibiotic prophylaxis is required to prevent systemic infection from invasive dental procedures. Unless advised otherwise by the physician, the American Heart Association's standard regimen to prevent endocarditis (http://www.heart.org/) is an accepted option.
- ***Infection:*** If the patient presents with an active infection, such as a purulent periodontal infection or an abscessed tooth, antibiotics should be given to the patient before and after dental treatment to prevent systemic infection. Confirm the choice of antibiotic and the dosage with the patient's physician.
- ***Excessive Bleeding:*** Several factors can cause bleeding problems in organ transplant candidates, such as organ dysfunction or their current medications. Many may be taking anticoagulants, and some may have a decreased platelet count. Patients with end-stage liver disease may have excessive bleeding because the liver is no longer producing sufficient amounts of clotting factors. Before treatment, assess the patient's bleeding potential with the appropriate laboratory tests and take precautions to limit bleeding.

Consult with the patient's physician about whether antifibrinolytic rinses or vitamin K interventions are appropriate. The physician also may decide to temporarily decrease the patient's level of anticoagulation before extensive dental surgeries. Some patients are only suitable for surgery in a hospital setting or dental offices designed to handle emergency medical situations.

- ***Medication Considerations:*** Patients preparing to undergo organ transplantation usually take multiple medications. These include anticoagulants, antihypertensive medications (beta blockers, calcium channel blockers, diuretics), and other drugs. Be aware of the side effects of these medications, which range from xerostomia and gingival hyperplasia to orthostatic hypotension and hyperglycemia, and their interactions with agents used in oral procedures.

Precaution is essential when prescribing medication to patients with end-stage kidney or liver disease. Many medications commonly used in dental practice, including NSAIDs, opiates, and some antimicrobials, are metabolized by these organs and are not removed from circulation normally in patients with markedly reduced kidney or liver function. Prior to dental treatment, consult the patient's physician on appropriate drug selection, dosage, and administration intervals.

- ***Other Medical Problems:*** Patients with end-stage organ failure may have other major medical conditions. A person with end-stage kidney disease, for example, may have diabetes and/or significant pulmonary or heart disease. Carefully review the medical history to determine what additional treatment considerations are indicated.

Whenever possible, all active dental disease should be aggressively treated before organ transplantation. Appointments should be scheduled the day after dialysis. The patient should be warned that oral health is important to successful outcome after organ transplant and more frequent appointments may be necessary to maintain oral health. The patient should bring a current list of all medications to each appointment.

During the period between determination of the need for the organ transplant and the transplant surgery, a team approach is needed to manage medical and oral care. Many of these individuals will be in very poor health, and oral care will mainly involve preventive care or oral emergency care. Transplantation of vital organs, including bone marrow, involves not only the surgical procedure but also a long period of immunosuppression. Questioning during the medical history review should include other organ systems that may be compromised because of the poorly functioning organ. For example, when chronic kidney disease is present, the client often has hypertension, diabetes, heart failure and ischemic heart disease, and secondary hyperparathyroidism. The chapters dealing with liver dysfunction, cardiovascular dysfunction, and kidney dysfunction can be consulted for management recommendations for the pretransplant issue. DM is discussed in this chapter.

Posttransplanted Organ

The client who had an organ transplant that was successful has improved physical health. According to the National Institute of Dental and Craniofacial Research,[21] patients should avoid dental treatment for at least 3 months following organ transplantation, except for emergency oral procedures. Dosage of immunosuppressive medications is highest in the early posttransplant period, and patients are at greatest risk for rejection of the transplanted organ and other serious complications during that time. Once the graft has stabilized, typically 3 to 6 months postsurgery, patients can be treated in the dental office with proper precautions.

Medical consultation should be completed before oral care is provided. The medical consult can give an understanding of the patient's general health and ability to tolerate treatment. Posttransplant patients vary widely in their ability to endure dental treatment and their healing capacity following invasive procedures. Antibiotic prophylaxis should be determined by the physician and the physician may adjust dosage of other medications before treatment.

- ***Infection:*** Patients who have undergone organ transplant surgery are at increased risk for serious infection. Bacterial, viral, and fungal infections are more common, especially immediately after surgery. The decision to premedicate with antibiotics for invasive dental procedures and selection of the appropriate regimen should be done in consultation with the patient's physician.
- ***Medication Considerations:*** Organ transplant recipients may be taking one or more medications that affect dental treatment. Immunosuppressive agents can cause gingival hyperplasia, poor healing, and infections and may interact with commonly prescribed medications. Anticoagulant medications may contribute to excessive bleeding problems, and those taking steroids may be at risk for acute adrenal crisis. The patient's physician may want to adjust these medications before an invasive dental procedure.

Management

All new dental disease should be treated after the transplant has stabilized.

- Check BP before beginning treatment. Know baseline levels for each patient and call the physician immediately if BP exceeds accepted normal ranges. Do not treat a patient when this problem is present.
- Examine the mouth thoroughly for dental infection, since immunosuppressive medication

can hide signs of a problem. As a result, infections may be more advanced than they appear. Treat all infections aggressively.

- Be aware of the patient's bleeding potential and take appropriate steps to manage excessive bleeding.
- Watch for signs of adrenal insufficiency with surgical stress in patients taking steroids. Although this emergency is rare, increased doses of steroids at the time of extensive dental procedures may be needed. A person experiencing this condition may become hypertensive, weak, feverish, and nauseated and should be transported immediately to a hospital for treatment.
- When the dentist plans to prescribe a drug the patient's physician should be consulted to ensure proper drug selection and dosing.
- Advise your patients to follow a conscientious oral hygiene routine and emphasize the importance of oral health before and after transplantation. Suggest an antimicrobial rinse when appropriate.

Oral Complications

Side effects from immunosuppressive drugs to prevent organ rejection are among the most frequent oral health problems affecting transplant recipients. Common immunosuppressive agents and their side effects include:

- ***Cyclosporine:*** Changes in liver/kidney function, hypertension, bleeding problems, and poor wound healing are among the adverse effects of this potent agent. This drug also interacts with a number of other drugs. Gingival hyperplasia occurs in some patients; incidence varies and is dependent on the individual patient's drug regimen. Children tend to be more susceptible to gingival overgrowth than adults. Emphasize conscientious daily oral hygiene to all patients.
- ***Tacrolimus:*** An immunosuppressive agent used increasingly in place of cyclosporine, tacrolimus causes less gingival overgrowth but is associated with oral ulcerations and numbness or tingling, especially around the mouth.
- ***Azathioprine:*** Bone marrow suppression and related complications such as stomatitis and opportunistic infections are significant side effects of this drug. A decrease in white blood cell counts and excessive bleeding may occur.
- ***Mycophenolate mofetil:*** This immunosuppressant is commonly used as an alternative to azathioprine. Adverse effects include decreased white cell counts, opportunistic infections, and gastrointestinal problems.
- ***Corticosteroids:*** Hypertension and high blood glucose (steroid-induced diabetes) are among the numerous side effects of these drugs, along with increased risk for infection, poor wound healing, and depression. Adrenal suppression may occur, making invasive dental and medical procedures more difficult for your patient. Corticosteroids may also mask the early signs of oral infection. The trend toward using lower doses of corticosteroids in combination with other immunosuppressants for posttransplant maintenance therapy has helped mitigate these side effects.
- ***Sirolimus:*** Side effects of this antirejection drug can include hypertension, joint pain, low white cell count, hypercholesterolemia, and oral ulceration.

Several complications associated with marked immunosuppression manifest in the mouth, including oral candidiasis, herpes simplex/herpes zoster, hairy leukoplakia, aphthous ulcers, and uncommon viral and fungal infections. Progressive periodontal disease, delayed wound healing, and excessive bleeding may also become problems for these patients.

Notify the patient's physician if these signs of marked immunosuppression are seen. In some cases, the dosage of antirejection agents prescribed for patients may need to be reduced. This may help control opportunistic infections and other oral complications. However, there will be patients who must be maintained on high-dose immunosuppression to prevent organ rejection. Treatment of oral opportunistic infection is necessary in any transplanted patient.

Immunosuppression can lead to development of malignancies. Posttransplant patients should be screened for oral malignancies at every appointment. Kaposi sarcoma, lymphoma, and squamous cell carcinoma of the lip are among the oral malignancies that sometimes occur in organ transplant patients. Malignancies can occur decades earlier in transplant recipients than in people who are not immunosuppressed.

If a patient's body begins to reject a transplanted organ, only emergency dental care may be provided. Talk with the patient's physician about management principles and antibiotic prophylaxis before treatment.

Management for issues identified from the client's responses will be dealt with by consulting the chapters that discuss the specific medical issue. Any warnings provided to the client by the transplant physician must be considered and implemented.

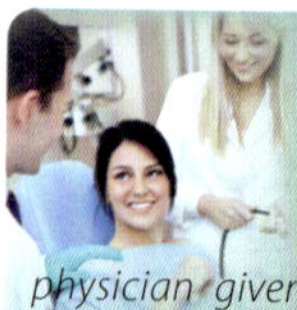

Follow-up Questions

"Do you have residual problems following your transplant? Has your physician given you any special instructions about receiving oral care?"

A medical consultation form should include any questions regarding what the client has told you, to verify understanding of the information. It is not uncommon for the client to become confused or understand physician recommendations incorrectly. Oral maintenance care may need to be scheduled quarterly rather than semiannually, depending on the health of the periodontal tissues. An oral cancer examination should be completed at every appointment due to the increased risk for cancer associated with immunosuppressant therapy.

Self-Study Review

14. Individuals with RA may have other autoimmune diseases. Prophylactic antibiotics are strongly recommended for these clients.
   a. Both statements are false.
   b. Both statements are true.
   c. The first statement is true, and the second statement is false.
   d. The first statement is false, and the second statement is true.

15. From the following list, identify the oral effects associated with posttransplant medications.
   a. Hemorrhage
   b. Poor wound healing
   c. Gingival hyperplasia
   d. Oral ulcerations
   e. Candidiasis
   f. Oral malignancies
   g. Hairy leukoplakia

Emergency Prevention

Emergency situations specific for the client with an organ transplant would involve the general health of the client. For the client waiting for a transplant the risks are much greater. When assessing the health of the client, vital signs should be taken during each appointment since the cardiovascular system can be affected by other organs. The risk of excessive bleeding should be considered when the failed organ could cause blood dyscrasias. Awareness of possible emergency situations that are possible with the specific medical health for the client is essential. Medical consultation might include a question about the risk for a medical emergency for the specific client's health status.

CHAPTER SUMMARY

This chapter detailed information related to managing clients who have a history of cancer therapy, DM, SLE, organ transplantation, and arthritis. Because these conditions involve immunosuppression, the clinician must be prepared to prevent and treat the condition itself as well as the effects of systemic treatment. Anticipating potential emergencies associated with these medical conditions is an essential component of treatment planning and delivery.

Review

1. Define the following terms: hyperglycemia, hypoglycemia, and osteoradionecrosis.
2. List three signs of undiagnosed diabetes.
3. Differentiate type 1 and type 2 DM.
4. Identify three disease conditions that involve persistent swollen glands or unexpected weight loss.

Case Study

Case A

Mrs. Meredith Swanson is a 55-year-old client who presents for an oral health evaluation. She reports a recent diagnosis of squamous cell carcinoma of the mandible and is scheduled for surgery and radiation therapy. The oncologist recommended that she undergo a comprehensive oral health evaluation before initiating cancer therapy. She is not undergoing any orthodontia and does not wear removable or fixed appliances. Vital signs include pulse 74 bpm, respiration 18 breaths/min, BP 130/60 mm Hg, right arm, sitting.

1. What steps should the dentist and dental hygienist take to perform a comprehensive oral health evaluation for this client?
2. List four benefits of providing oral care as part of a cancer pretreatment regimen.
3. What suggestions would you recommend if the client develops xerostomia associated with radiation therapy?
4. What questions should you ask the oncologist to prevent adverse emergency situations?
5. If the client presents for a follow-up appointment during cancer therapy and reports a platelet count of 40,000 platelets/mm^3, should treatment be postponed? Why or why not?
6. If the client develops oral mucositis, should chlorhexidine be used for treatment?

Case B

Mr. Peterson, a 38-year-old client, presents for a dental hygiene appointment. He reports a recent diagnosis of type 2 DM. He has been a client of the practice for 10 years, and dental records indicate that his oral health status is excellent. The client states that he is presently taking Glucotrol daily, has modified his diet, and exercises 3 to 4 days per week. He indicates that he is concerned about his oral health and is trying to adhere to his physician's recommendations. His blood glucose level taken just prior to coming to the appointment was 70 mm/dL. Vital signs include pulse 62 bpm, respiration 12 breaths/min, BP 118/64 mm Hg, left arm, sitting.

1. What follow-up questions should you ask based on the client's report of a recent diagnosis of DM?
2. During the course of the appointment, the client begins to experience perspiration, confusion, and lethargy. These signs represent what condition?
3. What management would you provide for the client who experiences perspiration, confusion, and lethargy?
4. What strategies could be used to prevent this type of emergency?

Chapter Eleven

Medical Conditions Involving the Cardiovascular System

Objectives

After completing the self-study chapter the reader will be able to:

- Identify examples of cardiovascular disease and explain the pathophysiology of each condition.
- Identify the clinical applications of information related to the client with cardiovascular diseases.
- Describe potential cardiovascular emergency situations, measures to prevent the occurrence of the emergency, and the management of the emergency should it occur.
- Identify oral healthcare procedures that may precipitate a migraine attack and information that helps prevent precipitation of migraine headache.

Key Terms

Angina pectoris: pain or pressure in the chest area often radiating to the left arm and caused most often by lack of oxygenated blood to heart muscle as a result of atherosclerosis of the coronary arteries

Atherosclerosis: plaques of cholesterol, lipids, and cellular debris in the inner layers of the walls of large- and medium-sized arteries

Bacteremia: the presence of bacteria within the bloodstream

Cerebral: having to do with the brain

Cerebrovascular accident: a stroke

Coronary: having to do with the heart, particularly the coronary arteries

Differential diagnosis: the determination of which one of several diseases may be producing the symptoms; possible diagnoses are recorded in order of probability, based on their prevalence and likelihood of causing the signs and symptoms

Dyspnea: shortness of breath or difficulty in breathing

Functional capacity: the ability to complete various physical activities, a measure of cardiac risk assessment

Ischemia: lack of oxygen to a tissue, usually as a result of blocked blood flow

Orthopnea: an abnormal condition in which the person must sit or stand to breathe deeply or comfortably

Stenosis: a constriction or narrowing of an opening or body passageway

MEDICAL CONDITION

INTRODUCTION

Cardiovascular disease (CVD) includes abnormal function of blood vessels and disease of the heart muscle. It can be congenital or acquired during the aging process. Those clients reporting risk factors for CVD (smoking, family history of CVD, diabetes mellitus, increased serum cholesterol levels, increased body weight, sedentary lifestyle) are at an increased risk for cardiac disease and cardiac-related emergency situations. CVD includes a variety of conditions ranging from hypertension to stroke to heart attack. It often leaves the client unable to respond to stressful situations. This inability to respond to stress is the main factor in precipitation of medical emergency situations in the dental office. When blood vessels are affected, conditions include **atherosclerosis**, **coronary artery disease**, and aneurysm (thin blood vessel walls, likely to rupture). Conditions related to disease in the heart muscle include myocardial infarction (MI; heart attack), heart failure (HF), and heart rhythm disorders. **Angina pectoris** is a situation that involves both blood vessel constriction or **stenosis** and heart muscle response.

DETECTION OF CVD

Cardiac disease may be present while the client is unaware of it. An example is hypertension, a condition that has no symptoms and is referred to as "the silent killer." Because of this fact the official American Dental Association (ADA) policy on screening for hypertension recommends that blood pressure be evaluated at the initial and annual recall dental appointments in both children and adults as a screening tool to identify undiagnosed CVD. A recent survey in 14 US states found that less than one-third of adults are aware of all five warning signs and symptoms of MI.[1] The authors explained that around 50% of all cardiac deaths occur within 1 hour of symptom onset, generally before individuals reach the hospital. This makes the identification of the warning signs very important to reducing death. It is logical when the client reports a history of CVD that precautions will be included in the oral healthcare treatment plan. However, when the client is undiagnosed, a situation exists in which unexpected emergency situations can occur. Vital sign measurements are the best clinical tool in the dental office to identify undiagnosed CVD.

"Please (X) a response to indicate if you have or have not had any of the following diseases or problems: CVD. If yes, specify below type of condition: angina, arteriosclerosis, coronary artery disease, chest pain upon exertion."

PATHOPHYSIOLOGY DISCUSSION

The conditions in the question above relate to the formation of atherosclerotic plaque deposited on the inner aspect or within the blood vessel walls, leaving them unable to fully dilate and respond to physiologic signals. The plaques may enlarge to the extent that the lumen of the affected blood vessel is narrowed or occluded, reducing the amount of blood to tissues supplied by the vessel. Pressure from the blood flow at the area of the obstruction can, over time, result in a ballooning and a thinning of the vessel wall. This leads to formation of an aneurysm in the vessel wall that can rupture. Another situation that reduces blood flow to tissues occurs when the atherosclerotic plaque breaks open (unstable plaque) and platelets form a clot to cover the damage. This causes a further narrowing or occlusion of the lumen of the blood vessel. The reduction of oxygenated blood to **coronary** tissues that follows this event results in a heart muscle response of pain, called angina or angina pectoris.

Angina Pectoris

Several events are likely to result in angina pectoris. When the heart rate increases, such as that which occurs during stress or exercise, the increased cardiac muscle function requires additional amounts of oxygenated blood. This is referred to as "increased cardiac workload." Diseased blood vessels compromised by atherosclerosis may be unable to dilate and supply the additional blood to cardiac tissue. Another situation that can result in reduced blood flow to coronary blood vessels (and cause angina) is when the blood flow is diverted to other areas of the body, such as after eating a large meal. Angina has been reported to occur after eating a heavy meal. Angina is characterized by pain in the chest that arises as a result of inadequate oxygenation of muscle tissue. It has been described as a "cramping, suffocating pain or pressure" in the chest area. Other signs include a sensation of numbness or tingling that may radiate to the shoulders, arms, jaws, or throat. It has been reported that craniofacial pain (jaw, teeth) can be the only symptom of cardiac ischemia (6% of cases) and should be considered in the **differential diagnosis** of toothache and orofacial pain.[2]

Either side of the body can be affected, but the most common area of discomfort is the left shoulder and arm. Angina is an important sign that indicates the presence of coronary artery disease and cholesterol-narrowed arteries, conditions that present an increased risk for an emergency during treatment. Clients who are experiencing frequent attacks, even though medication is taken to prevent them, are at an increased risk for a medical emergency. In addition, angina that is not relieved by rest has an increased risk.

Types of Angina

There are several types of angina. Stable angina is described as a condition resulting from coronary artery disease, usually triggered by physical exertion, that lasts from 1 to 15 minutes and is relieved by rest or the administration of sublingual nitroglycerin medication. Variant angina (also called vasospastic angina or Prinzmetal angina) is described as a sudden spasm of coronary arteries that narrows the artery and temporarily stops blood flow to part of the heart muscle, and is not associated with intravascular cholesterol plaques. It occurs at rest and exposure to cold and hyperventilation can induce a spasm. It is relieved by nitroglycerin. Unstable angina (now called acute coronary syndrome) is a sudden onset of pain (not relieved by rest) from blockage that reduces blood flow to cardiac muscle (often from intravascular clots) that can last up to 30 minutes and can lead to MI. Unstable angina is the result of severe, obstructive coronary artery disease. It poses the greatest risk for an adverse situation because of its unpredictability and possible progression to MI.[3]

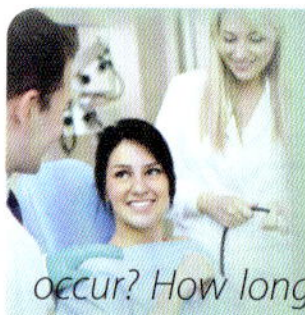

Follow-up Questions

"What usually causes your angina episode? How often does angina occur? How long does it last? Do you use nitroglycerin to manage the pain? Does rest help to relieve the pain? Have you ever needed to call for emergency assistance because of angina? Have you ever had a heart attack?"

Controlled angina is described as having an absence of signs or experiencing angina in situations when it would be expected, such as during excessive exercise. If the pain is relieved quickly after rest, it is considered to be less likely to progress to MI. Reports of an anginal event not relieved by rest, lasting 10 minutes or more, and requiring sublingual nitroglycerin or emergency medical assistance implies reduced control of the disease and carries an increased risk during stressful oral healthcare procedures.[2] When the client is at rest and develops chest pain in the dental office, activation of the emergency medical system (EMS) should be considered. Angina that culminated in a previous heart attack is a serious event that suggests an evaluation of **functional capacity** is needed before oral procedures. Severe chest pain accompanied by nausea or vomiting is a sign that an MI might be occurring.

APPLICATION TO PRACTICE

Determine whether angina is a current problem and what form of angina the client experiences. Question the client about the level of functional capacity (refer to Chapter 1) and ensure the client meets the 4 metabolic equivalent (MET) level of functional capacity.[3] Question the client to determine whether the symptoms usually resolve with rest or the client must take nitroglycerin to relieve the pain. Determine the frequency and pattern of attacks (e.g., at rest or only on exertion). Have the client bring the personal supply of nitroglycerin to the dental appointment. Check the expiration date on the bottle to verify the drug is active. This will influence the decision to treat or delay treatment (or have the office emergency supply of nitroglycerin available) and will guide management procedures should the client experience symptoms of angina during oral procedures. All clients reporting a history of CVD must have vital signs measured and assessed before initiating oral procedures and at every subsequent appointment. Because of these risks, it would be poor judgment to initiate treatment in a client with blood pressure values ≥180/110 mm Hg.[4] Failure to measure the blood pressure and pulse rate prevents the clinician from gaining important information needed to make proper clinical decisions. Generally, when angina is diagnosed the physician will prescribe rapid-acting nitroglycerin tablets for the client to carry at all times, and used if angina develops and is not relieved by rest. Other medication may be prescribed by the physician to *prevent* (rather than treat) anginal attacks (calcium channel blockers, long-acting nitroglycerin, others). These are not effective for relieving acute attacks. Questioning the client about the reasons medications are being taken may identify drugs prescribed for angina prophylaxis. If the client reports a history of recent anginal pain lasting longer than 15 minutes, and not relieved by rest, this is an indication of uncontrolled disease, especially if antianginal drugs are being taken. For these clients a medical consultation should be completed to determine the ability of the client to withstand the stress of elective oral care. The physician should be informed of the procedures planned and whether local anesthesia with vasoconstrictor will be used. The cardiac dose of 0.04 mg of vasoconstrictor should be used (no more than two cartridges of 1:100,000 epinephrine, or four cartridges of 1:200,000).[5] Local anesthetics with a vasoconstrictor should be used with caution in clients taking nonspecific β-blocker drugs (propranolol) and in poorly controlled anginal disease.[4]

POTENTIAL EMERGENCIES

Pain or pressure in the chest area causing anxiety in the client during treatment can be a frightening event, because one never knows whether it will resolve (stable angina) or progress to a life-threatening condition. Routine care should be limited to clients with stable angina who meet the 4 MET level of functional capacity, and for whom the pattern of symptoms has been unchanged for 2 months or in whom symptoms result after a predictable amount of exertion that are relieved by rest or nitroglycerin.[3]

Prevention

Treatment plan modifications to prevent an emergency situation include a stress reduction protocol (Box 11-1). Treatment plan modifications to respond quickly should angina occur include having nitroglycerin available during the appointment. Elective treatment should be delayed for the client with unstable angina or when a change in the pattern of symptoms has occurred in the previous few weeks. Monitor the vital signs at each appointment before deciding to continue with treatment. Do not treat the client with blood pressure values ≥180/110 mm Hg.[3–5]

Box 11-1

Stress Reduction Protocol

- Short appointments
- Be on time for appointment to reduce anxiety
- Use adequate measures to prevent pain during treatment
- Consider use of pretreatment antianxiety medication

Request the client to bring the personal prescription of nitroglycerin to the appointment. A stress reduction protocol should include measures to reduce pain or anxiety during treatment. Use the cardiac dose of vasoconstrictor. Local anesthetics without a vasoconstrictor may not provide adequate levels of pain control. Additionally, the dentist may decide to prescribe antianxiety medication (Valium®, Xanax®) to be taken before the appointment to reduce stress levels. Plan for short appointments at a time when the client is well rested. Watch the client during treatment for any signs of discomfort or stress. Oxygen should be easily available within the operatory if angina occurs during treatment.

Management

If angina occurs during the oral healthcare appointment, reposition the client to an upright position and reassure in an attempt to reduce anxiety. Provide 100% oxygen via an oxygen mask and ensure the client can breathe easily.

A flow of 4 L/ min via nasal cannula or 10 L/min via face mask minimizes the possibility of inadequate oxygenation.[5] Measure the blood pressure and the pulse for deviations from normal, paying attention to the regularity of the pulse. If pain persists, allow the client to place his or her own nitroglycerin tablet under the tongue and monitor the blood pressure after each dose of nitroglycerin. If systolic blood pressure is below 100 mm Hg, do not administer additional nitroglycerin as the vasodilating action of the drug could cause a severe loss of blood pressure.[5] Place no more than three sublingual tablets of nitroglycerin during a 10-minute period. Pain usually resolves within 5 minutes. If the pain is not relieved in 10 minutes, summon the EMS assistance (911). Provide basic life support and be prepared to institute cardiopulmonary resuscitation (CPR) if the event proceeds to cardiac arrest. When EMS arrives, provide information on vital sign values and qualities and a brief history of the emergency. Record the events of the emergency in the client's dental record (Box 11-2). For the client with no prior history of chest pain (marked "no" on health history) but if chest pain occurs during treatment, the EMS should be activated when chest pain persists for more than 2 minutes and before emergency kit nitroglycerin is administered.[5] In this case, the clinician does not know whether the client is experiencing angina or is having a heart attack, as both manifest as chest pain.

Box 11-2

Management of Angina in Client with History of Angina

- Reposition to upright position
- Reassure client, maintain composure
- Measure blood pressure and pulse, record values and qualities of pulse
- If systolic blood pressure is >100 mm Hg, place nitroglycerin sublingually
- Provide 100% oxygen
- Readminister sublingual nitroglycerin as needed (maximum three tablets in 10-minute period)
- If pain is not relieved in 10 minutes, summon 911 emergency medical system (call immediately in client with no history of angina)
- Record events of emergency in dental record

"Please (X) a response to indicate if you have or have not had any of the following diseases or problems: damaged heart valves, congenital heart defects, heart murmur, mitral valve prolapse, rheumatic heart disease."

These conditions all involve valvular heart disease, are associated with HF, and in some cases are at high risk for developing infective (or bacterial) endocarditis. Conditions that require antibiotic prophylaxis before oral procedures were discussed in Chapter 8. In the past, mitral valve prolapse, heart murmur, and rheumatic heart disease were recommended to have antibiotic prophylaxis before oral procedures, but these conditions were eliminated in the most recent guidelines. Heart murmur is a sign of a diseased cardiac valve. A replaced (prosthetic) cardiac valve is considered to be at risk for infection from **bacteremia**. Some developmental (also referred to as congenital) cardiac abnormalities are considered to be at high risk (refer to Chapter 8), although most other cardiac abnormalities have less risk for infection. It is not possible to identify which client will develop endocarditis or which invasive dental procedure may lead to the infection. There are currently no controlled human trials in clients with structural heart disease to definitively establish that antibiotic prophylaxis provides protection against endocarditis after invasive dental procedures. In fact, most cases of endocarditis are not associated with recent dental treatment.

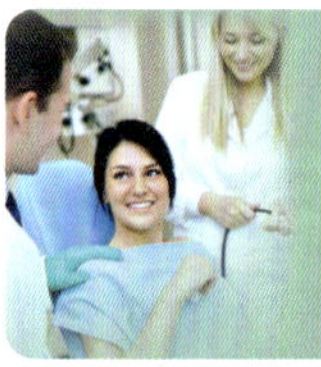

Follow-up Questions

"Have you been told to have antibiotics prior to dental treatment? Are you taking anticoagulant medications?"

The client who reports being told that a "heart murmur" existed at one time but that he or she "grew out of it" may have a transient physiologic murmur, called a functional heart murmur. An example of a functional murmur is one that occurs during pregnancy, but after the birth of the child it resolved to normal. Functional heart murmurs are not indicated for antibiotic prophylaxis. Clients who have cardiac valve replacements are indicated for antibiotic prophylaxis prior to most oral procedures and take anticoagulant medications (i.e., warfarin) to prevent clot formation around the valve replacement. They are generally kept at international normalized ratio (INR) values up to 3.5, which pose a low risk for excessive bleeding (refer to Chapter 9).

APPLICATION TO PRACTICE

Valvular cardiac disease has no specific clinical implications, with the exception of a cardiac valve replacement. Congenital heart defects are clinically important only if they are in the selected group of conditions that are to be considered for antibiotic prophylaxis or if the damage to cardiac function causes reduced functional capacity below the 4 MET level. A physician consultation should be completed to determine specific medical recommendations prior to oral procedures. The AHA has recommended against antibiotic prophylaxis before dental procedures for nonvalvular devices, such as stents, patches, and vascular grafts.[6]

Artificial Heart Valve with Anticoagulant Therapy

The earlier discussion related to an increased risk for bacterial endocarditis applies to the client with an artificial heart valve. In addition, the client with a prosthetic cardiac valve usually is taking anticoagulant therapy (Coumadin®), and INR values should be determined when procedures are planned that involve bleeding. Increased bleeding that may occur can often be managed with digital pressure. Rinses containing tranexamic acid or aminocaproic acid may be used to promote clotting after oral health care that involves bleeding.[5]

Self-Study Review

1. Jaw pain may be associated with angina or MI due to cardiac ischemia.
   a. Both the statement and reason are correct and related.
   b. Both the statement and reason are correct, but NOT related.
   c. The statement is correct, but the reason is NOT.
   d. The statement is NOT correct, but the reason is correct.
   e. NEITHER the statement NOR the reason is correct.

2. The form of angina that poses the greatest risk of emergency is:
   a. stable angina.
   b. variant angina.
   c. acute coronary syndrome.
   d. all forms pose equal risk.

3. The recommended cardiac dose of vasoconstrictor in local anesthesia is:
   a. 0.01 mg.
   b. 0.02 mg.
   c. 0.03 mg.
   d. 0.04 mg.

4. The maximum dose of nitroglycerin sublingual tablets that should be administered during a 10-minute period is:
   a. 1 tablet.
   b. 2 tablets.
   c. 3 tablets.
   d. 4 tablets.

5. What percentage of cardiac deaths occur within 1 hour of onset of symptoms?
   a. 20
   b. 30
   c. 40
   d. 50

6. Signs of bacterial endocarditis include unexplained fever and lethargy. These signs tend not to occur when prophylactic antibiotics are given before dental procedures are performed.
   a. Both statements are true.
   b. Both statements are false.
   c. The first statement is true, and the second statement is false.
   d. The first statement is false, and the second statement is true.

7. Elective oral healthcare procedures should be postponed when the blood pressure values are greater than 180/110 mm Hg. If the client takes Coumadin, an INR value of 4.5 is acceptable for reducing the risk of hemorrhage during dental treatment.
   a. Both statements are true.
   b. Both statements are false.
   c. The first statement is true, and the second statement is false.
   d. The first statement is false, and the second statement is true.

POTENTIAL EMERGENCIES

The most likely medical emergencies in the client with cardiac disease involve inability to respond to stress during treatment. In addition, there is a risk for increased bleeding in the client taking anticoagulant drug therapy (Coumadin®, INR >3.5). Signs of bacterial endocarditis would not be evident until several weeks after oral procedures so would not be an immediate emergency situation.

Prevention

Monitoring the vital signs and functional capacity to assess control of cardiac disease, requesting information about the medical recommendations regarding the need for antibiotic prophylaxis, and determining whether excessive bleeding is likely to occur during treatment are the main issues to consider. Follow the recommended protocols based on the client's cardiac condition and previous history of infective endocarditis. For instances in which the healthcare provider is unsure whether the cardiac condition requires antibiotic prophylaxis, seek medical consultation with written medical recommendations related to the need for prophylactic antibiotics (the fax machine is very useful for these written recommendations). This written recommendation should be placed in the client's chart. For clients with cardiac disease and hypertension, do not provide elective oral health care when blood pressure values are greater than 180/110 mm Hg. If warfarin (Coumadin®) is being taken, request INR values and determine whether the client is at risk for uncontrolled bleeding. Instruct the client to call the dentist if signs of endocarditis (unexplained fever, lethargy) develop after oral procedures, even if the antibiotic prophylactic regimen was taken. There are reports of endocarditis developing in clients who received antibiotic prophylaxis before dental procedures.[7]

Management

If the client shows signs of cardiovascular stress (perspiration, nausea, shortness of breath, pressure in the chest area), institute basic life support to maintain an open airway and to ensure that breathing and circulation are adequate. Provide 100% oxygen as needed. If rest does not resolve cardiovascular stress, call for EMS to transport the client to the hospital for medical evaluation. Excessive bleeding problems that occur during treatment may be resolved with digital pressure or local hemostatic agents (Gelfoam®, oxidized cellulose) as discussed in Chapter 9.

"Please (X) a response to indicate if you have or have not had any of the following diseases or problems: congestive HF or HF."

PATHOPHYSIOLOGY DISCUSSION

HF is defined as a clinical syndrome characterized by dyspnea and fatigue and signs of edema on physical examination.[8] It is a clinical diagnosis based on the medical history and physical examination of the client. New guidelines on the management of the condition dropped the term "congestive" from the name because the term "HF" better reflects the spectrum of heart diseases.[8] Individuals without congestion symptoms may still have a severely abnormal heart. The ADA health history includes the former term "congestive HF" because the majority of individuals with HF will manifest disease on the left side of the heart and have congestion in the lungs as a result of pressure within the left side of the heart, which forces fluid from the circulation into the lungs. When the left ventricle is compromised by disease so that it no longer can function to full capacity to pump blood from the heart, the condition is called HF. The result of HF is a reduced output of oxygenated blood as a result of the failure of left ventricular function, with, eventually, kidney function becoming compromised as a result of the reduced cardiac output. The heart rate may increase to supply the body's needs for oxygenated blood. When the left ventricular contraction fails to empty all blood, ventricular enlargement and stretching of cardiac muscle fibers results, making them less efficient. With time, the muscle stretches and loses its ability to function properly. Cardiovascular conditions that lead to a "failing heart" include MI, arrhythmias, congenital heart disease, and valvular abnormalities. Hypertension is commonly found in the client with HF. The American College of Cardiology and the American Heart Association classification for HF is used to guide dental treatment decisions.[8]

Class A: at risk for HF due to presence of hypertension, coronary artery disease, diabetes, alcohol abuse, or history of rheumatic heart disease or cardiomyopathy; no limitation of physical activity, absence of dyspnea, fatigue, or heart irregularities, or palpitation with normal physical activity.

Class B: structural heart disease associated with development of HF, but have not progressed to HF; mild symptoms of fatigue, palpitation, or dyspnea with normal physical activity, comfortable at rest.

Class C: structural heart disease and symptoms of HF; marked limitation of activity; normal physical activity produces increased symptoms described in class B, but client is comfortable at rest.

Class D: advanced structural disease and marked symptoms of HF at rest despite medical therapy; symptoms are present even when client is at rest, and mild physical activity increases symptoms.

The traditional clinical manifestations of HF represents stages C and D, which manifest impairment of either the left or right ventricle.

Right Ventricular Heart Failure

When the right side of the heart fails, pressure is produced in tissues that feed blood to the right ventricle (e.g., lower extremities). Edema can develop in the feet, ankles, and lower legs. This is usually treated with diuretics. As the condition worsens, the client may experience extreme fatigue and develop cyanosis of mucous membranes (lips, nail beds). The client with symptoms of right-sided congestive HF can be identified in the extraoral examination.

Left Ventricular Heart Failure

When the left side of the heart fails, edema collects in the lungs, causing **dyspnea**. This pulmonary fluid collection causes the client to have difficulty breathing when placed in a supine position, a condition described as **orthopnea**. The client may be unable to tolerate being placed in a supine position because of an inability to breathe easily. Those clients who have a history of awakening from sleep and being short of breath have a greater degree of disease. Generally the left side of the heart fails first, followed soon thereafter by the right side.

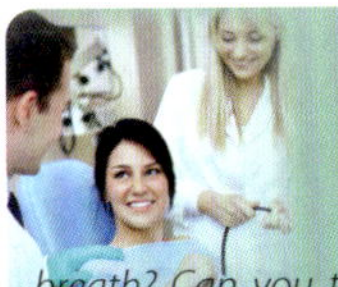

Follow-up Questions

"Do you need several pillows to sleep? Do you awaken from sleep short of breath? Can you tolerate being placed in a supine chair position for treatment? Can you walk up a flight of stairs without stopping to rest? How often do you see your physician to monitor your HF?"

Questioning should reveal the client with poorly controlled HF, who requires medical consultation before treatment. Consultation must determine the degree of disease control and the client's ability to tolerate receiving oral procedures. The client who requires an upright position to sleep, who awakens from sleep with respiratory difficulty, or who is unable to accomplish skills requiring minor exertion poses an increased risk for a medical emergency during treatment. An inability to climb a flight of stairs or carry in a bag of groceries without shortness of breath or fatigue may reflect poor functional capacity (less than 4 METs), which carries an increased risk for an emergency during oral procedures. The client who is symptomatic (dyspnea, fatigues easily) and who is not receiving medical care to control symptoms of HF poses a risk in treatment. The risk of treating a client with symptomatic HF is that symptoms could worsen, resulting in a fatal arrhythmia, stroke, or MI.[5] The client with mild dyspnea or fatigue can be treated in the dental office, but should be monitored for signs of acute pulmonary edema leading to cardiac failure.

APPLICATION TO PRACTICE

Elective dental treatment can be provided for clients in classes A and B. Class C clients require medical consultation before oral procedures and may need to receive treatment in a hospital setting where emergency equipment is available. Class D clients should not receive elective treatment until HF is better controlled. Emergency dental treatment should be provided in a hospital setting.[5] The client with a history of HF may have hypertension, coronary artery disease, or valvular disease. Evaluation of the client should be directed at identifying those cardiac problems that may coexist and managing them accordingly. Vital signs should be monitored at each appointment. The pulse and respiration rates are often increased.[4]

Attention should be paid to respiration sounds as that may indicate poorly controlled disease (pulmonary edema). The client who experiences orthopnea, extreme fatigue, or nocturnal dyspnea should only be treated after medical management to improve disease control. HF clients often request alteration of the chair position to a semiupright position. This improves the ability to breathe easily. Use a stress reduction protocol, plus supplemental oxygen when indicated. Nitrous oxide can be used in nonsymptomatic clients.[5] First-line medications for HF include diuretics to reduce fluid collection. All medications should be investigated for potential side effects and dental drug interactions that may affect the oral care treatment plan. Orthostatic hypotension is an example of a drug side effect that can result in an emergency situation. Vasoconstrictors in local anesthetics may be contraindicated in the poorly controlled client (determine at medical consultation).

POTENTIAL EMERGENCIES

Acute pulmonary edema is a potential life-threatening emergency situation. The onset of symptoms occurs quickly with a dry cough as the initial symptom, followed by wheezing. As the event progresses, the client feels suffocated and is anxious. Respiration increases as the client struggles to breathe, leading to hyperventilation. For the HF client who is controlled with medication, the clinician should monitor for signs of orthopnea and provide positioning to support breathing.

Prevention

When assessment of respiratory or voice sounds reveals sounds representative of congestion, with a respiration rate of more than 20 breaths/minute, the client should be referred for medical evaluation. Elective oral care should be deferred until disease control has been established. Emergency dental care should be completed in a hospital setting. Use of vasoconstrictors is contraindicated in poorly controlled clients.[5] A semiupright chair position is recommended for individuals with controlled HF who request it. Even though the client may prefer a more upright position, this does not mean that pulmonary edema is present. The absence of fluid in the lungs (noiseless respiration) and a respiration rate within normal limits are signs of disease control. In terms of drug side effects, follow the protocol for prevention of orthostatic hypotension at the end of the appointment by allowing the client to sit upright for a few minutes to allow for a physiologic increase in the blood pressure. Blood pressure can be measured before releasing the client from the dental chair to ensure that blood pressure levels are adequate to prevent loss of consciousness. If digitalis is being taken, monitor for an exaggerated gagging reflex. Vasoconstrictors in local anesthesia should be used in low concentrations (cardiac dose).

Management

Acute pulmonary edema is a life-threatening condition in which fluid collects in the alveolar spaces of lungs, causing extreme difficulty in breathing. The client experiencing acute respiratory distress will cough and may experience hyperventilation. Mucous secretions may be produced by the coughing and should be expectorated. Placing the client in an upright position to ensure an open airway is essential. Provide 100% oxygen at 10 L/min with a face mask, as needed. The client generally will remain conscious.[5] At the onset of respiratory distress, summon the 911 EMS and provide basic life support to the client. Vital signs must be monitored every 5 minutes and recorded in the record. The client may experience anxiety and should be reassured, in an effort to reduce cardiac distress. Reduction of stress and placement in an upright position to support breathing will reduce the cardiac workload and help reduce symptoms until the EMS response team arrives. Sublingual nitroglycerin may also help reduce cardiovascular symptoms.

"Please (X) a response to indicate if you have or have not had any of the following diseases or problems: heart attack."

PATHOPHYSIOLOGY DISCUSSION

Heart attack or MI is most often caused by atherosclerosis in coronary arteries, vasospasm, or thrombotic blockage of coronary arteries that fail to supply sufficient blood supply to the heart muscle. Other etiologic factors include muscle degeneration (myopathy) and complications producing scarring and failure of the muscle to function normally.[4] This cardiac **ischemia** leads to ventricular dysrhythmia and fibrillation. It is the single leading cause of death in the United States. Stress can lead to an increased heart rate and increased workload on the cardiac muscle. If disease has compromised the heart muscle and atherosclerosis or blood clots stop the flow of oxygenated blood, the affected heart muscle can die. This is a brief description of what occurs in a heart attack. The heart muscle is left damaged, and the process is more likely to occur again within the next month.[3,5] For this reason, oral care is contraindicated for the first month after a heart attack to allow the condition to stabilize.[5] Signs of MI include a squeezing sensation in the chest; pain in the chest that may radiate to the arms, neck, back, or jaw; difficulty in breathing; perspiration; nausea; vital sign abnormalities (hypertension, dysrhythmia); and a feeling of impending doom.[4]

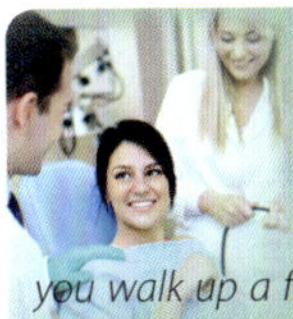

Follow-up Questions

"How long has it been since your heart attack? How is your health now? Can you walk up a flight of stairs without having to stop and rest? Can you walk a block without becoming short of breath? What medications are you taking?"

Follow-up questions relate to client recovery from the cardiac event and gaining a 4 MET level of functional capacity, restoration of normal cardiac function, and determining the risk of a cardiac event during oral treatment, as well as anticoagulant medications that must be investigated.

APPLICATION TO PRACTICE

Do not provide elective oral health care during the 1-month period following a heart attack. Determine whether adequate functional capacity (such as walking up a flight of stairs, walking a block without becoming short of breath, etc.) has been regained.[3] Written consultation with the client's physician is advisable for potentially stressful procedures.[4] Monitor the vital signs before and after the appointment to determine the degree of hypertensive risk. Investigate drugs being taken to determine side effects that may influence treatment. Use a stress reduction protocol with short appointments and procedures to prevent pain to reduce added stress. For stressful oral procedures, the dentist may prescribe a drug to reduce anxiety, to be taken before the appointment. Use the cardiac dose of vasoconstrictor in local anesthesia (no more than two cartridges of 1:100,000 vasoconstrictor); inject slowly using an aspirating syringe.[4]

POTENTIAL EMERGENCIES

Acute MI (AMI) is possible. As with all CVD the client may be unable to respond to the physiologic requirements on the cardiovascular system in stressful dental procedures. If anticoagulant medication is taken, increased bleeding may result.

Prevention

Delay elective treatment until after the 1-month period following a heart attack to allow for recovery from the event. Request a medical clearance asking if adequate functional capacity has been regained and if there are contraindications for dental treatment. Do not provide treatment when blood pressure values are excessive. Follow all procedures to reduce stress during the provision of services. Observe the client for signs of a heart attack and stop treatment if signs occur. Call 911 immediately if signs of MI occur in a client who has not reported a history of CVD or previous MI. Investigate medications being taken, paying attention to dental considerations for drug actions and adverse effects.

Management

If chest pain develops during the appointment, oral procedures should be terminated and the conscious client positioned to an upright position. If rest does not eliminate signs that indicate AMI is occurring, activate the 911 EMS. Because chest pain mimics that seen in angina, it is difficult to differentiate between these symptoms. For this reason, initial management is usually directed toward rest and relieving chest pain. This is accomplished by having the dentist provide sublingual nitroglycerin (up to three doses during a 10-minute period). If the pain is not relieved by 10 minutes, the client may be suffering a recurrent heart attack and the 911 EMS should be activated. Provide 100% oxygen and monitor vital signs. Have the client chew a 325-mg aspirin tablet, or crush a tablet of aspirin, and have the client swallow the granules with water. Provide basic life support until the EMS team arrives, particularly adequate oxygenation. If the heart stops beating before the arrival of the EMS team, start CPR procedures and continue until the EMS team arrives. The 2010 AHA recommendations advise either compression only or traditional CPR if the operator feels qualified.[9]

Self-Study Review

8. For which classes of HF can dental and dental hygiene care be provided without the need for a medical clearance?
   a. Class A
   b. Class B
   c. Class C
   d. Class D
9. Edema of the feet, ankles, and lower legs is indicative of:
   a. right-sided congestive HF.
   b. left-sided congestive HF.
   c. orthopnea.
   d. compromised kidney function.
10. The leading cause of death in the United States is attributed to:
    a. angina pectoris.
    b. congenital heart disease.
    c. congestive HF.
    d. MI.
11. Elective oral health care after MI is contraindicated for 1 month:
    a. Because congestive HF may occur in this time period.
    b. To allow the heart a chance to repair itself.
    c. To reduce the chance of blood clot formation.
    d. To reduce the chance of bacteremia.
12. If a client is suspected of having an MI, which of the following medications should be administered as part of emergency management?
    a. Sublingual nitroglycerin
    b. Aspirin
    c. Inderal
    d. Beta-blocker

After the release of the client to the EMS team, record the events of the emergency and the procedures followed in the dental record.

"Please (X) a response to indicate if you have or have not had any of the following diseases or problems: high blood pressure, low blood pressure."

Blood pressure is the force against which the heart must pump to perfuse the body with blood. Systolic pressure is the pressure in the blood vessels when the heart contracts and pumps blood. Diastolic pressure is the pressure in the vascular system when the heart is filling. In the recent Joint National Commission for Hypertension (JNC8) guidelines, hypertension is defined as blood pressure at or above a systolic measurement of 140 mm Hg or a diastolic measurement at or above 90 mm Hg. This disease directly increases the risk of MI, HF, stroke, renal failure, and atherosclerosis. Data from the 1999–2000 National Health and Nutrition Examination Survey (NHANES) indicated that the prevalence of hypertension increased to 29% in the United States after being at or below 25% for the last 30 years. The Centers for Disease Control report a prevalence of 28.6% in 2009–2010. The NHANES Survey is taken every 10 years to examine America's health. From the data reported, 58 million people have high blood pressure and many individuals affected were unaware of their condition. Both agencies suggest many diagnosed individuals were not receiving adequate medical treatment to reduce blood pressure levels. Treatment for hypertension includes reducing risk factors for hypertension (stop smoking, lose weight, reduce cholesterol serum levels, exercise, and so forth) and taking effective antihypertensive drugs.

PATHOPHYSIOLOGY DISCUSSION

The cause of hypertension is unknown, but it is related to lifestyle behaviors, such as smoking, being overweight, and having high cholesterol blood levels.[10] Other factors include having diabetes and being of the male sex, of African-American race, of increased age, and in poor physical condition. Although the cause is unclear at this time, it is known that atherosclerosis plays a major role by narrowing the lumen of the blood vessels and by reducing the ability of the smooth muscle of the blood vessel to dilate. The kidneys play a role by secreting substances, like vasopressin, that promote vasoconstriction (which increases pressure within arteries) and by retaining fluid in the body, thereby increasing peripheral resistance within the blood vessel (results in increased pressure within blood vessel). Sodium restriction has been suggested as a means to reduce fluid retention, leading to reduced blood pressure. As one has determined after reading the information in Chapter 1, hypertension is an indication of CVD and is found in many non-CVDs (diabetes, hyperthyroidism).

Low Blood Pressure

Low blood pressure occurs as a result of increased blood loss, leading to shock, or as a result of taking vasodilating medications. Medications that lower blood pressure are the most likely cause of hypotension in the dental client. The dental client with low blood pressure may experience loss of consciousness or fainting when arising from the dental chair after treatment. Using the protocol to prevent orthostatic hypotension after oral health care would be appropriate in this situation.

APPLICATION TO PRACTICE

Measurement of blood pressure as a screening device to identify the client with CVD is recognized as the standard of care before dental procedures and is suggested as a responsibility of dental clinicians.[10] The relevance of measuring blood pressure is discussed in Chapter 1 of this self-study. Because hypertension is most often not accompanied by symptoms, blood pressure should be monitored regularly. It is an essential factor in determining whether to continue with elective treatment or to send the client for medical evaluation. A blood pressure value higher than 180/110 mm Hg is an indication of severe CVD, and the client should be referred for immediate medical evaluation. Elective dental procedures are not recommended when blood pressure is in this category.[3,4] Increases in blood pressure caused by anxiety (white coat hypertension) can be lowered with nitrous oxide and oxygen analgesia. Nitrous oxide will not lower blood pressure from hypertensive disease.

"Please (X) a response to indicate if you have or have not had any of the following diseases or problems: pacemaker or implanted cardiac device."

Implanted cardiovascular devices are becoming the standard care for arrhythmia and other rhythm disturbances (such as a prolonged QT interval) within the heart. They are being used for managing symptoms of HF in some cases. Before the introduction of these devices individuals whose heart rates were slow often developed syncope and unconsciousness. Other individuals would develop rapid heart rates, leading to MI. The technology has developed in the recent past to design smaller device sizes and to extend battery longevity in implanted devices, such as pacemakers and implanted cardiodefibrillators (ICDs). These devices are designed to mimic the natural heart rate, in that they sense spontaneous cardiac depolarization and inhibit pacemaker output, allowing units to work only when required and thereby extending battery life to 10 or more years.[11]

The advent of small wireless implantable loop recorders which are implanted subcutaneously close to the heart resulted in a major breakthrough in diagnostic cardiology. These devices continuously monitor the electrical activity of the heart, store rhythm disturbance information, and provide information on cardiac events. The demand pacemaker (also referred to as "pacemaker") is the fundamental unit in use today for treating bradycardia. When the individual experiences inappropriate atrial tachycardia, the ICD provides a stimulus to slow the heart rate.

A pacemaker is an electrical device attached to the heart muscle to regulate the rhythm of a slow heart rate. Some individuals with a pacemaker may also have an ICD device. The purpose of the ICD is to deliver a shock to regulate heart rhythm during tachyarrhythmia. More than 2 million pacemakers are in use worldwide and over 400,000 ICDs.[12] Pacemakers with current technology are shielded and may have defibrillators to assist in maintaining heart rhythm function. Shielding protects some pacemakers from microwave electrical energy and from dental equipment that gives off electromagnetic energy, such as ultrasonic devices. The manufacturers of the pacemaker units in the United States have reported no interference between ultrasonic scaling equipment and pacemaker units.[13]

PATHOPHYSIOLOGY DISCUSSION

Pacemakers are placed to manage arrhythmias, symptomatic sinus bradycardia, and symptomatic atrioventricular (AV) block. Pacemakers work in a variety of ways, but in general, are not attached directly to cardiac muscle. They are implanted under the skin and have wires that are inserted through a vein and connected within the chambers to attach to cardiac muscle. The electrical component in the pacemaker senses the regularity of the heartbeat and stimulates the heart to normalize the heart rate. The units are about the size of a silver dollar and are placed in the upper shoulder area on the nondominant side.[14] The pacemaker acts like a computer in that it collects and stores information on cardiac rhythm events. The device uses this information to adjust the heart rate and, through sensing, deliver the most appropriate pacing therapy for the patient. Infective endocarditis rarely occurs from pacemakers. Therefore, it is not among the cardiovascular situations that are recommended for antibiotic prophylaxis to prevent bacterial endocarditis. A recent in vitro study (not with human subjects) determined whether electromagnetic interference with implantable pacemaker/ICD units was possible during the use of a variety of dental equipment.[15] Ten different devices, including an ultrasonic scaler, were tested. Only one ultrasonic bath cleaner interfered with two of the ICD units tested, and only up to a distance of 12.5 cm. This occurred both during continuous use and intermittent operation of the ultrasonic bath unit. All other equipment tested failed to produce interference. The authors concluded that normal clinical use of dental electrical equipment does not have significant effects on the ICDs tested. Other dental equipment that may cause electromagnetic interference with some types of implanted cardiac devices include electrocautery units and electric pulp testers.[5] The American Academy of Oral Medicine recommends avoiding use of external electromagnetic devices, such as electrosurgical units and transcutaneous electrical nerve stimulator (TENS) units, when the client has a pacemaker.[4]

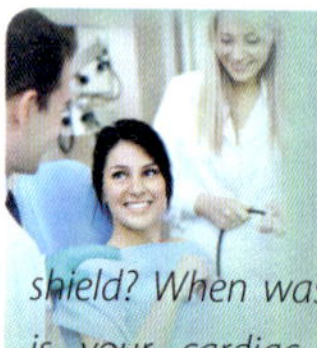

Follow-up Questions

"When was your pacemaker implanted? Does the pacemaker have a shield? When was the function last checked? How often is your cardiac condition and pacemaker medically evaluated? Has your physician warned you about dental equipment that may interfere with your pacemaker? Has the device regulated your heart rate?"

Due to the better technology in units manufactured within the past 10 years, most devices worn by cardiac patients will be shielded and will resist the possibility of electromagnetic interference. Units implanted in the 1990s or before could be disrupted by electromagnetic interference. It is important to determine whether enough time has elapsed to determine the function of the pacemaker to control a cardiac arrhythmia and bring the disease into a controlled state. Although there is no official recommendation in this regard, the client should be questioned to determine whether medical evaluation is being conducted on a regular basis. Most clients will be seeing the cardiologist or physician on a quarterly basis to monitor disease control and pacemaker function. Newer pacemaker devices are shielded against most electrical interference.

APPLICATION TO PRACTICE

In the past, pacemakers were considered to be a risk factor for infective endocarditis, but recent recommendations do not recommend antibiotic prophylaxis for the client with a pacemaker. Because heart rhythm abnormalities are a main reason for implantation of a pacemaker, the clinician should note qualities of the pulse (regularity, strength). If abnormalities are discovered the client should be referred for medical evaluation and treatment rescheduled until the physician releases the client for oral procedures.

POTENTIAL EMERGENCIES

There may be a low risk for the ultrasonic bath cleaner within 12.5 cm from the pacemaker unit to interfere with the function of the shielded pacemaker. This could interrupt the operation of the pacemaker and stimulate a cardiac arrhythmia. This equipment should not be placed closer than 3 feet to the client with a pacemaker/ICD is in the operatory.

"Please (X) a response to indicate if you have or have not had any of the following diseases or problems: stroke."

PATHOPHYSIOLOGY DISCUSSION

A stroke, or **cerebrovascular accident** (CVA), occurs when oxygenated blood fails to nourish tissues in the brain. This is called **cerebral** ischemia. A prolonged ischemic event in the brain can result in loss of neurologic function. There are three main causes of stroke: arterial thrombosis, such as a clot forming over a ruptured area of atherosclerosis; an embolism, such as a blood clot that dislodges from a remote site and occludes a blood vessel; and hemorrhage after a rupture in an aneurysm affecting the blood vessel.[16] These result in the two main types of stroke, occlusive or ischemic stroke and cerebral hemorrhage. Atherosclerosis in a blood vessel promotes all of these events. Hypertension is commonly found in the stroke victim and is a result of atherosclerosis. Signs of stroke may include severe headache (more commonly in the hemorrhagic type), having visual abnormalities, confusion, slurred speech or inability to speak, numbness, and losing the feeling on one side of the body.[4] Headache associated with acute stroke generally starts on the first day of the stroke and tends to be continuous, according to a recent study.[17] In more than half of the study patients, the headache appeared to be a reactivation of a previous headache. In this study of 124 individuals, preliminary diagnosis was that 61% experienced ischemic stroke and 39% had hemorrhagic stroke. Headache began on the first day of stroke in 86% of the patients, was more severe on the first day, and lasted an average of 3.8 days. Around 40% of individuals also experienced nausea and vomiting. The authors concluded that in this group of individuals headache appeared to be an entity that was reactivated by a brain insult, and not specific for stroke. Unequal pupil size is another sign of a stroke. A stroke-in-evolution causes symptoms for several hours and continues to worsen. The intellect often remains intact and the affected individual can respond to questioning. Signs and symptoms depend on the site, duration of occlusion, collateral circulation, and severity of the stroke.[4] Oral signs associated with a stroke include slurred speech, weak palate, and difficulty in swallowing. Clients who have a history of a stroke should not receive elective dental treatment for 6 months after the event to allow the brain to recover.[5]

Transient Ischemic Attack

A transient ischemic attack (TIA) is often referred to as "mini-stroke" and is a warning sign of a stroke. Sixty percent of strokes seen after a TIA in individuals with intracranial atherosclerotic disease occur within 90 days of the index event.[18] The risk of an early stroke (within 3 to 4 months) after a TIA is comparable to the risk seen after a prior stroke and should have the same 6-month period before elective oral procedures are planned. A TIA results from temporary ischemia of a localized area of the brain produced by blockage of a blood vessel (usually by a clot) or another event that narrows carotid arteries in the neck or a large artery in the brain.[5] This blood vessel disturbance requires immediate treatment to prevent a subsequent stroke. It is rapid in onset and has the same signs as a stroke but the client recovers quickly, usually within 10 minutes. A similar event, called a reversible ischemic neurologic deficit (RIND), does not clear within 24 hours, but eventually recovery does occur. Unilateral numbness (face, arm, leg) is a significant sign, as well as speech disturbances, usually resolving within 10 to 60 minutes. Having a TIA is a strong predictor for experiencing a CVA over the next 6 months. To respond to this risk, the client who has had a TIA will often be placed on anticoagulant therapy for a short time after the event.

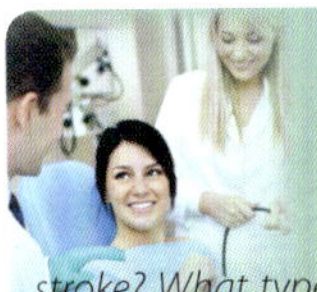

Follow-up Questions

"Did you have a TIA or a stroke? How long has it been since you suffered the stroke? What type of stroke did you have? Do you have a resulting loss of function in any part of your body? What medications are you taking? Are you recovered and has your physician given you any warnings about having a dental appointment?"

A positive response to this question requires the need to determine whether the condition was a TIA or a stroke and information about the recovery from the event. Many individuals recover following a TIA, but are placed on anticoagulant therapy for several months, to prevent ischemic stroke. If the TIA event resolved and 1 year has passed without another incident the risk is low.[5] Most clients will be taking anticoagulant medications that will need to be investigated in terms of their risks for increased bleeding during oral procedures. Neurologic deficiencies may have resulted that affect the ability to perform effective plaque removal. Speech impairment may have resulted, affecting the client's ability to communicate.

APPLICATION TO PRACTICE

When either stroke or TIA is reported on the health history elective dental treatment should be delayed for a 6-month period. For the client taking anticoagulant medications (Coumadin®), the INR value should be determined before procedures that can result in bleeding. When antiplatelet medications are taken (aspirin, Plavix®), bleeding should be monitored during treatment as there are no reliable laboratory tests to predict hemorrhage. If the stroke resulted in paralysis or loss of neurologic function, retraining in all aspects of daily oral care may be necessary. Power-assisted toothbrushes, flossing aids, antiseptic mouthrinses, and daily fluoride therapy may be needed for caries, gingivitis, and plaque control.[16] Short, mid-afternoon appointments and monitoring of blood pressure should be planned for post-CVA clients as blood pressure is lowest in the afternoon.[4] A stress reduction protocol should be implemented, including good pain control. Use of nitrous oxide analgesia is acceptable so long as good oxygenation is provided.[5] The single greatest risk factor leading to stroke is hypertension. For this reason, the vital signs should be monitored at every appointment. Dental medications that should be used with caution include central nervous system depressants (opioids), no gingival retraction cord with epinephrine, and no more than two 1.8-mL carpules of 2% lidocaine with 1:100,000 epinephrine.[4]

POTENTIAL EMERGENCIES

The most likely medical emergencies during oral health care for a client with this history would include increased bleeding from anticoagulant drug therapy. In clients with excessively high blood pressure, there is a risk of having another stroke during treatment.

Prevention

Monitor the blood pressure and do not provide elective treatment when the values are excessive (≥180/110 mm Hg). Follow a protocol for stress reduction. Assure that the 6-month recommendation for delaying elective treatment is followed. If hypertension is not controlled with medication, request a medical clearance from the client's physician regarding the client's ability to withstand the stress of dental treatment. This should be completed before providing oral care. Obtain laboratory values for anticoagulant medication (INR) to determine the risks for uncontrolled bleeding, and delay dental procedures involving bleeding when the INR exceeds the recommended values.

Management

If the client experiences signs of a stroke, stop the procedure and place the client in a comfortable position with the head slightly elevated.[4] In most cases, the victim will remain conscious and be able to answer questions. Four simple questions can be used to determine if a client is presenting with signs of a stroke. Ask the individual to smile, raise both arms, speak a simple sentence, and stick out the tongue. In 2013, the American Heart Association and American Stroke Association (AHA/ASA) updated 2009 guidelines for management of acute ischemic stroke.[19] Guidelines call for activation of the 911 EMS immediately when signs indicate acute stroke. Basic life support should be provided, ensuring the airway is open and providing ventilatory assistance, as needed. Supplemental oxygen is not recommended in the 2013 AHA/ASA guidelines in nonhypoxic patients with acute ischemic stroke.[19] The 2013 AHA/ASA guidelines recommend having the patient chew a 325-mg aspirin tablet within 24 to 48 hours to reduce the risk of death.[19] This can be included in the dental office protocol for emergency management of acute stroke. In the past, it was speculated that aspirin could increase the risk for intracranial bleeding but a review of the literature found the risk to be very low. Give the client 100% oxygen if respiratory distress occurs, monitor the vital signs, and record the values. The blood pressure is usually elevated, but the heart rate may be normal or elevated.[4] The stroke event must be treated quickly to reduce the loss of neurologic function so quick activation of the EMS is essential. At the hospital, tests will determine if the stroke is hemorrhagic or ischemic. If a clot blocks circulation in the brain, thrombolytic agents must be administered within 3 hours to prevent irreversible damage.

ROLE OF PERIODONTAL DISEASE IN CVD

Evidence suggests a weak association exists between periodontal disease (PD) and CVD, including stroke. Associations are greater for stroke than for coronary artery disease.[20] The AHA appointed a committee composed of members of the dental and medical communities to complete a systematic review investigating the strength of evidence for these associations. The conclusions were that although there is evidence of an independent association, there is no evidence that PD causes CVD and no evidence that periodontal treatment reduces symptoms of CVD.[21] This review highlighted significant gaps in current scientific understanding of the interactions between oral health and atherosclerotic vascular disease (ASVD). For this reason, authors recommended practitioners withhold "statements that imply a causative association between PD and specific ASVD events or claim that therapeutic interventions may be useful".[21]

"Please (X) a response to indicate if you have or have not had any of the following problems: severe headaches or migraines."

Severe headache is a symptom, rather than a disease. It can indicate a variety of problems, ranging from tension to experiencing a cerebral hemorrhage. For those clients who report a positive response to this question, try to determine the cause of the condition and follow the appropriate protocol for the causative factor. Bruxism and clenching may be causative factors in severe headache.

PATHOPHYSIOLOGY DISCUSSION

This discussion will focus on the migraine headache, commonly called a "vascular headache." The cause or causes of migraine are poorly understood, and several theories prevail. In this condition, blood vessels in the head are thought to enlarge and press on nerves, causing pain. Another theory is that they constrict and block blood flow to parts of the brain. Signs that accompany the migraine headache can include visual disturbances and numbness. Women are more prone to migraine than are men, and a certain personality type (compulsive, perfectionist, success-oriented) seems to be more susceptible to this kind of headache. The cause of migraine is unknown, but several factors may contribute to the condition, such as sharp reduction in caffeine, food allergies, interruption in eating or sleeping habits, and emotional stress. A tendency toward having migraine may also be inherited. The predominant symptom is a sharp, incapacitating pain on one or both sides of the head. Paleness, sweating, nausea, and sensitivity to light may accompany the pain. Treatment consists of drug therapy, ranging from analgesics and sedatives to antimigraine drugs. A common antihypertensive, antianginal drug (propranolol [Inderal]) has been used with success in some clients to prevent migraine.

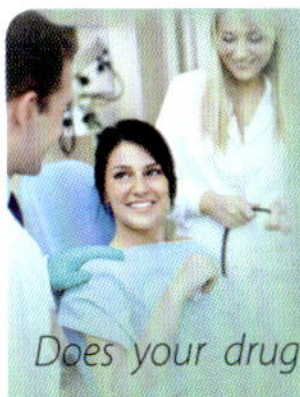

Follow-up Questions

"When was your last migraine and how often do they occur? Have you ever had a migraine during dental treatment? Does your drug therapy control the condition? Do you know what triggers your migraine?"

The risk for experiencing a migraine attack is increased in the client who has recently experienced migraine headaches. Those clients taking preventive antimigraine medications, and who are uncontrolled, pose an increased risk for an event. The triggering event may involve situations that could occur during oral health care.

APPLICATION TO PRACTICE

The most logical application to treatment plan modification is to question the client to determine whether any dental procedure in the past precipitated a migraine. For example, if the overhead dental light is unavoidably directed into the client's eyes and has caused a migraine, one would ensure this does not occur. Other applications to practice would involve examining the occlusion for evidence of bruxism and investigation of side effects or dental drug interactions with drug therapy to prevent or treat migraine. A drug reference would identify potential side effects to consider during and after treatment. β-Blocking and calcium-channel blocking drugs may be taken to prevent migraine and can result in side effects that may impact the treatment plan (e.g., orthostatic hypotension). They may interact with local anesthetic agents containing epinephrine.

POTENTIAL EMERGENCIES

Initiation of sharp headache pain and activation of migraine symptoms is the most likely emergency situation. The headache indicative of a hemorrhagic or ischemic stroke would need to be ruled out.

Prevention

Question the client to identify procedures planned during the provision of oral health care that may precipitate a migraine. Monitor the vital signs and oral cavity for potential medication side effects.

Management

If migraine occurs during oral health care, treatment should be stopped and rescheduled. Allow the client to rest in a dark room. The client may request that someone be called to drive him or her home. If symptoms indicate the headache is related to stroke, the EMS should be activated immediately and management procedures for acute stroke initiated.

Self-Study Review

13. The leading cause of hypertension is:
  a. unknown.
  b. obesity.
  c. high cholesterol.
  d. aging.

14. A blood vessel disturbance of the brain for which the client recovers within 5 minutes is referred to as a(n):
  a. cerebral hemorrhage.
  b. occlusal stroke.
  c. transient ischemic attack.
  d. arterial thrombosis.

15. From the following list, identify the signs of a cerebrovascular accident.
  a. Severe headache
  b. Unequal pupil size
  c. Slurred speech
  d. Numbness
  e. Profuse sweating
  f. Visual disturbances
  g. Difficulty breathing

16. Clients taking a beta-blocker or calcium-channel blocking medication for migraine headaches may be vulnerable to what condition during oral health treatment?
  a. High blood pressure
  b. Orthostatic hypotension
  c. Syncope
  d. Nausea and confusion

CHAPTER SUMMARY

This chapter provided a focus for addressing emergency situations related to cardiovascular conditions. Understanding methods to prevent and manage these emergency situations will enable the oral health professional to handle events appropriately. The next chapter will discuss patients with special needs involving neurologic conditions and their clinical applications.

Review

1. Define the following terms: dyspnea, ischemia, and orthopnea.
2. Identify an oral health practice that might precipitate a migraine headache.
3. List the cardiac conditions that do not require antibiotic prophylaxis before oral health treatment.
4. List four oral health treatment procedures for which antibiotic prophylaxis is indicated for those clients at high or moderate risk for endocarditis.

Case Study

Case A

Major Taylor presents to the practice for an amalgam restoration on tooth number 30. He is a 45-year-old man with a history of hypertension and elevated cholesterol, which is being treated with Norvasc and Lipitor. He is overweight, but proudly reports that he is on a weight management program and has lost 14 pounds in the past 3 months. Vital signs include pulse 70 bpm, respiration 14 breaths/min, blood pressure 160/80 mm Hg, right arm, sitting.

1. During the course of treatment, the client places his hand over his chest and complains of a crushing pain and difficulty breathing. What two cardiac conditions might be causing these symptoms?

2. The client is placed in an upright position. If angina is suspected, what steps would you take to treat this client?
3. If the client does not respond to the above treatment efforts and loses consciousness, and a pulse cannot be felt, what interventions would you do to manage this emergency?
4. If the client returns for a dental examination 6 months later, what follow-up questions would you ask concerning his coronary condition?
5. If the client reports a coronary artery bypass graft was performed, is antibiotic prophylaxis required for oral prophylaxis and restorative care? Why or why not?

Case B

Bernard Heny, a 78-year-old client, presents for an oral prophylaxis. He reports a recent onset of several TIAs. He is taking 325 mg of aspirin daily in the morning. The client states that other medications were prescribed, but he cannot afford them. Vital signs include pulse 78 bpm, respiration 18 breaths/min, blood pressure 150/86 mm Hg, right arm, sitting.

1. What is the most likely medical emergency that could occur during oral health treatment?
2. What other type of medication could have been prescribed for an individual with a recent history of TIA?
3. During the course of treatment, the client develops slurred speech, difficulty swallowing, and severe headache. What other signs and symptoms characterize a CVA?
4. What emergency management steps would you take to handle the above situation?
5. Should aspirin be administered to this client as part of emergency care?

Chapter Twelve

Medical Conditions Involving Neurologic Disorders

Objectives

After completing the self-study chapter the reader will be able to:

- Identify the types of seizure disorders and determine the risks for medical emergency situations in each type of seizure.
- Describe the management of seizures during oral health care.
- Describe the clinical implications of treating the client who reports a history of fainting or blackouts.
- Determine clinical implications for clients who suffer from sleep disorder and chronic pain.
- Identify treatment implications, drug effects, and follow-up questioning for a client with a mental health disorder.
- Describe oral management strategies for clients who present with Parkinson's disease or Alzheimer's disease.

Key Terms

Absence seizure: a type of generalized seizure with a variety of symptoms in which the person is unaware of the seizure, but does not fall to the floor, and usually occurs in childhood

Congenital: occurring at birth

Electroencephalogram: a graphic chart of the brain wave pattern

Generalized seizure: a type of seizure that affects the entire brain, includes tonic-clonic seizures and absence seizures

Idiopathic: cause of condition is unknown.

Postictal: the time immediately following a seizure.

Psychotherapeutic drugs: drugs that are prescribed for their effects in relieving symptoms of anxiety, depression, or mental disorders

Seizure: a hyperexcitation of neurons in the brain leading to convulsions or abnormal behaviors

Status epilepticus: continuous seizures that occur without interruptions, a life-threatening event

Tonic-clonic seizure: a prolonged contraction of muscles followed by rhythmic contraction and relaxation of muscle groups

MEDICAL CONDITION

INTRODUCTION

The conditions in this chapter include situations that involve emotional anxiety, impaired consciousness, or loss of consciousness during oral procedures. Neurologic disturbances involve a variety of situations ranging from mood disorders to stroke to epilepsy. Some special needs conditions (cerebral palsy, traumatic brain injury, etc.) have coexisting neurologic conditions, such as seizure disorder. This discussion will focus on **seizure** disorders because medical emergency situations can arise in clients with a history of seizure. Sleep disorders, mood disorders, and chronic pain situations have a low risk for medical emergency situations but may involve modifications in the oral care plan. Fainting is often a stress-related event and is the most common medical emergency in dentistry, although due to loss of consciousness it has been associated with epilepsy disorders. It has been discussed in Chapter 3.

"Please (X) a response to indicate if you have or have not had any of the following diseases or problems: neurological disorders, epilepsy, fainting spells, or seizures. Specify condition."

Epilepsy is a common neurological spectrum of disorders affecting over 2 million Americans. It has a wide range of severities and seizure types. The term is used to describe a variety of disorders of the brain that are characterized by recurrent seizures.[1] A seizure is not a disease, but rather, it is a *sign* of disease which manifests as a disturbance of movement, feeling, or consciousness.[2] Seizures are generally sudden and result from excessive electrical discharges in the brain that override normal brain function or loss of inhibitory function. A seizure may involve the loss of consciousness or awareness of the seizure and may or may not result in convulsions. Epilepsy is also called "seizure disorder," and the abnormal neurologic activity in the disorder leads to different types of seizures. Some forms of seizure disorder are described by the client as "fainting spells." More than 2 million Americans have epilepsy.[3] It is more common in children, with another peak occurring in the elderly.[2,3] The health history must be examined for a history of events related to seizure. Clients must be questioned to determine if seizure activity is recent and if antiseizure drugs are being taken. Questioning should attempt to identify triggers for seizure. Signs and symptoms of seizure must be recognized in order to manage the emergency situation that can develop.

PATHOPHYSIOLOGY DISCUSSION

Epilepsy is a disorder characterized by sudden surges of disorganized electrical impulses in the brain. The pathogenesis includes a disruption of neurological function that maintains the balance between excitation and inhibition of brain electrical activity. There is a loss of inhibitory activity or an overproduction of excitatory activity which results in the foci of the seizure. These cells create a burst of abnormal electrical signals that spread to adjacent areas of the brain, creating events that result in a seizure.[2] Seizures can be mild (manifested by a prolonged blank stare) or severe (causing violent convulsions). Symptoms vary according to the type of seizure experienced. Not all seizures have convulsive movements. Causes of epilepsy are usually divided into two categories: acquired and **idiopathic**. The National Institute of Neurological Disorders and Stroke defines an epilepsy diagnosis only if the individual has experienced two or more seizures. Box 12-1 includes the etiologies of epilepsy. Although seizure is required for a diagnosis of epilepsy, not all seizures imply presence of the disease. Seizures caused by high fever or from conditions that do not disrupt electrical disruption in the brain (e.g., eclampsia during pregnancy) are examples of seizures that are not associated with epilepsy.[3]

Box 12-1

Etiologies of Epilepsy

Genetic – the direct result of a known or presumed genetic defect(s) in which seizures are the core symptom of the disorder

Structural/metabolic – a distinct structural or metabolic condition or disease has been demonstrated to be associated with increased risk of developing epilepsy. It can be acquired or genetic in origin. Often when of genetic origin a separate disorder is interposed between the gene defect and the epilepsy

Unknown – nature of underlying cause is unknown

(Adapted from Berg AT, Schaeffer IE. New concepts in classification of the epilepsies. Epilepsia 2011;52(6):1058–1062.)

Acquired (Secondary) Epilepsy

Causes of acquired epilepsy include high temperature, head injury, brain tumor, drug toxicity, cerebral palsy, or malformations of blood vessels in the brain. Acquired epilepsy occurs most often after the age of 65.[3] The increased incidence in the elderly is associated with brain-related trauma such as stroke, brain tumors, and Alzheimer disease. Systemic conditions that can cause epilepsy include infection, hypertension, diabetes, electrolyte imbalances, dehydration, and lack of oxygen.[2] Other causes are chronic use of, and withdrawal from, drugs such as heroin, cocaine, and drugs that depress the central nervous system (CNS), such as chronic use of alcohol.

Idiopathic (Primary) Epilepsy

Until the age of 25, the cause of most seizures is unknown and includes approximately 70% of all cases. Primary seizure disorders tend to occur between the ages of 2 and 5 years and again at puberty. The condition tends to occur in families, supporting a genetic factor in the etiology.[1,4]

Types of Seizure

The International League Against Epilepsy (ILAE) revised the classification system for epilepsy disorders in 2011. It is currently being updated using an evidence-based approach to develop the classification.[5] The 2008 Task Force report[6] provided a detailed list of seizure types; however, the recommendations presented in the 2011 ILAE document suggest abandoning some vocabulary (e.g., focal, generalized) as advances in imaging technology and better understanding of the role played by genetics has revealed the former terms to be artificial. In reality, seizures can progress from one area of the brain to more widespread involvement.[5] Seizures are classified according to the presented symptoms. The former classification separated seizures into focal and generalized types depending on the extent of brain involvement.[4] The focal seizure affects a localized area of the brain, whereas the **generalized seizure** affects a larger area of the brain and electrical excitation generally spreads over a wide area of the brain. The 2011 ILAE recommended no specific classification to replace the use of "focal seizure," so for the purpose of clarity, this chapter will use the former descriptions.

Focal Seizures

Focal seizures are the most common type experienced by people with epilepsy, occurring when abnormal electrical activity involves only one area of the brain.[3]

There are two kinds of focal seizures: simple, in which the person remains conscious; and complex, in which consciousness is lost or altered. Although the 2011 ILAE report eliminated the term, nothing in the report precludes describing seizures according to these features.

- Simple focal seizures are confined to a small area of the brain, characterized by feeling a tingling sensation in the arm, finger, or foot; perceiving a bad odor; seeing flashing lights; or speaking unintelligibly while remaining conscious. Typically, this seizure type does not progress into a generalized seizure, but the discussion on classification includes that rarely these seizures progress to a generalized seizure.[4] Although the person remains aware of the environment and remembers the experience, he or she may be limited in how to interact while it is in process.[3]
- Complex focal seizures can involve one side of the brain or extend to both lobes of the brain; characterized by episodes of "automatic behavior" in which the client remains conscious (although consciousness can be impaired and there is no memory of the seizure)[2] but sits motionless or moves or behaves in strange, repetitive, or inappropriate ways; and can progress to a convulsive seizure if the epileptogenic

stimulation crosses to involve both lobes of the brain. The ability to speak, for example, may be lost. The Epilepsy Foundation describes focal seizures as able to progress through several stages that reflect the spread of abnormal neuronal firing to different areas of the brain, allowing the seizure to develop into a generalized seizure (www.epilepsyfoundation.org).

Generalized Seizures

Generalized seizures affect both sides of the brain and cause loss or alteration of consciousness either briefly or for a longer period of time.[3] Generalized seizures are categorized into several types including tonic-clonic convulsive seizures (and variations), myoclonic, absence (formerly called petit mal), and atonic (also referred to as drop attacks).

- **Tonic-clonic seizures** (formerly called *grand mal*) have a variety of symptoms. These include "crying out," stiffening of muscles, becoming unconscious and falling to the ground, loss of urinary and bowel control, and having muscle spasms or thrashing movements of the limbs. The tonic phase is characterized by stiffening of limbs that is followed by the clonic phase characterized by jerking of the limbs and face. Bladder and bowel control may also be lost. During the tonic phase, breathing may decrease or cease, producing blue (cyanotic) lips, nail beds, and face. Breathing typically returns during the clonic phase, but can be irregular.[3]

Spasm of the jaw muscles can cause the victim to bite the tongue and bloody saliva may be observed. An "epileptic cry" is often associated with the tonic-clonic seizure. It is not a cry from pain but occurs from air being forced through the contracting vocal cords. The seizure generally lasts from 1 to 3 minutes. Following the seizure (called the **postictal** phase), the individual will be fatigued and confused and want to sleep after recovery from the seizure. A warning sign, or aura, is sometimes found with this type of seizure. It can include headache, drowsiness and yawning, or a tingling sensation. Not all clients have an aura, however. When continuous seizures occur (seizure that lasts more than 5 minutes or recurs in a series of three or more seizures),[2] with one seizure followed by another seizure, this is a life-threatening event called **status epilepticus**. There are six characteristics of a seizure episode which require a contact with the 911 emergency medical service.[2] These include (1) seizures that continue for more than 5 minutes without the individual regaining consciousness between attacks, (2) breathing difficulties after a seizure, (3) persistent confusion or unconsciousness for more than 5 minutes following the seizure, (4) injuries sustained during the seizure, (5) a first seizure in an individual with no past history of seizures, and (6) seizure occurring in a pregnant patient or one with diabetes (Box 12-2). Some individuals experience only the tonic phase of the seizure, while others exhibit only the clonic phase.

- Myoclonic seizures: This form of generalized seizure is generally a rapid, brief contraction of body muscles, usually occurring simultaneously on both sides of the body. Clients often describe them as sudden jerks or clumsiness. This type of seizure does not pose an emergency situation, although when the clinician is working in the mouth and a myoclonic seizure occurs, the instrument could lacerate oral soft tissues.
- **Absence seizures** (formerly called *petit mal*) are characterized by a brief impairment of consciousness and jerking, staring, or spastic muscle movements (fluttering eyelids) of the eyes, which begin and end abruptly, lasting only a few seconds.[3,6] Alterations in sensation and impaired consciousness without falling to the floor are common. There are no warning and no aftereffects from this type of seizure. They generally pose no risk of medical emergency. Diagnosis of this form of epilepsy is by the pattern of electrical brain wave activity on an **electroencephalogram (EEG)** that has a "spike

Box 12-2

Seizure Conditions Requiring EMS Or 911 Contact

Seizures that continue for more than 5 minutes without the regaining of consciousness between attacks (status epilepticus)
Breathing difficulties after a seizure
Persistent confusion or unconsciousness for more than 5 minutes
Injuries sustained during a seizure
A first seizure and no history of prior seizure
Seizure during pregnancy or in person with diabetes

(Adapted from CDC, Epilepsy 2009. MMWR 2009;58(42):1183 and Jacobsen PL, Eden O. J Contemp Dent Pract 2008;9:54–62.

and dome" brain wave pattern. It is characterized by periods of staring into space, rhythmic blinking of eyes, and "daydreaming" in which the client has a brief lapse of consciousness (does not fall to the floor) but is completely unaware of having a seizure. It is most common in children.[1,3,6] In the atypical absence seizure, motor signs and changes in muscle tone can occur, followed by postictal confusion. Absence seizures often resolve as the individual matures, but some develop into a tonic-clonic seizure.

- Atonic generalized seizures produce an abrupt loss of muscle tone. The seizure can cause head drop, loss of posture, or sudden collapse.[3] This form of seizure is often resistant to drug therapy and poses a risk for recurrent seizure during oral care.

It is important to determine the cause and type of seizure experienced by the client. Stress is one of the most important factors to provoke seizures so stress-related factors should be eliminated before beginning treatment.[6] Seizures associated with no convulsive movements are not life-threatening and can be managed more easily. The tonic-clonic convulsive seizure is the most difficult seizure to manage. Epilepsy cannot be cured and is generally controlled with anticonvulsant medication. In this situation, drugs are taken to *prevent* seizures. If a seizure occurs, it can mean the client is not taking the medication as prescribed or it can mean the drug regimen may need to be changed. A recent study assessed overall adherence to medication therapy and reported that adherence was 79.4% after the initial 5 days of diagnosis and initiation of drug therapy.[7] For this reason, questioning regarding adherence to taking anticonvulsive medication is essential to determine the risk of a seizure during oral care. Some clients who are seizure-free for several years are taken off anticonvulsant drugs. This poses no increased risk for precipitating a seizure during oral procedures. When the client reports having seizures although anticonvulsant medication is being taken, the risk for a seizure during the appointment increases. Knowing what happens at the beginning or just before a seizure helps the oral healthcare professional recognize the onset of an episode and institute management procedures quickly. If the client has had a seizure during oral procedures, it is important to identify what precipitated the seizure so those activities can be avoided.

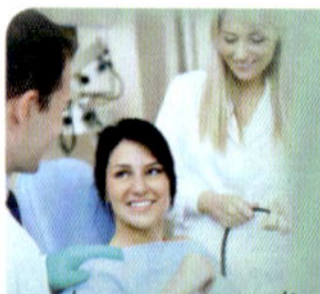

Follow-up Questions

What type of seizure do you have? When was your last seizure? Have you taken your medication today? Do you know when a seizure is coming on? What usually happens in your seizure? Have you had a seizure during dental treatment? Are there any special things I should avoid during your treatment which may precipitate a seizure?"

APPLICATION TO PRACTICE

Elective oral care should not be provided for the client who has a history of recent seizure activity until a medical consultation to determine disease control has been completed. For those clients who appear to be controlled, elective treatment can be provided, but the clinician should watch for signs of an unexpected seizure. Some anticonvulsant medications can have oral side effects. Phenytoin (Dilantin®), a common antiseizure drug, may cause overgrowth of gingival tissue (known as gingival hyperplasia [GH]). This situation requires strict plaque control to reduce the rate of gingival enlargement, although the practice does not prevent GH.[1] Some drugs used to control seizures may cause dry mouth. The oral examination should be used to identify the oral complications (e.g., caries, candidiasis) when xerostomia occurs chronically, or every day. Daily fluoride rinses or gels are recommended to prevent dental caries. Oral yeast infection is treated with antifungal medication prescribed by the dentist.

POTENTIAL EMERGENCIES

The most serious emergency to manage is the tonic-clonic, convulsive seizure. The absence seizure, myoclonic seizure, and simple partial seizures do not cause significant management problems. The absence seizure lasts for a brief time and resolves, with the client being restored to normal consciousness. The complex focal seizure may progress to a tonic-clonic seizure in some cases. Determination of a history of recent convulsive seizure is the most reliable way to predict an emergency situation during oral care.

Prevention

Three fundamental principles guide the clinician to prevent a seizure during treatment.[6] (1) Thorough questioning of the client should determine whether seizures are controlled with medication and if the client takes the medication regularly. The client should have been seizure-free for several months to be considered controlled. (2) Know conditions that may provoke a seizure. When the client reports that certain procedures likely to occur during oral care have precipitated a seizure in the past (e.g., use of the ultrasonic scaler, flicking the overhead dental light in the eyes, medicinal odors), these situations should be avoided. (3) Recognize signs of seizure and provide supportive care. For those clients who experience an aura before the seizure, request that the client alert the clinician when the aura is felt. Positioning the client out of the way of the dental equipment may prevent injury during the seizure. Conscious sedation, (use of nitrous oxide therapy), may be used to reduce anxiety.[6]

Individuals who have experienced seizure during oral procedures are likely to experience seizure again. When a seizure occurs during an appointment for oral care, record a description of the event in the dental chart for future reference. If it can be determined that some event in the oral procedure precipitated the seizure, a description of the event should also be explained in the written record. Box 12-3 includes factors to consider before starting oral procedures.

Box 12-3

Factors to Consider before Treatment

- Date of last seizure and frequency of seizure activity
- Consciousness and respiratory state during seizures
- Physical condition after seizures
- If an aura is felt before a seizure
- Factors provoking seizures, including seizure during oral treatment
- Stress reduction protocol, use of nitrous oxide
- History of status epilepticus

(Adapted from Mehmet et al. Surg Sci 2012;3:47–52.[6])

Management

Nothing can be done to stop a seizure once it has begun. The management of a seizure during oral procedures is related to the type of seizure that occurs. For those seizures that result in nonconvulsive alterations in perception (e.g., simple focal seizure, absence seizure), the seizure will occur and resolve. After the seizure, as the client recovers, question the client to determine whether someone can be called to take the client home. This is because having a recent seizure increases the risk for another seizure. Appointments should be planned for morning hours and sessions kept short to reduce stress.[6] During a seizure, the practitioner should remain calm and reassure the client showing empathy for the condition. Continuing oral care should be rescheduled to allow the client to return when seizures are controlled with medication. When convulsive seizures develop, the goal as described above is to prevent the client from injury during the seizure. When the client warns the clinician of an impending seizure, move the client to the floor (if the seizure has not started). Roll the person on the side to prevent choking on oral fluids or vomitus. Keep the airway open, if necessary, by gripping the jaw gently and tilting the head back. Do not restrict the person from moving unless it is apparent that he/she is in danger of suffocating. If possible, place a pillow under the head to avoid impact with the floor. Do not put anything into the mouth during the seizure. If the seizure begins in the dental chair, move the bracket tray and arms of the dental chair so that the client does not come into contact with them during the seizure. Do not attempt to place anything between the teeth. After the seizure, ensure an open airway and do not leave the client in a position in which oral secretions could be aspirated and cause suffocation. When the client completes the seizure and regains consciousness, move him or her to an area, such as the recovery room, to recover. Note how long the seizure lasted and the symptoms that occurred so that this information can be given to EMS personnel and for recording in the client's treatment record. Monitor the client during this time for additional seizures. The client will be confused until recovery is complete. Arrangements must be made to transport the client home. If continuous seizures occur, activate the 911 system because status epilepticus can lead to fatality. Diazepam (Valium), an anticonvulsant drug given by the intravenous route, is the preferred treatment to resolve status epilepticus. If an intravenous line cannot be inserted, the dentist can inject the drug intramuscularly. When a seizure occurs during an appointment for oral care, record a description of the event in the dental chart for future reference. If it can be determined that some event in the oral procedure precipitated the seizure (such as local anesthetic injection), a description of the event should also be explained in the written record (Box 12-4).

"Please (X) a response to indicate if you have or have not had any of the following diseases or problems: blackouts or fainting spells."

Box 12-4

Management of Tonic-Clonic Seizure

Recognize signs and symptoms of convulsive seizure

Remove instruments from mouth

Move to floor prior to seizure onset, if possible

If seizure occurs during treatment, place chair back to supine position

Turn client to side in order to minimize aspiration of secretions

Remove dental equipment that may result in injury to client during convulsion

Use passive restraint only to prevent client from falling from the dental chair

Maintain open airway, if necessary gently move jaw to tilt head back

Do not place anything into the client's mouth

Note how long the seizure lasts, what symptoms occurred

Record information in the treatment record after seizure resolves

(Adapted from Rados C, FDA Consum 2005;39:31–35 and Jacobsen PL, Eden O. J Contemp Dent Pract 2008;9:54–62.[2, 3])

Self-Study Review

1. Causes of acquired epilepsy include all of the following EXCEPT one. Which one is the EXCEPTION?
   a. High temperature
   b. Idiopathic causes
   c. Head injury
   d. Drug toxicity
2. Tingling sensations in the arm, seeing flashing lights, and perceiving a bad odor are signs of a(n):
   a. simple focal seizure.
   b. tonic-clonic seizure.
   c. myoclonic seizure.
   d. absence seizure.
3. Loss of consciousness, loss of urinary control, thrashing movements of the limbs, and an aura are signs of a(n):
   a. simple focal seizure.
   b. tonic-clonic seizure.
   c. myoclonic seizure.
   d. absence seizure.
4. The most life-threatening type of seizure is:
   a. complex partial seizure.
   b. absence seizure.
   c. generalized convulsive seizure.
   d. status epilepticus.
5. The preferred treatment to resolve status epilepticus is to:
   a. move the client away from areas of injury.
   b. place a pillow under the client's head.
   c. activate the 911 emergency medical system.
   d. administer diazepam [Valium].
6. When a client reports having seizures even while taking anticonvulsant medications, the risk for a seizure during an oral healthcare appointment increases because the seizure disorder is not controlled.
   a. Both the statement and reason are correct and related.
   b. Both the statement and reason are correct, but NOT related.
   c. The statement is correct, but the reason is NOT.
   d. The statement is NOT correct, but the reason is correct.
   e. NEITHER the statement NOR the reason is correct.
7. The epileptic cry occurs when the
   a. brain perceives changes as painful.
   b. diaphragm contracts to force air from lungs through vocal cords.
   c. muscles contract causing sudden painful sensations.
   d. seizure crossed and involves both sides of the brain.

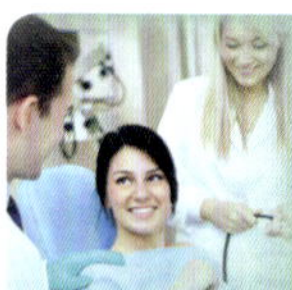

Follow-up Questions

"What caused you to faint or have blackouts? How often does it happen? Have you seen a physician about it?"

Fainting (syncope) is a loss of consciousness that can be caused by a variety of situations, such as fear and anxiety, neurologic disease, or an irregular heartbeat. The client may describe losses of consciousness as having "blackouts." Psychogenic episodes of fainting were discussed in Chapter 3. Blackouts may be a sign of epilepsy. Questioning to determine the cause of the positive response may influence treatment considerations. For clients who have not sought medical evaluation for blackouts or fainting spells, referral to a physician to determine the cause is necessary before oral treatment.

APPLICATION TO PRACTICE

Because the loss of consciousness that may be described by the client as "fainting or blackout" can result from a variety of causes, it is essential to determine the cause of the event. The clinician should request that the client seek medical evaluation to determine the cause of the fainting or blackout. Blackouts and loss of consciousness are associated with an amnesia event in epilepsy. If loss of consciousness was connected to a psychogenic stress response, the clinician should consider whether events in the planned oral health care may precipitate another episode.

POTENTIAL EMERGENCIES

A loss of consciousness or seizure related to the cause of the fainting or blackout episode is the most likely emergency situation.

PREVENTION AND MANAGEMENT

Prevention relates to the cause of the event. For stress-related syncope, refer to Chapter 3, stress-related emergencies discussion. Prevention and management of epileptic seizure is described above.

"Please (X) a response to indicate if you have or have not had any of the following diseases or problems: sleep disorders."

PATHOPHYSIOLOGY DISCUSSION

Sleep disorders include apnea, insomnia or sleep disturbance, and narcolepsy.

Sleep Apnea

This condition is associated with being overweight (adults) or anatomical interference with breathing (mainly children), which interrupts or causes absence of breathing during sleeping. It generally is not life-threatening but can cause exhaustion as a result of lack of restful sleep. Some clients can suffer cardiovascular problems and respiratory problems because of a build-up of carbon dioxide levels in the blood. Generally, the spouse or parent recognizes the problem. Signs are loud snoring, followed by silence (when breathing stops), then a loud choking or gasping as the sleeper partially awakens, clears the air passage, and resumes breathing. As a result, persons with sleep apnea are likely to be drowsy during the day, have decreased memory and attention span, and feel irritable as a result of lack of sleep. Losing weight is recommended to resolve the disorder. Other therapies include surgical treatment in the soft palate area. In children, the condition is not associated with obesity, but appears to be a disorder in the breathing control center. Removal of enlarged tonsils and adenoids that may obstruct the airway is often completed. The condition may result in breathing difficulty during oral procedures.

Insomnia

This condition is associated with the inability to sleep during normal sleeping hours when there is no apparent reason to be awake. It ranges from restlessness to complete sleeplessness. The most common cause is psychological or emotional problems, such as depression and anxiety. Bipolar disorder and including manic-depressive disorder is characterized by variation in mood with elation followed by depression. Days may pass with little or no sleep. Speech is often rapid and loud, with abrupt changes in ideas or topics. It may be difficult to get the client to concentrate on oral care information during the appointment due to both the mental disorder and the lack of sleep.

Narcolepsy

This is a disorder in which a person suffers an irresistible, uncontrollable desire to sleep. The cause is unknown. The client may lapse into a deep sleep during waking hours, often at inappropriate times. The episode lasts only a few minutes, after which the person awakes feeling refreshed but is likely to fall asleep again a few hours later. The diagnosis is confirmed by observation in a sleep laboratory or by EEG studies. This condition is treated with CNS stimulant drugs.

The most logical application to the oral healthcare plan in a client who has a sleep disorder is to determine the cause of the problem and the current therapy to resolve signs and symptoms.

Follow-up Questions

"Have you seen your physician about the problem? Do you know what causes you to have sleeplessness? Are you taking medication to help you sleep? Has it caused breathing difficulty or any problem during dental treatment?"

Drugs are often used to keep the client alert and reduce the desire to sleep, or the opposite, to help the client fall asleep at night. Side effects from medications could affect oral tissues.

APPLICATION TO PRACTICE

A history of disease-associated problems during oral health care should be investigated. Determine what the problem was, what procedure precipitated it, and how it was resolved. The treatment plan should deal with managing the clinical signs of sleep deprivation (falling asleep during treatment, snoring) and avoiding respiratory obstruction. Clients may be difficult to deal with because of emotional agitation seen with this condition. If the client frequently misses appointments, a system to remind the client the day of the appointment might help to alleviate this problem. Medications to help the client sleep may have oral side effects that can result in oral complications. Amphetamines are often used to treat narcolepsy. Because vital signs can be affected by the medication, monitor blood pressure and pulse values.

POTENTIAL EMERGENCIES

Emergency situations associated with sleep deprivation could involve airway obstruction by the tongue. Clients who fall asleep during oral health care have a relaxation of the tongue and jaw so that the normal responses to fluid collections in the throat may be inhibited. Choking can occur.

Management

The client who chokes during treatment should be rolled to the side to allow secretions to be cleared from the airway.

"Please (X) a response to indicate if you have or have not had any of the following diseases or problems: chronic pain."

PATHOPHYSIOLOGY DISCUSSION

Pain is an unpleasant or uncomfortable sensation that can range from mild irritation to excruciating agony. It is probably the most commonly reported symptom bringing a client for an unplanned dental visit. Oral pain is associated with a variety of causes, such as oral infection and mucosal ulceration. Acute pain is differentiated from chronic pain by the symptoms and time of onset. Acute pain is often a sharp pain that occurs quickly, and chronic pain is milder and develops slowly, lasting for a long duration. Chronic pain occurs on a long-term basis, such as pain associated with arthritis, and is usually relieved with pharmacologic therapy, such as analgesics, muscle relaxants, or antianxiety agents. New guidelines identify acetaminophen as the first choice for pharmacologic treatment of osteoarthritis.[8] Use of nonsteroidal analgesics (e.g., naproxen, ibuprofen, others) on a long-term basis should be avoided.

Osteoarthritis can affect the temporomandibular joint (TMJ), resulting in crepitation during jaw movements, such as eating. Determining the cause for chronic pain can be difficult. It can result in anxiety, discomfort, and loss of sleep for those affected.

Follow-up Questions

"What is causing your pain? What areas of your body are affected? Are you hurting today? Are there dental procedures that cause the pain to be worse?"

When chronic pain is unrelated to oral disease, the clinician will determine the effect on the oral care plan. Chronic muscle or joint pain in the back may require using an alternative chair position. The client must be questioned to determine whether positioning during oral procedures would exacerbate the pain.

APPLICATION TO PRACTICE

This discussion will be limited to oral pain situations. Finding the cause of chronic pain is helpful to determine whether a procedure planned during oral care could exacerbate additional discomfort. Some clients cannot endure putting cold water into the mouth when they have sensitive teeth. One condition, trigeminal neuralgia, may have a specific area on the face that, when touched, causes a stabbing pain to occur. When the cause of chronic pain is caused by an infected tooth, resolution can result simply by removing the infection. This is done by tooth removal or by endodontic therapy. Osteoarthritis of the TMJ is often painless.

POTENTIAL EMERGENCIES

Exacerbation of pain during treatment can result in fainting or other stress-related emergency situations.

Prevention

Finding out why the client responded in a positive manner on this question helps to design a treatment plan that will avoid causing additional discomfort during oral procedures. Avoid procedures that may cause a painful response.

Management

The relief of pain is directly related to the cause. In cases of oral infection, debriding the area and cleaning out the infection will often resolve pain. Analgesic medications may be recommended during the postoperative period.

Self-Study Review

8. The most common reason for fainting is:
   a. anxiety.
   b. irregular heartbeat.
   c. hypotension.
   d. stress

9. Sleep disorders may cause what type of problem during oral health care?
   a. Decreased memory
   b. Breathing difficulty
   c. Drowsiness
   d. Irritability

10. Some clients with sleep apnea can have both cardiovascular and respiratory problems because carbon monoxide builds up in the blood.
   a. Both the statement and reason are correct and related.
   b. Both the statement and reason are correct, but NOT related.
   c. The statement is correct, but the reason is NOT.
   d. The statement is NOT correct, but the reason is correct.
   e. NEITHER the statement NOR the reason is correct.

11. An irresistible urge to sleep refers to:
   a. sleep apnea
   b. insomnia
   c. narcolepsy.
   d. sleep disorder.

12. The most common symptom that induces clients to seek dental treatment is bleeding. This symptom can be managed through regular dental treatment and meticulous home care.
   a. Both statements are true.
   b. Both statements are false.
   c. The first statement is true, and the second statement is false.
   d. The first statement is false, and the second statement is true.

"Place (X) a response to indicate if you have or have not had any of the following diseases or problems: mental health disorder, if yes, specify type."

This question is added to the American Dental Association (ADA) Health History Form to identify the client who may demonstrate unusual behavior, or show lack of interest in oral care, whose medications may have significant oral side effects, and to alert the clinician to have empathy for and understanding of psychiatric disease. In the author's experience, situations have included the following:

1. A client who would only let one dentist in the office administer the local anesthetic (he thought no one else knew how to find his nerves).
2. A client who was noncompliant with the antipsychotic medication became belligerent during health history questioning about his diabetes control and told the student he would not drink the juice if it was offered.
3. A client who came to the dental office to have all restorations removed because he believed someone had placed receivers under the restorations to spy on his behavior.

These may be extreme examples, but they are offered as an example of the strange behaviors that may alert the clinician to the psychiatric client. Depression is a commonly reported mental health disorder that may adversely affect the client's motivation to practice oral hygiene on a regular basis.

PATHOPHYSIOLOGY DISCUSSION

Disorders of mental health include a wide variety of conditions. The American Psychiatric Association identifies more than 200 types of mental disorders. These include conditions that may last for a short time (situational depression) to long-term conditions, such as Alzheimer disease, bipolar disorder, schizophrenia, or psychosis. The medications given to reduce symptoms of mental disorders all have xerostomic side effects and generally must be taken over long time periods. This results in oral conditions associated with chronic xerostomia (e.g., caries and candidal infection). Given the shift in treatment regimens from institutionally based facilities to community-focused alternatives, oral care providers are likely to have patients with various forms of psychiatric disorders present for oral care. One group consists of clients with bipolar disorder, which can include manic-depressive disorder. Bipolar disorder is one of the most treatable forms of psychiatric illness, and many individuals with this condition have regular employment and are part of daily society. Symptoms of schizophrenia represent an exaggeration or distortion of normal situations, such as delusions and hallucination.[9] Examples of delusions are the belief that one's thoughts and actions are being controlled by an outside force and the belief that others can read one's thoughts.[9] Many mental health disorders cannot be cured and are managed with pharmacotherapy. Some disorders are **congenital** in nature (Down syndrome) or are acquired as the individual matures. In some cases, communication must be completed with a caregiver rather than the actual patient. When one experiences a disorder of mental health, the perception of reality may be altered. The individual does not reason situations out in a normal manner (disturbance in thinking, feeling, and acting). As a result, misunderstanding of questions asked during medical history review or of procedures necessary during treatment may precipitate the client to behave in an abnormal manner. Some clients may become aggressive and belligerent, causing uncomfortable situations. It is difficult to deal with these situations. The clinician may feel a loss of control of the situation and be unsure how the client will behave. Showing genuine desire to help the client, and demonstrating a sincere acceptance of the mental and emotional state, may enhance the appointment experience. The clinician must gain trust and establish rapport with the client to have a more successful experience during treatment. This discussion will focus on the outcome of a mental disorder as it relates to management during oral health care and potential management situations as a result of drug effects.

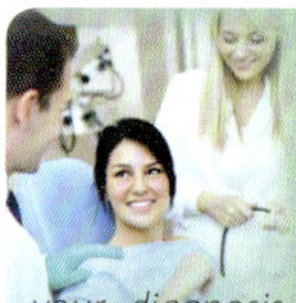

Follow-up Questions

"How are you feeling? Did you take your medications today? When was your diagnosis and how long have you been taking the medication? Do you have any concerns about our treatment today? Are you experiencing dry mouth from your medications?"

The clients with psychiatric disorders take medications that allow them to participate in society, such as going to work and meeting dental appointments. It takes 3 to 4 weeks for many psychotherapeutic medications to show an improvement in relieving symptoms of the disease. Behavioral problems during the oral healthcare appointment are more likely to develop when the client is uneasy about what will occur during the appointment. Developing rapport and trust with the client will help alleviate the risk of these problems. Xerostomia is a common side effect of psychotherapeutic medications. When medications have been taken for a long time, the client may not be aware of reduced salivary flow as oral sensation has accommodated to the effect. Other side effects relevant to oral care include fine hand tremors (lithium), nausea or abdominal discomfort, and rarely, blood dyscrasia.[10]

APPLICATION TO PRACTICE

With the development of more effective medications and current policies of deinstitutionalization, more individuals with mental disorders are likely to be seen in private dental offices. Effective communication, including explaining what procedures will be completed (before you initiate them, e.g., warn the client), may help alleviate any concerns the client may have about treatment. Occasionally, clients will make inappropriate comments, and (depending on the comment) it is best to change the subject to focus on the oral health of the client. In some cases, the more one can allow the client to have some control over planning of oral healthcare procedures, the better the communication between the clinician and the client. In many cases, the client's desires can be accommodated without causing an unacceptable level of care. Gaining the trust of the client and communicating a sincere desire to assist with the current oral health problem will promote a successful appointment experience. Consultation with the psychiatrist treating the client to obtain the psychiatrist's opinion as to the client's medicolegal competence to sign a consent form for the proposed treatment has been suggested.[9,10]

Other conditions likely to affect oral health care include advanced dental disease and oral side effects of pharmacologic products used to manage symptoms of the mental health disorder. The causes include situations in which the disease impairs the ability to plan and perform oral hygiene procedures, as well as drug side effects.[9] The mental disorder may result in the client having poor habits in oral hygiene, promoting periodontal disease. Most psychotherapy drugs result in xerostomia. Because clients generally take these drugs for months to years, this oral side effect can result in increased caries and candidiasis. Caries often manifests in a cervical, or class V, decay pattern (Fig. 12.1). Tardive dyskinesia occurs with some of the older antidepressant medications. Tardive dyskinesia causes the client to have involuntary movements, such as tongue protrusion, facial tics, and uncontrolled movements of the mouth and jaw.[9] Some **psychotherapeutic** agents can have cardiovascular side effects, such as orthostatic hypotension. Lithium is associated with fine hand tremors. Often the client with a mental health disorder will take a combination of psychotherapeutic agents, rather than a single drug. Interactions with drugs used during oral procedures should be investigated. Local anesthetic agents containing epinephrine should be used with caution, with aspiration technique and in low concentrations.[10]

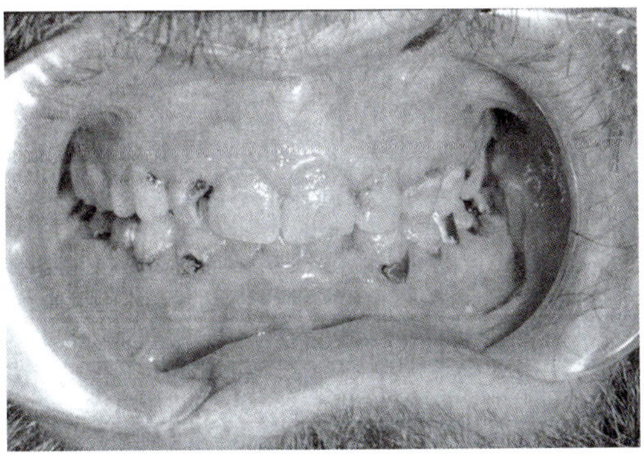

Figure 12.1 ■ Cervical caries in client on long-term antidepressant medications.

Nonsteroidal anti-inflammatory drugs, such as ibuprofen, can increase plasma levels of lithium and should be avoided. Refer to a drug reference to determine potential side effects of medications, drug interactions, and the appropriate dental considerations. A frequent, quarterly maintenance schedule for oral prophylaxis, fluoride therapy, and oral hygiene instruction (which includes the caregiver, if appropriate) should be considered for the client with a mental health disorder who has oral disease.

Management

Problems with clients who report a positive response to this question may involve behavior management situations and inappropriate verbal comments. These will be managed according to the specific situation, trying to allow the client to have some control over appointment procedures. Through encouragement, persuasion, and education about improved oral health, the practitioner can enhance the self-esteem of the client. Orthostatic hypotension management would include prevention of this condition after treatment by raising the chair back slowly and having the client sit for a few minutes before dismissing from the dental chair. Chronic xerostomia is managed by recommending home fluoride therapy on a daily basis. Dental treatment may need to be modified because of the client's impaired ability to think logically and the effects of psychiatric medications. The oral healthcare provider must understand the disease process so that effective communication is enhanced, both with the client and the client's caregivers and the treating psychiatrist.[9,10]

Self-Study Review

13. Individuals with a mental health disorder may become belligerent or uncooperative during oral health care as a result of:
    a. misunderstanding procedures to be performed.
    b. feeling a loss of control.
    c. side effects of medication management.
    d. poor oral habits.

14. Oral effects of psychotherapy medications include all of the following EXCEPT one. Which one is the EXCEPTION?
  a. Xerostomia
  b. Caries
  c. Candidiasis
  d. Bleeding

15. One of the most treatable forms of mental illness is:
  a. depression.
  b. bipolar disorder.
  c. schizophrenia.
  d. alzheimer disease.

"Place (X) a response to indicate if you have or have not had any of the following diseases or problems: neurological disorder. If yes, specify"

This section will include a discussion of Parkinson disease and Alzheimer disease, both progressive brain disorders. People are living longer with today's advanced medical options and therapies, and the number of elderly clients is increasing. In order to provide comprehensive care, dental hygienists need to recognize and understand diseases and conditions associated with aging.

PATHOPHYSIOLOGY DISCUSSION

Parkinson Disease

Parkinson disease (PD) is a progressive disorder of the CNS resulting in reduction of dopamine production in the brain. The condition develops over time, and the symptoms occur late in the disease process. Signs and symptoms are tremors of the face and hands (pill-rolling activity of fingers), stiffness and a shuffling gait, and loss of facial expression muscles. Falls are common with this condition, and orthostatic hypotension affects about 50% of those affected. Impairment of memory and concentration occurs in varying degrees, along with mood disturbances and sleep disturbances. This neurodegenerative disorder is a common disease affecting the elderly, with over a million people in the United States estimated to be affected.[11] The primary etiology of PD is unknown, although most cases are believed to result from genetic and environmental factors (genetic mutation, stroke, brain tumor, exposure to contaminants) that lead to degeneration of neurons in the CNS.[11]

There is no good drug therapy to cure this disorder, and medications are prescribed to reduce the symptoms of the tremors, mainly carbidopa/levodopa (Sinemet®). Physical therapy is prescribed to help the client learn how to safely rise from a chair and ambulate (stairs, around furniture, etc.).

Alzheimer Disease

Alzheimer disease (AD) is defined as a progressive brain disorder that gradually destroys memory and the ability to reason, to learn, to make judgments, to communicate, and to carry out daily activities.[12] Dementia is associated with aging, and dementia from AD affects over 3 million people in the United States. AD destroys neurons in the brain producing changes in the structure referred to as beta-amyloid plaques and neurofibrillary tangles. These changes disrupt the neuronal transport of information leading to the signs and symptoms of the disease. Research to determine how these plaques and tangles can be prevented is currently ongoing. The etiology is related to the form of the disease in that early-onset AD is genetically related. Most cases occur before the age of 60 years.[12] The late-onset form of AD is the most common form, and the etiology is unknown but is related to the loss of cholinergic neurons.[11] It is a condition that mainly affects the elderly, between 70 and 80 years of age. As the disease progresses, the client will have difficulty remembering information, have problems in performing activities of daily living (e.g., getting dressed, brushing teeth, remembering how to use the toilet), become unable to recognize family members, and have oral problems, such as difficulty swallowing. Symptoms are managed with medications, with varying degrees of success.

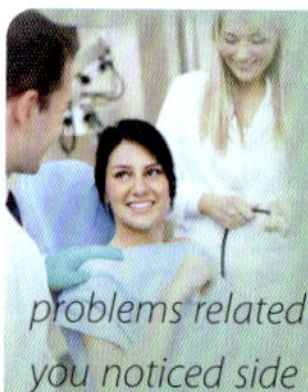

Follow-up Questions

"Do you have any limitations I should consider regarding your oral care? What problems related to your mouth can I help you with? Have you noticed side effects from your medications that affect your mouth? Is there someone here to help you get home?"

APPLICATION TO PRACTICE

Parkinson's Disease

Muscular defects and tremor can contribute to poor oral hygiene. Both the ability to hold and manipulate the toothbrush should be assessed. A power toothbrush may be helpful when deficiencies are observed in manipulation with the hands. Power brushes have large handles that are easier to grasp than a normal toothbrush and may be helpful. Burning mouth syndrome is reported by some individuals with PD. Excess salivation and drooling is possible, and swallowing difficulty may be present. Fungal infection is commonly reported.[13] In contrast, xerostomia can result as a side effect of medications used to control the disease symptoms. Orthostatic hypotension is common in PD. Drug side effects should be investigated in a drug reference and managed according to oral effects present. For example, daily fluoride products should be recommended when caries is present. Xylitol gum can help stimulate salivation and provide an anticaries effect as well. Taste disturbances have been reported in PD. Bowel dysfunction may require bathroom breaks during an appointment.[13]

Management

The initial patient evaluation must include the nature, control, severity, and stability of the disease. To reduce the likelihood of a fall in the dental setting, the client should be assisted while entering and leaving the operatory and when sitting in the dental chair or leaving the dental chair. The client should sit upright at the end of the appointment for several minutes to allow the blood pressure to rise physiologically to avoid orthostatic hypotension. If the client is cognitively impaired, oral health instructions can be written. The practitioner should have the client perform oral hygiene procedures while being observed and instruction provided to enhance efficacy. Appointments should be planned several hours after medications have been taken to take advantage of the time the medications are working. Appointments should be planned for the time of day the client is less symptomatic. When oral tremors are problematic, mouth props may be helpful to stabilize the jaw. The main drug interaction with medications used to manage PD may interact with epinephrine in local anesthetics, and the dose should be limited to no more than 2 cartridges of 1:100,000. Orthostatic hypotension and rigidity must be monitored. Maintenance appointment scheduling should be more frequent, according to the oral condition, and those who provide personal care and assistance should be informed of the oral hygiene needs for the client, and instructed in their performance.

Alzheimer's Disease

Even in the early stages of AD, the affected individual may need assistance with personal oral care.[12] The practitioner must assess the oral condition, the dexterity of the client, and determine the most appropriate interventions. Routine procedures, such as taking blood pressure, could cause the client to feel anxious when not forewarned about the procedure. Procedures should be explained in simple language, such as "I'm going to check your teeth." Smiling, direct eye contact, and gentle touching help to communicate nonverbally.[12]

Oral health instructions must involve the primary caregiver, as the client may need to be reminded it is time to brush the teeth. Communication with the client who has AD is challenging. Chaining, bridging, and rescuing are communication techniques useful in managing the client with AD or dementia.[14]

Chaining involves starting a task and assisting the client to finish the task, such as brushing the teeth. Bridging uses the client's senses, such as sight and touch, to help them understand the task. The client may want to feel the prophy cup before allowing it to be placed within the mouth. Rescuing is a process when the client refuses to complete the task, which allows another individual to finish the task.

Management

Consent forms can be signed by the caregiver if the physician has determined the client to be unable to understand consent for treatment.[12]

Frequent maintenance visits should be planned. Appointments should be scheduled when there is low activity in the office in order to reduce the stress of crowded rooms. Oral hygiene products (fluoride gel or paste, salivary lubricants, antimicrobial products) and power toothbrushes should be considered. Drug oral side effects must be determined and product recommendations made as needed. Antidepressant and antipsychotic medications are commonly prescribed for individuals with dementia. When the client is no longer able to talk, the caregiver may know how to communicate with the client. Oral care requires patience, understanding, and providing a relaxed environment for the client. The caregiver should be in the operatory with the client to provide reassurance and reduce fear. Oral care providers should use a calm tone of voice, speak slowly, avoid sudden movements, and ensure a painless appointment.

Self-Study Review

16. Clients with Parkinson disease have a higher incidence of falls due to orthostatic hypotension occurring from medications used to treat the disease.
    a. Both the statement and reason are correct and related.
    b. Both the statement and reason are correct, but NOT related.
    c. The statement is correct, but the reason is NOT.
    d. The statement is NOT correct, but the reason is correct.
    e. NEITHER the statement NOR the reason is correct.
17. Alzheimer disease is a progressive brain disorder that gradually causes memory changes and the ability to reason. New medications are reversing these effects by removing beta-amyloid plaques in the brain.
    a. Both statements are true.
    b. Both statements are false.
    c. The first statement is true, and the second statement is false.
    d. The first statement is false, and the second statement is true.
18. Excessive salivation and xerostomia are both found in clients with Parkinson disease. Salivation is associated with the disease itself, while xerostomia is a side effect of medications used to treat the disease.
    a. Both statements are true.
    b. Both statements are false.
    c. The first statement is true, and the second statement is false.
    d. The first statement is false, and the second statement is true.

MANAGING CARE FOR PATIENTS WITH SPECIAL NEEDS

Individuals with special neurological needs have unique issues related to management of oral care. Individuals with special needs disabilities face limited access to care. In addition, there is limited preparation of oral care professionals to serve this population. Oral procedures may require hospitalization. The high cost of dental treatment in hospital settings and the low rate of dental insurance coverage add to the access to care issues. The Affordable Care Act (Obamacare) includes provisions that increase the opportunity for all individuals to obtain private dental insurance coverage (Box 12-5 for URLs).

Box 12-5

Web Resources for Special Needs Patients

Oral Health for Children with Special Needs July 2012 [http://www.mchoralhealth.org/highlights/cashcn.html]

Affordable Care Act. Help for Children with Special Needs 2011 [http://nmcohpc.net/resources/CSHCN%20Brief.pdf]

Southern Association of Institutional Dentists and Special Care Advocates in Dentistry(http://saiddent.org/modules.php)

National Maternal and Child Oral Health Services and modules for management [http://www.mchoralhealth.org/SpecialCare/index.htm]

American Academy of Pediatric Dentistry. Guideline on Management of Dental Patients with Special Healthcare Needs [http://www.aapd.org/media/Policies_Guidelines/G_SHCN.pdf]

NIDCR Guidelines. Developmental Disabilities and Oral Health. Practical Oral Care for Autism [http://www.nidcr.nih.gov/OralHealth/Topics/DevelopmentalDisabilities/PracticalOralCarePeopleAutism.htm]

National Institute of Neurological Disorders. Spina Bifida Fact Sheet [http://www.ninds.nih.gov/disorders/spina_bifida/detail_spina_bifida.htm]

National Institute of Neurological Disorders has a wide variety of conditions providing guidance [http://www.ninds.nih.gov/disorders/disorder_index.htm]

Depending on the disability, there could be difficulties in patient positioning, communication, and behavior problems. There are many disorders included in label of "special needs." It is difficult in a text of this type to provide a recommendation for each individual group. For this reason, the reader is directed to find management recommendations from a reliable website (Box 12-5). The National Maternal and Child Oral Health Services prepared a series of modules for guidance on managing oral care for children with special needs. The series of five modules is designed to provide oral health professionals with information to help ensure that young children/individuals with special needs have access to health promotion and disease prevention services that address their unique oral health needs in a comprehensive, family-centered, and community-based manner. Modules include an overview of oral problems found in various special needs conditions, optimum oral healthcare educational needs, how to monitor oral health, strategies to prevent oral disease, and strategies for child behavior guidance (Box 12-5). The Southern Association of Institutional Dentists also has training modules on dental management for a variety of neurological conditions.[15]

SCHEDULING APPOINTMENTS

The initial contact with the dental practice allows both the patient and the clinician an opportunity to address the child's primary oral health needs and to confirm the appropriateness of scheduling an appointment with the practitioner. Along with the child's name, age, and chief complaint, the receptionist should determine the presence and nature of the presenting dental need. When appropriate, the name(s) of the child's medical care provider(s) for consultation is useful. Following the oral examination, the clinician can determine the need for an increased length of appointment and/or additional auxiliary staff needed to accommodate the patient in an efficient manner. The need for increased appointment time as well as customized services should be documented for future appointments. During treatment, it is imperative that information is protected and practitioners are familiar and comply with Health Insurance Portability and Accountability Act (HIPAA) and Americans with Disabilities Act (AwDA) regulations applicable to dental practices. HIPAA ensures that the patient's privacy is protected and AwDA prevents discrimination on the basis of a disability.

Dental home

Patients with special needs who have a dental home are more likely to receive appropriate preventive and routine care. The dental home provides an opportunity to implement individualized preventive oral health practices and reduces the child's risk for preventable dental/oral disease. When patients reach adulthood, their oral health care needs may extend beyond the scope of the pediatric dentist's training. The parent/patient should receive education to prepare the patient and parent on the value of transitioning to a dentist who is knowledgeable in adult oral health needs. The transition to a dentist knowledgeable and comfortable with managing the specific healthcare needs can promote access to oral care. In cases where this is not possible or desired, the dental home can remain with the pediatric dentist and appropriate referrals for specialized dental care can be recommended as needed.

PATIENT ASSESSMENT

An accurate, comprehensive, and up-to-date medical history is necessary for medical management and effective treatment planning. Information regarding the chief complaint, history of present illness, medical conditions and/or illnesses, medical care providers, hospitalizations/surgeries, anesthetic experiences, current medications, allergies/sensitivities, immunization status, review of systems, family and social histories, and thorough dental history should be obtained. An attempt should be made to communicate directly with the patient during the provision of oral care. When this is not possible, a parent, family member, or caretaker may need to be present to facilitate communication and/or provide necessary information.

Many children with special needs may have sensory issues that can make the dental experience challenging.[15,16] This issue should be considered as equipment is planned for use and be prepared to modify the traditional delivery of dental care to address the unique needs. Cerebral palsy can predispose the client to movement during procedures, and safety can be an issue when sharp instruments are used.[17] If the patient/parent is unable to provide accurate information, consultation with the caregiver or with the patient's physician may be required. Caries risk assessment provides a means of classifying caries risk at a point in time and, therefore, should be applied periodically to assess changes in an individual's risk status. An individualized preventive program, including a dental recall schedule, should be recommended after evaluation of the patient's caries risk, oral health status, and oral physiotherapy abilities.

INFORMED CONSENT

All patients must be able to provide signed informed consent for oral treatment or have someone present who legally can provide this service. Informed consent/assent must comply with state laws and, when applicable, institutional requirements. Informed consent should be documented in the dental record through a signed and witnessed form.

BEHAVIOR GUIDANCE

Behavior guidance of the patient can be challenging. Because of dental anxiety or a lack of understanding of dental care, children with disabilities may exhibit resistant behaviors. These behaviors can interfere with the safe delivery of treatment. Communication with caregivers can provide valuable information for a successful appointment. Protective stabilization can be helpful in patients for whom traditional behavior guidance techniques are not adequate. When protective stabilization is not feasible or effective, sedation or general anesthesia may be the behavioral guidance armamentarium of choice. When in-office sedation/general anesthesia is not feasible or effective, an outpatient surgical care facility might be necessary. Physician consultation may clarify options for delivering care.

PREVENTIVE STRATEGIES

Individuals with special needs may be at increased risk for oral diseases. Clinical guidelines for recommendation of products to prevent caries identify fluoride, sealants, and nutritional guidance as the primary strategies to prevent caries. Education of parents/caregivers is critical for ensuring appropriate and regular supervision of daily oral hygiene. Power toothbrush technology may be useful. A noncariogenic diet and advice to refrain from between-meal snacks should be discussed for long-term prevention of dental disease. When a diet rich in carbohydrates is medically necessary (e.g., to increase weight gain), the dentist should provide strategies to mitigate the caries risk by altering frequency of and/or suggesting good snacks (popcorn, fresh fruit, nuts, cheese). As well, possible oral side effects (e.g., xerostomia, gingival overgrowth) of medications should be reviewed with the caregiver. All appointments should include an assessment of the oral hygiene effectiveness.

BARRIERS

Practitioners should be familiar with community-based resources for patients with special needs and encourage such assistance when appropriate. While local hospitals, public health facilities, rehabilitation services, or groups that advocate for those with special needs can be valuable contacts to help the practitioner and patient address language and cultural barriers, other community-based resources may offer support with financial or transportation considerations that can improve access to care.

INDIVIDUAL SPECIAL NEEDS GROUPS

Box 12-5 provides a variety of web-based links to provide access to special situations. The Southern Association of Institutional Dentists has a free web access to guidance for management of patients with neurological needs, such as intellectual disabilities or those institutionalized.[15] Modules for dental management for individuals with mental retardation, Down syndrome, cerebral palsy, maladaptive behaviors, mental illness, and for those with severe disabilities are available.

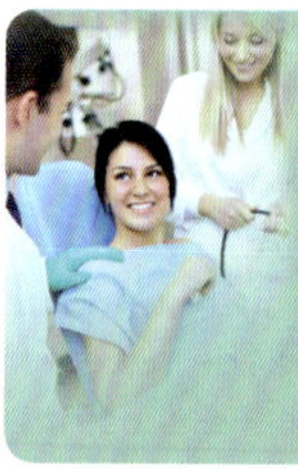

Follow-up Questions

"Do you have any special situations of which I need to be aware?" Follow-up questions will relate to situations related to the disability.

After investigating medical issues related to the disability, the practitioner would identify needed information to direct the treatment plan. Physician consultation may be necessary to supplement medical information. Treatment decisions will be based on safe treatment, pain control for the client, and strategies for communication and engagement of the patient. Autistic children may be more cooperative if allowed to complete an interesting activity or exploring their environment further prior to receiving treatment. Allowing the child to become familiar and comfortable in the dental office setting before the treatment begins is a strategy used successfully.[16] Prevention and management considerations relate to associated conditions with the special need. For example, individuals with traumatic brain injury often have seizures. Prevention and management strategies are the same as for seizure. Consultation with the parent or caregiver regarding individual medical problems would identify potential emergency situations.

CHAPTER SUMMARY

Medical conditions associated with neurologic disorders that have the potential to involve impaired consciousness or loss of consciousness during oral health care were reviewed. Medical emergencies such as seizures, syncope, orthostatic hypotension, and respiratory obstruction were discussed in terms of prevention and management strategies. Oral effects of neurological diseases were identified and preventive strategies identified. The next chapter will provide an overview of gastrointestinal disorders and respiratory disease or respiratory obstruction issues.

Review

1. Define the following terms: seizure, absence seizure, and tonic-clonic seizure.
2. Identify the two major etiologic categories of epilepsy.
3. List an example of an oral healthcare practice or procedure that can precipitate a seizure.
4. Differentiate insomnia from narcolepsy.

Case Study

Case A

Cameron Blakely, a 27-year-old hairstylist, presents for a restorative dental appointment. She reports that she is in good health and does not take any medications. She reports a prior history of seizure disorder as an early teenager, but has been seizure-free for 10 years. During the course of restorative therapy, the client becomes stiff and her jaw muscles begin to spasm. Her arms and legs thrash about, and the client then loses consciousness.

1. What type of seizure is described in this case scenario?
2. If the client were to experience an aura, what types of experiences would occur?
3. What steps would you take to manage this condition?
4. If continuous seizures were to occur, how would you treat this emergency?
5. Identify the seizure conditions that require EMS/911 contact?

Case B

Samantha Feldman, a 62-year-old housewife, presents for her dental hygiene appointment. She reports a history of mild hypertension, but is not taking any medications. She has reduced the salt in her diet instead. The client completes the dental hygiene appointment without incident. She leaves the office and returns 10 minutes later crying saying that her car was stolen, and accuses the dental hygienist of taking her car. She also says she cannot find her pocketbook, but is actually holding her purse in her left arm.

1. What condition does this client most likely demonstrate?
2. Is this client at risk for a medical emergency?
3. How would you handle this situation to avoid a medical emergency and to resolve the client's concerns?

Chapter Thirteen

Medical Conditions Involving Gastrointestinal Disorders and Respiratory Disease

Objectives

After completing the self-study chapter the reader will be able to:

- Describe the pathophysiology of various conditions involving the gastrointestinal system and determine the potential emergency situations that can occur in these individuals.
- Describe the management of the client with a gastrointestinal condition.
- Identify respiratory disorders that can result in a modification of the oral healthcare treatment plan and describe those modifications.
- Describe the management of the client with an airway obstruction.

Key Terms

Gastroesophageal reflux disorder: backflow of contents of the stomach into the esophagus

Perimylolysis: erosion of enamel and dentin as a result of chemical effects, usually affecting maxillary lingual surfaces

Status asthmaticus: a prolonged, severe asthma attack that develops quickly

MEDICAL CONDITION

INTRODUCTION

This chapter refers to disturbances of the gastrointestinal (GI) system and respiratory system. These medical conditions can be acquired or inherited (cystic fibrosis). Modifications related to the oral healthcare treatment plan may involve using a more comfortable chair position, maintaining an open airway, and recommendations to minimize adverse effects of the disease (or treatment for the disease) on soft tissue or tooth structure.

"Please (X) a response to indicate if you have or have not had any of the following diseases or problems: GI disease, GERD/persistent heartburn, ulcers."

Disorders of the GI system are numerous, including conditions such as peptic ulcers, heartburn, Crohn disease, irritable bowel syndrome, and diverticulitis. This discussion will concentrate on the most common conditions, namely **gastroesophageal reflux disorder** (GERD; and the persistent heartburn and increased risk for GI cancer that occurs in this condition), as well as peptic ulcer disease.

PATHOPHYSIOLOGY DISCUSSION

GERD

The most prevalent GI disease in the United States includes GERD, or persistent heartburn. This condition is characterized by the contents of the stomach flowing backward (called refluxing) into the esophagus, usually as a result of reduced function of the lower esophageal sphincter. Because the esophagus is not designed to accommodate gastric acids, the lining becomes irritated, inflamed, and ulcerated. Esophageal epithelium undergoes metaplasia with chronic irritation and is at an increased risk for malignancy. It is characterized by a complex clinical situation that may include lesions of the esophageal mucosa and lesions of a different nature and severity of the respiratory and oral mucosa.[1] Pain in the middle of the chest results from the inflamed esophagus, mimicking the symptoms of a heart attack. Nonspecific symptoms can include burping, cramps, flatulence, and a feeling of fullness in the stomach. The cause of the acid reflux is lack of function of the lower esophageal sphincter allowing backflow of acid to occur. Symptoms of GERD are exacerbated by eating large meals and by lying in a supine position. Individuals are urged to avoid eating for 4 hours before bedtime, eat small meals, and raise the head of the bed or use several pillows during sleeping to place the throat above the esophagus. Treatment also includes medications that reduce secretions of acid in the stomach (Prilosec®, Zantac®) or medications that increase the tone of the esophageal sphincter (Reglan®). Antacids (Tums®) are used for acute relief of symptoms.

PEPTIC ULCER

An ulcer is an erosion on the surface of tissue. When it occurs within the esophagus, stomach, and duodenum, it is referred to as a peptic ulcer. The main cause for peptic ulceration is related to infection by *Helicobacter pylori* bacterium. This bacterial infection breaks down the mucosal barrier that lines the intestines and normally provides protection against acid erosion. The bacterium can invade the mucosa and secrete enzymes that liquefy the barrier. This allows the strong acidic digestive juices of the stomach to penetrate into the underlying epithelium and digest the epithelial cells, thus diminishing the protective effect of the mucosal barrier.[2] Other factors include the presence of excessive amounts of acid produced by the stomach, ingesting large amounts of aspirin and aspirin-like compounds (such as ibuprofen or naproxen), smoking, and alcohol. Aspirin products exert a direct damaging effect on the lining of the stomach because of the acidic nature of the drugs and have been implicated as a contributing factor in some clients. Smoking is thought to increase stimulation of the stomach secretory glands, and alcohol tends to break down the mucosal barrier of the intestines.

Symptoms include burping, heartburn, severe pain radiating into the upper body, nausea and vomiting, and a burning sensation in the abdomen. The pain occurs either after eating or during the night when the stomach is empty. The increased acids irritate the unprotected nerve endings in the ulcer. Pain may subside after eating or drinking something or after taking an antacid product. Blood in the feces, making the stool black in color, is a sign of a bleeding ulcer. If left untreated, serious damage to the GI tract can result. Treatment includes combination antibiotic therapy to eliminate *H. pylori* plus drugs to reduce the secretion of acid (Prilosec, Zantac) or to reduce the acidity of the GI system (Tums). Most ulcers heal within 6 weeks of starting therapy.

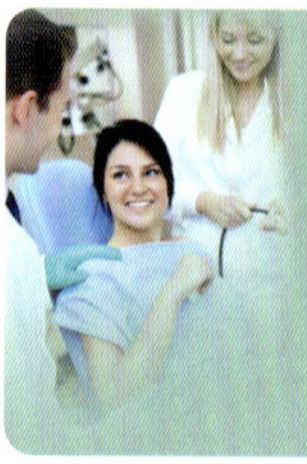

Follow-up Questions

"Has your medication controlled the symptoms of your condition? Can you tolerate being placed in a supine position?"

APPLICATION TO PRACTICE

Most clients with any form of GI disorder will prefer to be placed in a semiupright position in the dental chair. This diminishes the risk of refluxing stomach contents into the throat and provoking a coughing attack. Acidic medications, such as aspirin-like analgesics, are contraindicated in clients with GI disease. Dental pain is best managed with acetaminophen. Examination of the teeth for erosion from acid reflux and for increased risk of dental caries is recommended (Fig. 13.1). Clinical signs associated with erosion include raised amalgam restorations on occlusal surfaces of teeth. Teeth may have a smooth, shiny appearance, and the vertical dimension may be reduced secondary to the enamel erosion.[3] Fluoride therapy with daily, low-concentration sodium or stannous fluoride products is recommended to prevent dental caries. Rinsing the mouth with a weak sodium bicarbonate solution after the vomiting episode may reduce the acidity of oral fluids.[4]

Clients should be advised to avoid toothbrushing for at least an hour after a reflux episode. Drug interactions can occur between drugs used in dentistry and many drug products used to manage symptoms of GI disease. For example, penicillin needs an acid pH for fast absorption, and changing the pH of the small intestine with antacids may delay absorption of the antibiotic. As well, minerals in antacid products may prevent the absorption of tetracycline.

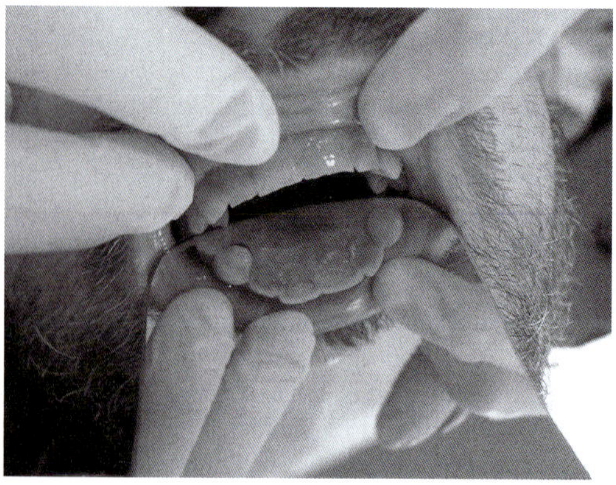

Figure 13.1 ■ Clinical photograph of lingual erosion in client with gastroesophageal reflux disorder. (From personal files of Frieda Pickett, RDH, MS.)

POTENTIAL EMERGENCIES

Choking during oral health care as a result of aspiration of reflux acids is the most likely emergency situation to occur.

Prevention

Place the client in a semiupright position for treatment. Schedule the appointment at least 3 hours after a meal or consult with the client for times when reflux symptoms would be least likely to occur. Inform the client to tell you whether short breaks during treatment (with return to an upright position) would help reduce symptoms of the condition.

Management

If the client refluxes during treatment, stop immediately and turn the head to the side so that the client is less likely to choke. The client can use a saliva ejector to remove contents from the mouth. Return the chair position to a full upright position, provide some water to clear the throat area, and let the client decide when to continue with treatment. In some cases, the client will need to be rescheduled for a time when symptoms are less likely to occur.

Self-Study Review

1. In GERD, reflux occurs as a result of:
   a. Increased esophageal motility.
   b. Reduced function of the lower esophageal sphincter.
   c. Lack of function of the vagus nerve.
   d. Increased stimulation of the stomach secretory glands.
2. Symptoms of GERD are exacerbated by:
   a. Eating small meals more frequently.
   b. Raising the head of the bed.
   c. Lying in a supine position.
   d. Avoiding eating meals before bedtime.

3. From the following list, select the symptoms of a peptic ulcer.
    a. Heartburn.
    b. Nausea.
    c. Cramps.
    d. Burping.
    e. Diarrhea.
    f. Vomiting.
    g. Gas.
4. The medication that is most likely to damage the lining of the stomach in individuals with GI disease is:
    a. Aspirin.
    b. Zantac.
    c. Reglan.
    d. Vitamin B.

"Please (X) a response to indicate if you have or have not had any of the following diseases or problems: malnutrition or eating disorder, if yes, specify type."

Malnutrition is uncommon in the United States. When it occurs, it is mainly a result of eating disorders. Malnutrition can reduce healing within the body. Bald, painful tongue and angular cheilitis are oral complications associated with reduced levels of B vitamins.

Eating disorders are more likely to be seen in an adolescent or young woman, although men can also have these conditions. Eating disorders include two main conditions, bulimia and anorexia nervosa. Xerostomia is reported to occur in the client with an eating disorder.[4]

PATHOPHYSIOLOGY DISCUSSION

This discussion will focus on the pathophysiology of the more common eating disorders.

Bulimia Nervosa

Bulimia is abnormal, excessive eating triggered by emotional factors. Victims of the disorder eat beyond the normal appetite requirements. It is thought that the bulimic individual is using gratification from food as an escape from personal problems. The condition is characterized by binging on specific foods (such as a gallon of ice cream at one time), then feeling guilty and forcing themselves to purge, such as vomiting. Not all individuals purge, but many do follow this practice. Some individuals attempt to prevent the absorption of calories from foods by overusing laxatives. Bulimia is more difficult to recognize than anorexia because individuals are usually of normal weight and do not appear to be ill. Treatment is difficult, but psychological counseling to help the client identify what triggers the emotional response to food and focus on healthy substitutes to provide satisfaction (nutritional counseling, exercise program) is successful with some clients. The most common oral finding associated with bulimia is erosion of the lingual surfaces of maxillary teeth and incisal areas of the mandibular teeth, a condition known as **perimylolysis** (Fig. 13.2). Other oral signs include increased dental caries, restorations that may appear raised because of erosion of the enamel around the margins, xerostomia, tooth sensitivity, impaired taste sensation, and enlargement of the parotid salivary glands.[4,5]

Anorexia Nervosa

Anorexia is another eating disorder most commonly found in young women. The individual with anorexia suppresses the desire to eat and

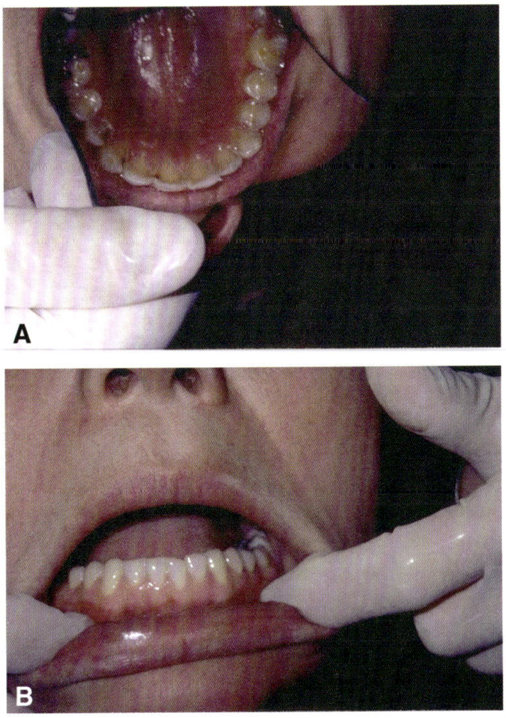

Figure 13.2 ■ Clinical photographs of perimylolysis (**A**) and chipping of lower anteriors (**B**) in bulimic client. (From personal files of Frieda Pickett, RDH, MS.)

starves oneself. The client continues to lose weight to the point of starvation and malnutrition. Some individuals have a bulimic-type anorexia, practicing features of both anorexia and bulimia. Causes are unclear, but one theory is that individuals with anorexia starve themselves because they mistakenly believe that they are fat and need to lose weight. Physiologic problems occur, such as loss of menstrual periods and the destruction of healthy muscle, bone, and organ tissues. Individuals with anorexia nervosa who did not seek medical treatment have died of cardiac arrest.

APPLICATION TO PRACTICE

Because anorexia nervosa can affect organ function, such as the heart muscle, the vital signs should be monitored to determine what effects have occurred in the cardiovascular system. Cardiac arrhythmia can result when an electrolyte imbalance occurs in the body. Vital sign abnormalities may also include a low pulse rate, hypotension, decreased respiratory rate, and low body temperature.[4] Any deviation from the normal vital sign limits should be reported to the client. Because cardiac arrhythmia is a frequent sign preceding a heart attack, this finding requires a referral for medical evaluation before stressful oral healthcare procedures (surgery, periodontal debridement). Examination of the oral cavity for erosion and enamel breakdown should be completed. When the clinician observes lingual erosion in the maxillary dentition, questions should be posed to determine the cause of the condition. It could relate to any condition in which gastric acids frequently enter the mouth, such as with GERD or frequent vomiting.[5] A dialogue might evolve, such as "I notice that your teeth are sensitive and you can see that the enamel is wearing from the backs of your teeth (or describe any symptom noticed). This often indicates excessive vomiting. Is this a problem for you?" Questioning the client with an eating disorder and receiving truthful responses may be uncomfortable for the client because of the emotional nature of the disorder. It is not unusual for a client to deny the eating disorder. The clinician must be sincere and empathetic and demonstrate acceptance of the client's privacy. Effective communication is best achieved after rapport is established and there is a trusting relationship between the client and the clinician. When the clinician suspects a medical condition (such as anorexia nervosa) that can result in significant deterioration of health, it is necessary to try to get the client to seek medical help for the condition. When signs of malnutrition are observed, such as cracking at the corners of the mouth, questioning might include a dialogue such as "I notice you have cracking at the corners of your mouth and your nails appear thin and brittle (or describe evidence of malnutrition observed). These may be signs of nutritional deficiency. Have you seen a physician about this?" The clinician should be prepared with a list of local resources to provide to the client.

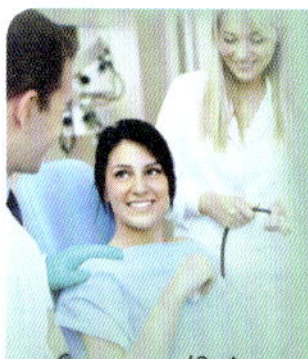

Follow-up Questions

"What is the cause of malnutrition in your body? Do you binge eat and vomit or purge? Do you brush your teeth afterward? Are your teeth sensitive, if so where? (Women) Are you having normal periods? Have you sought medical treatment for the condition?"

The usual chief complaint in the client with eating disorders that bring them for dental treatment is tooth sensitivity. Questioning and examination often discover that sensitivity is caused by loss of tooth structure from erosion or pain as a result of dental decay. It is common to discover the client brushes the teeth immediately after a purging episode, unaware that this practice is harmful to tooth enamel.[5]

The client who has physiologic changes in the body (abnormal menstrual periods) has been in the disease for a long time and needs immediate medical treatment. Death can result when major organs are damaged from eating disorder effects.

For individuals who experience an emotional response during the discussion, such as crying, management should include reassurance of the desire to help the client avoid serious consequences to health. If signs of an eating disorder are noted in a child, parents should be notified.[5] Eroded incisal and lingual surfaces of anterior teeth can be difficult to restore and may require modifications of restorative procedures. Restorative dentistry should be delayed until the disease is controlled and vomiting has ceased. All physical findings and recommendations should be recorded in the treatment record.

Self-Study Review

5. All of the following are oral manifestations of eating disorders EXCEPT one. Which one is the EXCEPTION?
    a. Caries
    b. Xerostomia
    c. Perimylolysis
    d. Periodontitis
6. One feature that distinguishes bulimia from anorexia nervosa is:
    a. onset of disease.
    b. fear of gaining weight.
    c. purging.
    d. normal weight.
7. Anorexia nervosa may be fatal because of cardiac changes such as hypertension due to an electrolyte imbalance.
    a. Both the statement and reason are correct and related.
    b. Both the statement and reason are correct, but NOT related.
    c. The statement is correct, but the reason is NOT.
    d. The statement is NOT correct, but the reason is correct.
    e. NEITHER the statement NOR the reason is correct.

"Please (X) a response to indicate if you have or have not had any of the following diseases or problems: asthma or respiratory disorders (emphysema/bronchitis)."

Respiratory disorders are important to investigate because they involve potential airway obstruction. Asthma is a chronic condition that can develop during childhood or during adult years. Emphysema and chronic bronchitis are associated with chronic obstructive pulmonary disease (COPD). Cystic fibrosis is a genetic-related disease that manifests as thick mucoid secretions occluding bronchioles and alveoli of the lungs.

PATHOPHYSIOLOGY DISCUSSION

This discussion will include asthma, COPD, and cystic fibrosis.

Asthma

Asthma is a respiratory disease that causes reversible airway obstruction and a reduced ability to expire or completely empty the lungs of gases. Inflammation is a component of the disease process and results in increased mucous secretions in the lungs and swelling in the bronchioles.[6] Clinical manifestations include cough, shortness of breath, chest tightness, and wheezing. The literature consistently identified asthma as one of the most common emergencies in dental practice, but does not suggest that outcomes are generally fatal.[7] The most common form, called extrinsic asthma, develops as a result of allergy to environmental pollutants. It generally occurs during childhood and may or may not extend into adult years. Stress-induced asthma or an allergic response to a dental material may result in exacerbation of symptoms of asthma during oral healthcare procedures. When an asthmatic episode occurs, symptoms develop because of constriction of bronchioles compounded by a narrowed airway space when mucus collects on the inner lining of the respiratory tree area. This narrowed airway causes a reduced ability to exhale air from the lungs. Inflammation results in mucous secretions collecting on the lining of bronchioles and narrowing the airway space. Oral complications associated with asthma medications include dry mouth, candidiasis, and an increased dental caries rate.[6]

Chronic Obstructive Pulmonary Disease

COPD is a group of diseases that includes emphysema and chronic bronchitis, characterized by obstruction of airflow out of the lungs and shortness of breath. As much as 75% of the physiologically active surface area of the alveoli can be lost in severe cases of emphysema, causing the alveoli to coalesce, resulting in a loss of total surface area for gas exchange. The alveolar walls become thickened and inflamed and are unable to efficiently transmit oxygen and carbon dioxide.[7] There is also a loss of elastic fibers in the lung, making exhalation less effective. The bronchitis component of COPD impairs airway flow because of excessive, tenacious mucus production, and individuals are susceptible to pulmonary infections, for example, pneumonia. Although individuals can have either chronic bronchitis or emphysema in COPD, it is more common to have both components of the disorder concurrently.[7]

The most common cause is smoking, and the adverse effects of smoking are more damaging when the individual begins smoking at a young age.[7]

Clients with severe COPD can develop pulmonary hypertension, increasing the risk for cardiac arrhythmias.[6] Emphysema results from irreversible destruction of alveolar spaces within the lungs, resulting in airway collapse.[6,7]

This disease cannot be cured and is managed by bronchodilating drugs and corticosteroids to reduce inflammation. Bronchitis often occurs with emphysema. It involves the collection of inflammatory secretions that may become infected with microorganisms. All of these features make the client with COPD at risk for airway obstruction and respiratory infection. It has been suggested to administer oxygen at a low flow rate (3 to 4 L/minute), if required during treatment.[7,8] Depending on the extent of disease, several medications are taken to manage symptoms of the disease. These include bronchodilating drugs, inhaled steroids, decongestants, antihistamines, cough suppressants, and expectorants to thin mucous secretions.

The client with COPD is thought to receive the drive to breathe from hypoxia. It has been theorized that if hypoxia is corrected, the client might stop breathing. It is unclear whether this actually occurs, and the current thinking is that supplemental oxygen should be provided (if a respiratory emergency occurs) using a manual bag-mask, if needed, to support ventilation.[7,9]

Cystic Fibrosis

Cystic fibrosis (CF) is the most common lethal inherited disease in Caucasians. Due to improved medical management, individuals with CF can live into their 60s. Cystic fibrosis is an autosomal recessive disorder, and most carriers of the gene are asymptomatic. Most patients with CF have severe chronic lung disease and insufficient excretion of pancreatic hormones.

The disease of exocrine gland function involves multiple organ systems but chiefly results in chronic respiratory infections, pancreatic enzyme insufficiency, and associated complications in untreated patients. Pulmonary involvement occurs in 90% of patients surviving the neonatal period. Cells in the liver and spleen can be affected by the genetic alteration. End-stage lung disease is the principal cause of death.

The diagnosis is based on typical pulmonary manifestations, GI tract manifestations, a family history, and positive sweat chloride test results. Newborn screening for CF is universally offered in the United States. As a result of the complex and multisystemic involvement of the condition and the need for care by specialists, treatment and follow-up care are often provided at specialty centers with multidisciplinary care teams.

Oral disease is described as a low level of dental caries and an increased incidence of periodontal disease with excessive calculus formation. Enamel defects are reported to occur in some patients.[10]

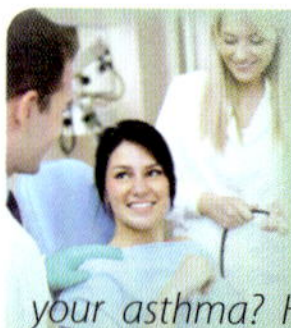

Follow-up Questions

For asthma: "When was your last acute asthma attack? What triggers your asthma? Have you been hospitalized for asthma? Do you have your bronchodilator or rescue inhaler with you? How often do you use the bronchodilator? Have you experienced asthmatic symptoms during dental treatment or after receiving a local anesthetic? What do you use for mild pain?"

For asthma, CF, or COPD: "Can you be seated in a supine position or do you prefer a more upright chair position? Have you had problems in oral care appointments?"

These questions will provide information on the history of acute attacks, on the availability of rescue medications should the client experience bronchoconstriction, the degree of disease control achieved by the drug therapy, and any precautions to consider during oral healthcare procedures. A history of a recent acute asthma attack, especially one involving hospitalization, places the client at increased risk for an asthmatic emergency during oral health care. Because 5% to 15% of asthmatics are allergic to aspirin, and may not be able to take nonsteroidal anti-inflammatory drugs (NSAIDs: ibuprofen, others), the clinician should recommend acetaminophen if oral procedures are expected to result in mild pain.[9] Clients with diseases that involve respiratory obstruction often prefer a semiupright position for oral health care.

APPLICATION TO PRACTICE

When a history of asthma, CF, or COPD is reported, respiratory sounds must be evaluated during vital sign assessment. Sounds during respiration mean there is an airway obstruction. Clients with mild, intermittent asthma use a corticosteroid spray and a short-acting inhaled bronchodilator for occasional use or for acute attacks.[6] The more medications used on a regular basis generally indicate uncontrolled disease or a more severe condition.[9] Severe asthma or COPD is usually treated with steroid tablets, as well as inhaled steroids. Although adrenal crisis from steroid therapy is uncommon, a stress reduction protocol and medical consultation to identify the need for additional steroid supplementation may be indicated (based on physician consultation).[7] Elective oral health care should only be provided for asymptomatic clients or for clients whose symptoms are well controlled. The clinician must be sure that the client has brought a bronchodilator to the oral healthcare appointment, in case acute asthma develops. It is best to use the client's personal bronchodilator, but if the client did not bring a bronchodilator, the clinician should retrieve a bronchodilator from the office emergency medical kit. Over-the-counter epinephrine inhalers are available for the office emergency kit or the dentist can order a prescription product, such as albuterol, for the kit. There is no absolute contraindication for the use of local anesthetics in individuals with COPD. However, local anesthetics with vasoconstrictors use sulfite as an antioxidant. Determine whether the client has an allergy to sulfites, and if so, a local anesthetic without a vasoconstrictor should be selected. Most clients with respiratory disease prefer a semisupine chair position. Breathing is easier in a more upright position. When medical consultation is indicated, the medical clearance form or a transcription of recommendations received from the physician should be placed in the permanent dental record. Oral health education should include:

1. A need to rinse the mouth after use of inhaled steroids to reduce candida infection.
2. The need for a home fluoride program to reduce dental caries.

POTENTIAL EMERGENCIES

Bronchoconstriction, airway obstruction, and choking leading to suffocation are the most likely emergencies. A condition called status asthmaticus is described as persistent life-threatening bronchospasm despite drug therapy. The client with this form of asthma should not receive elective treatment or should receive emergency treatment in a hospital setting. Instruments that produce significant aerosols, such as an ultrasonic scaler, are likely to enhance breathing difficulties in clients with respiratory difficulties. Mucus and secretions associated with cystic fibrosis can lead to choking.

Prevention

The main concern for the client with respiratory disease is to prevent acute bronchoconstriction or airway obstruction from mucus. The patient should be questioned concerning measures to take regarding chair positioning to avoid choking. Observation, listening to sounds during evaluation of respiration, and questioning of the client for asthma control before the treatment begins may prevent an acute attack. The most common dental situations to provoke an attack are:

1. After local anesthesia administration, in individuals who may have an allergy to cartridge components.
2. After tooth extraction, surgery, or general anesthesia due to stress relationships.

Selecting the appropriate local anesthetic agent is essential so that drugs used during the procedure would be unlikely to precipitate an asthma attack. Stress-induced asthma can occur, and the operator must monitor the client during treatment to assure good pain control and maintenance of an open airway. The best appointment time is in the late morning or late afternoon as this is the time when clients are least symptomatic.[11] When questioning reveals a client has **status asthmaticus**, it is prudent to have a medical consultation regarding prevention and management of asthmatic symptoms during oral healthcare procedures. In the client with other respiratory conditions, questioning regarding past experience during oral care may identify safe positioning. For the client with CF, both respiratory obstruction and GI discomfort may need to be addressed. Inhalers are often used to dilate bronchioles and mucolytic agents to reduce mucus formation in CF.

Management

If symptoms of bronchoconstriction occur, the clinician should terminate the procedure, place the client in an upright position, have the client use two "puffs" of the bronchodilator medication in the rescue inhaler device, and provide supplemental oxygen, as needed. Oxygen is not contraindicated for short-term use in medical emergencies that normally would include oxygen administration. The former belief that short-term oxygen use might cause the client to stop breathing is not based on evidence-based science.[7] If signs of severe bronchoconstriction are not relieved in 10 minutes, a second metered dose of the bronchodilator drug should be administered, the 911 emergency medical system should be activated, and the client transported to the hospital for further treatment and evaluation. In most cases, if only one dose of bronchodilator relieves the bronchoconstriction, the emergency medical system (EMS) is not necessary and 100% oxygen should be provided, usually at 4 to 6 L/minute.[7] The client will need to be rescheduled.

Individuals with severe asthma should not receive sedative or anxiolytic drugs due to the potential side effect that may depress respiration.

If choking develops, follow the emergency management for choking described in the discussion of reflux disease at the beginning of this chapter.

When emergency situations arise during treatment, the clinician should try to determine what precipitated the attack and make arrangements to avoid the causative factor in future appointments. The emergency situation should be described in the treatment record, identifying the causative factor (if known), listing of medications used by the clinician, the procedures used during management of the emergency, and the outcome of the emergency situation.

AIRWAY OBSTRUCTION FROM FOREIGN BODIES OR DENTAL MATERIALS

One situation that can result in airway obstruction that is unpredictable (and would not be included on a health history) is when a foreign body obstructs the airway during oral health care. Supine positioning of the client for oral health care promotes dental materials, teeth, or other objects placed within the mouth to fall to the pharyngeal area. This poses an increased risk for airway obstruction.

Airway Obstruction

Respiratory obstruction during oral health care can develop if a foreign body blocks the airway. Dental materials that have been implicated in blocked airways (although not a complete list) include crowns, inlays, cotton rolls, rubber dam clamps, and periodontal pack. Respiratory obstruction can be partial or total. In a partial obstruction, wheezing or a high-pitched crowing sound (called stridor) can be heard as the client attempts to breathe.[11,12] In this situation, the client will have some air exchange. Victims remain responsive, can cough, and usually can speak. Total obstruction of the airway is characterized by the complete absence of sound or soft, wheezing sounds as they try to inhale.[12]

They will not be able to speak or cough forcefully. Signs and symptoms of airway obstruction include agitation; placing the hand at the throat (universal distress signal); coughing, wheezing, crowing, or silence; and cyanosis of face and lips.[11]

Prevention

Use of the saliva ejector helps to remove oral fluids in the area of the throat. Careful observation to ensure that objects are not allowed to fall into the throat is important. When cotton rolls or rubber dam clamps are used, a preventive strategy to retrieve them easily is to tie dental floss around them. If the item obstructs the airway, it can be removed easily by pulling on the floss ligature. The rubber dam is used to prevent restorative materials from entering the oral cavity and pharyngeal area. Examination of the margins of restorations, especially crowns and inlays, to determine the security of the restoration before scaling is helpful to identify loose restorations.

Management

Simple choking is managed by bringing the head forward and allowing the cough mechanism to expel whatever caused the choking event.[12] Allow the client to assume a position that allows a forceful and effective cough.[11] If a dental material falls to the back of the throat, turn the client to the side quickly. Instruct the client to bend over the side of the dental chair arm so that the lips are lower than the throat. This may allow the object to fall forward and be removed by the client. If the object is not removed by bending the client over the chair and using gravity to allow the object to fall forward, a specialized device called Magill forceps can be used to remove objects that can be seen (Fig. 13.3). If these efforts fail, place the chair upright, have the client stand, and perform the Heimlich maneuver to dislodge the object. If the Heimlich does not remove the object and the client becomes unresponsive and unconscious, place the client on the floor and, using the tongue-jaw lift method, try to remove any object you see.[12] If no object can be seen, or if the object was removed and the client is not breathing, give rescue breaths. If rescue breaths are unsuccessful, reopen the airway and give rescue breaths again. This can be followed by abdominal thrusts according to procedures learned in the cardiopulmonary resuscitation (CPR) certification

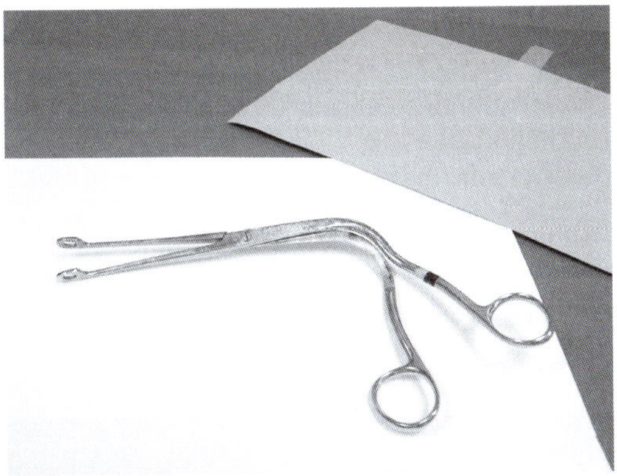

Figure 13.3 ■ Magill forceps.

course.[12] In all cases of foreign body airway obstruction, the object must be retrieved before the event is determined to be resolved. An aspirated object can lodge in the upper airway and not stimulate signs of aspiration. The object may be swallowed by the client. If the object is not retrieved, the client should have radiographic examination (usually at the hospital, where film and equipment are available) to determine whether the object is in the respiratory area or in the GI area. The medical personnel will determine strategies to remove the object in this event. In the dental office if the object cannot be removed, the EMS must be activated quickly to prevent asphyxiation and death. An invasive technique used by trained professionals involves puncturing the neck at the area of the larynx to supply oxygen, called the transtracheal technique.[11] Most dental professionals do not have the skills to perform the transtracheal technique to ventilate the client, although this technique is recommended in emergency management texts. In this technique, an incision is placed in the cricothyroid area of the neck, and a catheter is attached to an empty syringe just above the cricoid cartilage into the trachea. This technique is designed to get oxygen to the lungs when the obstruction occurs superior to the larynx.

Self-Study Review

8. Sounds during respiration signifies:
- a. Asthma.
- b. Cystic fibrosis.
- c. Airway obstruction.
- d. Bronchitis.

9. Asthma is characterized by a reduced ability to inhale. This is caused by inflammation and mucous secretions in the lungs and bronchioles.
- a. Both statements are true.
- b. Both statements are false.
- c. The first statement is true and the second statement is false.
- d. The first statement is false and the second statement is true.

10. A genetic disease associated with chronic lung infections is:
- a. Asthma.
- b. Cystic fibrosis.
- c. COPD.
- d. Emphysema.

11. Persistent life-threatening bronchospasm despite drug therapy describes:
- a. stress-induced asthma.
- b. intrinsic asthma.
- c. extrinsic asthma.
- d. status asthmaticus.

12. Preventing airway obstruction during oral health care can occur through all of the following EXCEPT one. Which one is the EXCEPTION?
- a. Use of a saliva ejector to remove excess oral fluids.
- b. Tying dental floss to cotton rolls or clamps.
- c. Use of a Magill forceps.
- d. Use of a rubber dam.

CHAPTER SUMMARY

Medical conditions related to GI diseases and eating disorders may present with similar oral health findings. Recognizing these conditions and offering supportive care will ensure a positive experience for clients. Understanding how respiratory obstruction can affect the delivery of oral health care will allow the clinician an opportunity to eliminate risks for respiratory emergency situations. The next chapter will include kidney disease and other miscellaneous conditions. It will end the medical disease discussion.

Review

1. Define the following terms: GI reflux and perimylolysis.
2. List the follow-up questions that should be asked for clients who report a history of GERD or peptic ulcer.
3. Identify the oral changes most likely to be seen in a client with a history of GI disease.
4. Identify the oral changes associated with bulimia nervosa.
5. Describe the difference between partial and total airway obstruction.
6. Identify ways to prevent respiratory obstruction.

Case Study

Case A

Laura Davidson presents to the office for a crown preparation procedure. She reports positive responses to a history of GERD and notes that she is taking acid reduction medication for this condition. Her vital signs are pulse, 68 bpm; respirations, 14 breaths/min; blood pressure, 100/68 mm Hg, right arm, sitting.

1. What is the cause of GERD?
2. List at least three symptoms of GERD.
3. What emergency situation is most likely to occur in the dental office setting for this client?
4. What prevention strategies should be used to avoid this emergency situation for this client?
5. If the client experiences reflux during treatment, how would you best manage this condition?

Case B

Catherine Kelly, a 19-year-old client, presents to the practice for caries restoration on the occlusal surface of tooth number 31. She reports a history of asthma and uses an albuterol inhaler as needed. She has seasonal allergies and takes Claritin or Allegra as recommended by her family practitioner. Currently, Ms. Kelly is not taking any medications and has not used her inhaler in 1 month. Her vital signs are pulse, 72 bpm; respiration, 12 breaths/min; blood pressure, 110/62 mm Hg, right arm, sitting. The dentist proceeds with restorative treatment and administers an injection of lidocaine 1:100,000 vasoconstrictor. While the dentist is drilling her tooth, the client reports that she is beginning to have difficulty in breathing and feels as though she is having an asthma attack.

1. What is the most likely cause of the asthma episode?
2. What treatment should be administered?
3. If severe bronchoconstriction occurs even with a second dose of bronchodilator, what treatment steps should be taken?
4. What documentation should you note in the treatment record about this emergency?
5. What prevention strategy should be used for future appointments?

Chapter Fourteen

Medical Conditions Involving Glaucoma, the Kidneys, and Thyroid Disorders

Objectives

After completing the self-study chapter the reader will be able to:

- Identify the client at risk for an attack of acute glaucoma and describe measures to prevent this during the oral healthcare appointment.
- List kidney conditions that cause a change in the oral healthcare plan and describe the medical management of the client and the prevention of infection after oral health care.
- Describe the dental management of the client on hemodialysis.
- Describe the dental management of the client with an organ transplant.
- Describe how to prevent thyroid storm in the uncontrolled hyperthyroid client.

Key Terms

Bradycardia: reduced heart rate, below 60 bpm

Ecchymosis: collection of blood under the mucosal layer

Euthyroid: pertaining to normal thyroid gland function

Glaucoma: a condition of the eye, characterized by increased pressure within the eyeball

Hemodialysis: the removal of wastes and other undesirable substances from the blood by means of a medical device

Renal: having to do with the kidneys

Tachycardia: increased heart rate, above 160 bpm

Uremia: the presence of excessive amounts of urea and waste products in the blood, occurs in renal failure

MEDICAL CONDITION

INTRODUCTION

This chapter includes a discussion of the conditions included on the American Dental Association (ADA) Health History form that have not been included in previous chapters. The discussion will focus on clinical implications for glaucoma, kidney disease, thyroid disease, and various special needs conditions; potential emergency situations; and prevention and management strategies for emergency situations.

"Please (X) a response to indicate if you have or have not had any of the following diseases or problems: glaucoma."

PATHOPHYSIOLOGY DISCUSSION

Glaucoma is a condition in which the pressure within the eye is increased. It is among the most common causes of blindness, occurs mainly in older individuals, and is diagnosed by means of an ocular examination. Pressure within the eye is increased when fluid cannot flow through the canal of Schlemm at the junction between the iris and the cornea.[1] There are two forms of glaucoma: open-angle glaucoma (affecting 95% of glaucoma cases), in which pressure gradually increases; and narrow-angle glaucoma, an acute situation in which pressure suddenly increases.[1]

Open-Angle Glaucoma

Symptoms in this common form of vision deterioration are so gradual that they often go unnoticed. For this reason, it is recommended that persons with a family history of the disease be screened annually at the age of 40. As the condition progresses, peripheral vision is lost; then, blurred vision with difficulty in adjusting to brightness and darkness is noticed. One symptom suggestive of chronic glaucoma is the perception of a halo surrounding a light when looking at a distant light while in the dark. The condition is only mildly painful. This form is treated with eyedrops that relieve intraocular pressure.[2] Because some medication causes constriction of the pupils (which can be misconstrued as a symptom of heroin overdose), clients may carry an identification card that describes the medical history, in case of emergency. The cause of glaucoma is unknown. If left untreated, partial or complete vision loss can occur. Clients with a history of cataracts can develop glaucoma.

Narrow-Angle Glaucoma

Acute glaucoma manifests as sudden, severe pain and abrupt vision blurring. It is a rare condition but must be treated quickly by emergency ophthalmic surgery to relieve pressure and prevent permanent blindness.

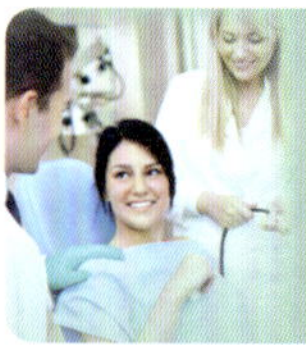

Follow-up Questions

"Have you ever experienced an acute glaucoma attack during oral care? Is your vision impaired by the disease?"

APPLICATION TO PRACTICE

If the client has suffered vision impairment as a result of glaucoma, this may affect the ability to perform effective self-care procedures. Assess the effectiveness of the client's techniques and make recommendations as needed. Provide protective eyewear during the appointment, and consider adaptations during the appointment for clients with limited sight. In the client with narrow-angle glaucoma, the dentist should avoid using drugs that can precipitate an attack, such as anticholinergic drugs.[2] In clients using medications to prevent an attack of glaucoma, there is generally a low risk for causing an acute attack during treatment. Use of a drug reference will determine the medication side effects relevant to oral health care.

POTENTIAL EMERGENCIES

Anticholinergics such as atropine (Banthine®), used in dentistry to reduce salivary secretions, can cause an acute rise in intraocular pressure and precipitate an acute painful attack in unrecognized cases of narrow-angle glaucoma.[2]

Prevention

In clients with narrow-angle glaucoma, anticholinergic agents (e.g., atropine, scopolamine) should not be used. There is no contraindication to using drugs used in dentistry in the client with open-angle glaucoma.

Management

The acute narrow-angle glaucoma attack must be treated quickly in a hospital setting. Activate the 911 emergency medical system to transport the client to a facility where ophthalmic surgery can be completed.

Self-Study Review

1. Symptoms of open-angle glaucoma include all of the following EXCEPT one. Which one is the EXCEPTION?
   a. Sudden, sharp pain.
   b. Blurred vision.
   c. Halo appearance surrounding a light.
   d. Loss of peripheral vision.
2. One drug that should be avoided in clients with narrow-angle glaucoma is:
   a. β-Blockers.
   b. Atropine.
   c. Glucocorticoids.
   d. Warfarin.
3. Treatment of open-angle glaucoma involves:
   a. use of eyedrops
   b. activation of 911 EMS
   c. ophthalmic surgery
   d. prescription eye glasses

"Please (X) a response to indicate if you have or have not had any of the following diseases or problems: kidney problems."

PATHOPHYSIOLOGY DISCUSSION

The kidneys are the organs that eliminate waste products (contained in urine) from the body and also serve to maintain proper water balance in the body. The kidneys are bean-shaped structures located in the posterior section of the abdomen. Their main functions are to filter wastes from the blood and to provide for reabsorption of essential chemicals back into the bloodstream. Disorders in the urinary system range from infection to **uremia** and end-stage **renal** disease (ESRD). Treatment depends on the stage of the disorder. This discussion will focus on chronic problems that may cause an alteration in the oral healthcare treatment plan, such as glomerulonephritis, ESRD (e.g., kidney failure) and hemodialysis, and organ transplant. Kidney infections will not be included because they are treated with anti-infective agents and are generally cured quickly with no residual effects. Management for the ambulatory client who has a chronic kidney disease (CKD) that requires modification of the treatment plan, and who is likely to present for oral health care in a dental office, will be included in this section.

End-Stage Renal Disease or Kidney Failure

Healthy kidneys clean the blood by filtering out extra water and waste products. They also synthesize erythropoietin, a hormone active in red blood cell production that carries oxygen to all parts of the body; and vitamin D, responsible for calcium absorption and bone health. When both kidneys fail, the body holds fluid, blood pressure rises, and harmful wastes build up in the body tissues. In addition, the production of red blood cells diminishes, leading to anemia. The most common causes of ESRD are diabetes, hypertension, and chronic glomerulonephritis.[3,4] Deterioration of the functional nephrons in the kidney (glomerulus, tubules, blood vessels) is the direct pathologic influence on renal failure.[3] Regeneration of nephrons does not occur. Deterioration continues until the nephrons are lost and signs of uremia appear. The failing kidneys cause fluid overload, hypertension, and cardiac complications. Approximately 50% of clients with ESRD die of cardiovascular complications.[3]

This condition often requires the affected person to be placed on dialysis or to have a kidney transplant. There are two forms of dialysis: hemodialysis and peritoneal dialysis. Hemodialysis uses a dialyzer, or unique filter, to cleanse the blood. The dialyzer filters out wastes and extra fluids. The cleaned blood flows from the venous access site in the arm to the dialyzer, is filtered, and then flows through a different set of tubes back into the body. Peritoneal dialysis is a procedure usually performed at home. In this method, a cleansing solution, called dialysate, travels through a surgically implanted catheter into the abdomen where the lining of the abdomen filters the blood. Fluid, wastes, and chemicals pass from tiny blood vessels in the peritoneal membrane into the dialysate. After several hours, the dialysate is drained from the abdomen, taking the wastes for the blood with it. This process takes 30 to 40 minutes and is repeated four times a day. The fluid in the peritoneum adds weight to the abdominal area, leads to acid reflux disorder, and the client may prefer to be seated in a semiupright position for oral care.

Infection in the client with CKD can lead to profound acidosis and be fatal.[3] Therefore, oral health information regarding the importance of maintaining healthy periodontal tissues and frequent maintenance to prevent oral infection or to identify oral infections early is important. Oral infections should be treated aggressively with antibiotics, with advisement from the nephrologist on which agents to use. Increased susceptibility to infection occurs as a complication of CKD, as a result of decreased chemotaxis and phagocytosis of leukocytes.

Blood abnormalities can include anemia, leukocyte and platelet dysfunction, and coagulation abnormalities. Hemorrhagic disturbances that result in increased bleeding are caused by abnormal platelet aggregation, decreased platelet function, and impaired prothrombin conversion to thrombin. Alveolar bone stability is compromised in ESRD and can predispose the jaw to fracture. Panoramic radiographs should be completed to identify osteolytic lesions in the jaws. ESRD results in an immunocompromised state and an increased risk for infective endocarditis. It has been proposed for individuals on hemodialysis that antibiotic prophylaxis should be considered prior to oral procedures that can cause a bacteremia.[4]

However, a recent systematic review on indications for antibiotic prophylaxis prior to oral procedures determined that there is no evidence that prophylaxis would prevent infection related to hemodialysis.[5] The authors state that of the more than 375,000 individuals with ESRD in the United States, more than 275,000 are receiving dialysis for chronic renal failure. The vascular access sites for hemodialysis equipment include grafts of synthetic materials or catheters. Grafts are usually placed below the skin in the antecubital fossa area and are punctured several times each week for dialysis. Repetitive needle punctures can result in infection from skin bacteria, mainly *Streptococcus aureus.* This infection can cause morbidity and mortality and hospitalizations, often despite aggressive antibiotic therapy. Infective endocarditis is a complication of vascular access infections, but there is no evidence that antibiotic prophylaxis will prevent the cardiac infection. Current American Heart Association guidelines for nonvalvular cardiovascular devices do not include hemodialysis shunts as a device requiring prophylaxis.[6]

Oral signs of uremia caused by kidney failure include odors in the mouth, metallic taste, dry mouth, enlarged parotid glands, mucosal pallor, stomatitis and oral ulceration, candidiasis, osteolytic lesions in the jaws, and petechial hemorrhages in oral soft tissues (Box 14-1).[3,7] Oral health care can be influenced by potential complications of kidney failure, which include anemia, abnormal bleeding, blood pressure changes, loss of jaw stability or risk of fracture, and the inability to eliminate drugs normally. Bleeding problems are principally due to abnormal platelet function and impaired prothrombin levels.[3] Although research is sparse investigating the role of periodontal infection and ESRD, one study of individuals with diabetes who had moderate to severe periodontal disease found that periodontal disease resulted in twice the incidence of ESRD and concluded that periodontitis is predictive for renal failure.[8] Because ESRD can affect multiple organ systems, medical consultation prior to stressful oral procedures is recommended. For the client whose disease is controlled by medical therapy and dialysis, the risk for complications during periodontal maintenance care is low.[3]

Box 14-1

Oral Manifestations of Chronic Renal Failure

- Bad odor in mouth and metallic taste
- Dry mouth, candidiasis
- Enlarged parotid gland
- Mucosal pallor
- Stomatitis, painful ulcerations
- Osteolytic lesions in bone, risk of fracture during treatment
- Petechial hemorrhages, gingival bleeding

(Adapted from DeRossi S, Glick M. Dental considerations for the patient with renal disease receiving hemodialysis. J Am Dent Assoc 1996;127:211–219.)

Glomerulonephritis

Each kidney contains more than a million filtering units called nephrons. Each nephron contains a network of tiny blood vessels (called a glomerulus) that are responsible for filtering blood. Inflammation (-itis) of this unit (glomerulus) interferes with the normal function of the kidney. Inflammation can be caused by different reasons, but most often it is caused by an autoimmune response to infections in other parts of the body. The most common sites of infection to cause this response in the kidney are infection of the throat, tonsils, or skin. Streptococcus bacteria are commonly implicated. The immune response to the streptococcal infection occurs as an inflammation of the capillaries in the glomeruli of both kidneys. The capillaries become congested, leading to enlargement of the kidney. Protein, which should remain in the blood, filters into the urine, and edema forms in the body. These two signs, edema and the presence of protein in urine, are the main indicators of the disease. If not resolved, the capillaries can form scar tissue and no longer hold blood, so that the areas of the kidney that they serve cease to function. This process continues to affect other parts of the kidney, and total kidney failure results. At this stage, the client is placed on dialysis and awaits a kidney transplant. During the acute stage of the infection, the client has headaches, mild fever, facial edema, and pain in the lower back. Antibiotics are the treatment of choice. In approximately 20% of clients, the condition becomes chronic. The client is not likely to seek oral health care in the acute phase, so the application to practice discussion will focus on the client with chronic glomerulonephritis. In the past, it was reported that individuals with a history of glomerulonephritis should have antibiotic prophylaxis prior to oral procedures; however, there are no official guidelines in this regard and no studies to demonstrate that prophylactic antibiotics prior to oral care prevents infection in the kidney.

Dialysis

One form of dialysis that can be accomplished at home is peritoneal dialysis. It does not require changes in the treatment plan, other than to affect decisions related to drugs the dentist plans to use as part of treatment. The type of dialysis that requires significant modification in the treatment plan is **hemodialysis**. Hemodialysis is the removal of wastes and other undesirable substances from the blood by means of a medical device. Two plastic tubes, one connected to an artery and one to a vein, are implanted in the client's arm or leg (Fig. 14.1). During dialysis, blood from the artery tube enters the dialysis machine and comes into contact with a thin membrane. Wastes from the blood pass through the membrane into circulating fluid on the other side of the membrane. Blood cells and other protein elements do not cross the membrane. The cleansed blood is then piped back into the patient through the vein tube. This process takes several hours and must be done several times a week.[3,7,9] The client is given heparin, an anticoagulant drug, to prevent clotting of blood during the hemodialysis process. In addition, the dialysis procedure can injure platelets, reducing the platelet count.[9] Oral complications reported in the hemodialysis client include mucosal **ecchymosis**, oral malodor, xerostomia, taste changes, and tongue and mucosal pain.[3] Dialysis diminishes many of the signs and symptoms of ESRD. An increased risk for bleeding is expected (due to platelet damage during the dialysis procedure) and can often be managed with digital pressure or topical hemostatic agents (e.g., thrombin, GelFoam®).

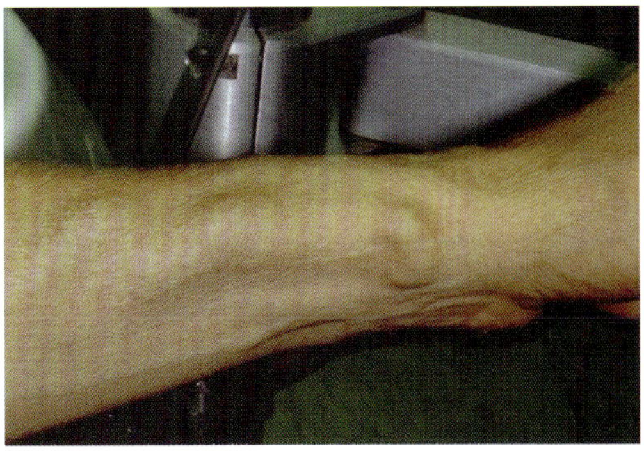

Figure 14.1 ■ Clinical photograph of implanted arteriovenous shunt.

Kidney Transplant

In terms of quality of life and long-term survival, transplant is the best treatment option for individuals with kidney failure. After a kidney is transplanted, it usually begins working immediately and dialysis is no longer needed. The kidney recipient is monitored after the transplant to ensure the new kidney is functioning and dosages of the immune suppressant drugs to prevent rejection are adjusted for efficacy. Oral care should be delayed for 6 months following the organ transplant.[3] The client who has received a kidney transplant will be taking antirejection drugs (cyclosporine, prednisone, others) that result in immunosuppression.[2,3]

Because the immune system does not fight infection normally, it should be treated early and aggressively with antibiotics. Wound healing will be slow. Adrenal function may be depressed as a result of antirejection medication. Excessive immunosuppression can result in oral infections, such as candidiasis, herpes simplex, herpes zoster, and hairy leukoplakia. Other oral lesions associated with immunosuppression include aphthous ulcers, malignancies (lymphoma, Kaposi sarcoma), and squamous cell carcinoma. Side effects of drugs used can include bleeding, infection, ulcerations, gingival hyperplasia (e.g., cyclosporine), and reduced salivation.[3] Other medications are often taken following a kidney transplant, such as antihypertensives. Coexisting medical conditions, such as diabetes, must be considered in the management of the individual with a kidney transplant. The client with a successful kidney transplant poses less risk for a medical emergency than the client with CKD.

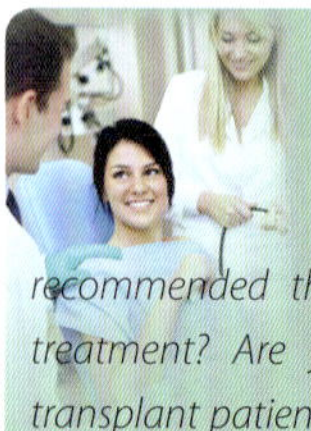

Follow-up Questions

"What type of kidney problem do you have? Has your physician recommended that you take antibiotics before dental treatment? Are you on hemodialysis? (for the kidney transplant patient). What drugs are you taking to prevent rejection of your kidney?"

APPLICATION TO PRACTICE

CKD predisposes the client to have a variety of complications during oral health care. The risk of cardiovascular problems, which mainly include heart attack and stroke, rises dramatically when CKD is present. For this reason, blood pressure should be monitored and treatment delayed until levels are ≤180/110 mm Hg. Medical consultation should include blood studies to identify potential bleeding problems and reduction in healing associated with the blood abnormalities discussed above. Lab tests should include the platelet function analyzer-100 (PFA-100) and the platelet count.[3]

During medical consultation, the nephrologist should be asked if prophylactic antibiotics should be considered when invasive oral procedures are planned (e.g., deep scaling, complicated periodontal debridement) and the physician should determine the drug dosage, agent used, and prepare the prescription.[3] Some drugs used in dentistry cannot be tolerated in the client with ESRD. Aspirin and nonsteroidal anti-inflammatory drugs (NSAIDs; such as ibuprofen [Motrin®]) are to be used with caution in moderate renal failure and are not recommended for clients with severe renal failure.[7] Acetaminophen (in low doses and for a short time), most antibiotics (except tetracycline), and lidocaine local anesthetic can be used.[3,7] Nitrous oxide and diazepam are antianxiety agents that can be used. Other central nervous system (CNS) depressants are to be used with caution and only after medical consultation.[3] Individuals on dialysis often take multiple medications to control hypertension, heart failure, or thickening of the blood (hypercoagulability). Adverse drug effects that can influence oral care should be investigated and monitored.

To reduce complications associated with ESRD, treatment plan modifications for the client with kidney disease include:

1. Appoint on the day following dialysis when the client is rested and the effects of heparin used during dialysis are no longer in the body.
2. Consult with the nephrologist or physician to determine whether there are potential complications that may affect the provision of oral care, such as the use of an air-polishing device or the need for antibiotic prophylaxis prior to oral procedures.
3. Determine the risk for increased bleeding or anemia by getting laboratory tests (e.g., platelet count, PFA-100, complete blood count) and monitor clotting during procedures.
4. Monitor the blood pressure for hypertension and using the arm that does not have the vascular access shunt for blood pressure measurement.
5. Take panoramic radiographs to identify bone abnormalities.
6. Avoid using aspirin or NSAID medications; acetaminophen, nitrous oxide, and lidocaine can be used for oral pain.

Bleeding episodes not resolved by digital pressure can be treated with local hemostatic agents, such as oxidized cellulose and tranexamic acid mouthrinses.[7] Many of the clients are on salt-restricted diets, and use of the bicarbonate of soda–based air-polishing device might be contraindicated. The best analgesic to recommend is acetaminophen, but in low doses. Schedule frequent continuing care appointments to monitor oral health status and reduce the risk for periodontal disease (Box 14-2).

Hemodialysis

For clients on hemodialysis, there are several other treatment plan modifications before oral health care. Most patients receive dialysis 3 days a week. To this effect, an artificial permanent vascular access is placed in the form of a catheter or surgically performed arteriovenous fistula.[9]

The pressure from the blood pressure cuff can cause the arteriovenous shunt to collapse, so blood pressure should be taken on the opposite arm.[7] Because it has been shown that when

Box 14-2

Treatment Modifications for ESRD

- Appoint on the day following dialysis when the client is rested and the effects of heparin used during dialysis are no longer in the body
- Consultation with physician to determine disease and treatment modifications
- Monitor vital signs to determine cardiovascular for blood pressure measurement use that does not include the hemodialysis shunt
- Consider increased risk for excessive bleeding; monitor blood coagulation levels with platelet count and PFA-100 laboratory studies
- Order complete blood count to identify anemia if extensive treatment is planned
- Avoid using aspirin or NSAID medications; acetaminophen, nitrous oxide, and lidocaine control can be used
- Use full series or panoramic radiographs to disease; determine bone stability and identify abnormal arm bone lesions
- Frequent maintenance schedule to prevent oral infection or identify infections early

PFA, platelet function analyzer; NSAID, nonsteroidal anti-inflammatory drug; CBC, complete blood count.

periodontal tissues are healthy the risk for bacteremia is reduced, excellent oral hygiene habits should be encouraged.[5] When dialysis occurs, the client may be given heparin to reduce the risk of clotting during the procedure. The effects last for a few hours after the procedure, so it is best to schedule maintenance visits the day after dialysis when the effects of heparin are no longer present and the blood waste products have been removed.[4,9] If oral procedures will involve significant bleeding, then laboratory tests should be requested to determine the risks of hemorrhage. Clients on chronic dialysis are prone to develop infections, so a frequent maintenance schedule is recommended to monitor oral health. Be aware that hemodialysis does not remove breath odor, xerostomia, taste disturbances, or mucosal pain associated with ESRD.

Renal Transplant

Dental management for the client who is post-transplant can be divided into three phases.[3]

The immediate period after the transplant procedure lasts for 6 months. During this time, antirejection medication doses are being adjusted and the transplanted organ is monitored for evidence of rejection. No routine oral care should be provided during this time. The next phase is the stable period where the organ is functioning and the medication is preventing organ rejection. During this period, the practitioner should consult with the transplant medical physician to coordinate care. The key points during this period include (Box 14-3):

Box 14-3

Treatment Modifications for Organ Transplantation

Emphasize the importance of maintaining periodontal health, control of biofilm and use of antimicrobial oral products, and effective oral hygiene devices

Schedule maintenance care every 3 to 6 months, according to client's periodontal needs

Identify oral infection early and treat effectively; immunosuppression from antirejection medications predisposes to candidiasis

Avoid excessive bleeding or trauma during oral care. Monitor blood pressure using physician recommendations for excessive values

1. Emphasize the importance of maintaining periodontal health through control of biofilm, use of antimicrobial oral products, and effective oral hygiene devices.
2. Schedule maintenance care every 3 to 6 months, according to client periodontal needs.
3. Identify oral infection early and treat effectively, remembering the client is immunosuppressed from antirejection medications and predisposed to candidiasis.
4. Avoid excessive bleeding or trauma during oral care.
5. Monitor blood pressure using physician recommendations for excessive values requiring referral to medical office.

The final phase is the chronic rejection period. During this period, oral care should only be provided after medical consultation and based on recommendations of the transplant care physician.

Antirejection drugs may be taken for life. The most common therapy is triple drug combinations with cyclosporine, prednisone, and mycophenolate mofetil (CellCept®). When cyclosporine is taken to prevent organ rejection, monitor the gingiva for the presence of hyperplasia, and inform the client that plaque removal must be completed daily to reduce the risk for enlargement. Drugs used in dentistry that can interact with immunosuppressive antirejection therapy are erythromycin and ketoconazole (an antifungal drug). Any antimicrobial agent needed should be prescribed only after consultation with the physician to avoid complications. Monitor blood pressure during each appointment to determine the control. Investigate side effects of all drugs taken and manage as indicated.

Chapter 10 includes organ transplant management recommendations in general.

Self-Study Review

4. All of the following are causes of ESRD EXCEPT one. Which one is the EXCEPTION?
   a. Hypertension
   b. Diabetes
   c. Hypothyroidism
   d. Chronic glomerulonephritis
5. Medication contraindicated in clients with severe ESRD includes:
   a. aspirin.
   b. antibiotics.
   c. acetaminophen.
   d. lidocaine.
6. From the following list, identify the oral signs of uremia caused by kidney failure.
   a. Metallic taste
   b. Malodor
   c. Hypersalivation
   d. Ulceration
   e. Enlarged parotid glands
   f. Candidiasis
   f. Petechia
7. The primary cause of glomerulonephritis is:
   a. inflammation.
   b. congestion of capillaries.
   c. autoimmune response to infection.
   d. edema and hemorrhage.
8. The purpose of administering heparin during hemodialysis is to:
   a. remove waste products.
   b. prevent infection.
   c. prevent clotting.
   d. fight infection.

POTENTIAL EMERGENCIES

There are no medical emergency situations specifically for having kidney disease. However, it should be noted that the risk for cardiovascular emergencies is increased. Cardiovascular disease is the number one cause for death in individuals with CKD. If increased bleeding occurs during therapy, it should be managed with digital pressure or hemostatic agents, using topically applied agents such as oxidized cellulose, thrombin, or tranexamic acid.

"Please (X) a response to indicate if you have or have not had any of the following diseases or problems: thyroid problems."

Uncontrolled hyperthyroidism, exacerbated by the stress response, poses a risk for a medical emergency. Therefore, oral healthcare procedures that are stressful should not be provided to the client with uncontrolled hyperthyroid disease. Those clients with undiagnosed thyroid disease or uncontrolled thyroid disease pose a potential medical emergency situation, called thyroid storm. The condition is more common in clients who know they have the condition, but in whom the disease is uncontrolled.[3] Controlled clients should have vital signs monitored to determine the degree of disease control but can receive oral care without adverse effects.

PATHOPHYSIOLOGY DISCUSSION

Thyroid gland disorders include a variety of conditions, such as thyroid cancer, hypothyroidism, hyperthyroidism, goiter, and autoimmune conditions that affect the thyroid gland, including Graves disease and Hashimoto thyroiditis.[3] Hashimoto thyroiditis leads to hypothyroidism and thyroid enlargement (e.g., nonfunctional goiter), whereas Graves disease leads to hyperthyroidism and enlargement of the thyroid (e.g., functional goiter). Therefore, the presence of a goiter is an indication for referral for medical evaluation. The thyroid gland is a two-lobed structure located at or below the thyroid cartilage in the neck. The gland produces three hormones (thyroxine [T4], triiodothyronine [T3], and calcitonin) that influence every tissue in the body.[2] The gland is regulated by the pituitary gland, which secretes thyroid-stimulating hormone (TSH) when thyroid hormone level is low. The pituitary stops secreting TSH when an adequate hormone level occurs. Thyroid hormones play a role in maintenance of body temperature, conversion of food and vitamins to energy, growth, and regulation of body functions.[3]

Low dietary intake of iodine is associated with an increased prevalence of thyrotoxicosis (hyperthyroidism), although this etiology only accounts for 20% to 40% of disease.[3] Graves disease is more common in women.

Hypothyroidism

This condition results because of an inadequate supply of thyroid hormones necessary for body needs. Several factors can decrease secretion of thyroid hormone. These include chronic inflammation of the thyroid seen in autoimmune-related situations (Hashimoto thyroiditis) or a deficiency of TSH from the pituitary gland.[3] The presence of a goiter, or enlarged thyroid gland, is a sign of Hashimoto thyroiditis. Hypothyroidism can result after pharmacologic treatment for hyperthyroidism through oversuppression of glandular function. Women are more likely to be affected, and pregnancy may trigger the hormonal imbalance. Myxedema is the condition caused by hypothyroidism in adults. Cretinism is hypothyroidism that occurs during childhood. Evaluation of reduced growth patterns is often the first clue to diagnosis in children. Signs of chronic hypothyroidism are anemia; **bradycardia**; sluggishness and fatigue; edema in the tongue, face, neck, and hands; depression; weight gain as a result of a reduced metabolic rate; dry skin and hair; and recurrent infections. The client is often intolerant to cold temperature. Uncontrolled hypothyroid clients are unusually sensitive to the effects of CNS depressant drugs, such as sedatives, opioid analgesics (e.g., codeine, Demerol®), and antianxiety drugs.[2] These drugs are used commonly in dentistry.

Hyperthyroidism

Hyperthyroidism is a general term that involves several different disorders with the common feature of excessive production of thyroid hormone. The two most common forms of hyperthyroidism are autoimmune-related Graves disease and toxic goiter.[3] In toxic goiter, nodules of thyroid tissue form and secrete abnormally large amounts of thyroid hormone independent of the TSH function in the pituitary. In Graves disease, the autoimmune reaction causes increased secretions of thyroid hormone (opposite of what occurs in Hashimoto thyroiditis). A common sign of Graves disease is bulging of the eyes. Signs of hyperthyroidism involve many vital organs and include increased body temperature and sweating (intolerance to hot temperatures), weight loss and increased basal metabolic rate (BMR), **tachycardia**, hyperactivity and nervousness, tremors, emotional instability, and hypertension (Box 14-4). The medical emergency situation (thyroid storm) involves a sudden development of increased body temperature and hypertension. Graves disease occurs most often in women between the ages of 30 and 40 and is associated with an extraoral sign of bulging eyeballs due to enlargement of fat and muscle within the orbit.[3] Toxic goiter affects those in middle age or the elderly. The uncontrolled hyperthyroid client is overly responsive to epinephrine, and local anesthetics containing epinephrine should not be used unless disease control is established.

Box 14-4

Signs of Thyroid Disease

Hypothyroidism	Hyperthyroidism
Hypotension to normal BP, bradycardia	Hypertension, tachycardia
Intolerance to cold	Elevated body temperature and heat intolerance
Intolerance to CNS depressant drugs	Intolerance to epinephrine
Edema of face, tongue, neck, goiter	Bulging eyes, goiter
Lethargic, fatigued, dry skin	Nervous, trembling, sweating

BP, blood pressure; CNS, central nervous system.

Treatment

Treatment for both hypothyroidism and hyperthyroidism includes drug therapy or removal of all or part of the thyroid gland.[2] Drug therapy for hyperthyroidism often results in a hypothyroid condition. The **euthyroid** or controlled client poses no additional risk during oral health care, although if thyroid hormone is taken the practitioner should be cautious and use vasoconstrictors in low concentrations.[2] Clients with controlled hyperthyroidism can tolerate small doses of epinephrine (no more than two cartridges of 1:100,000).[2] Side effects of the various drugs used in treatment should be investigated using a drug reference, along with oral examination, extraoral examination, and assessment of vital sign values.

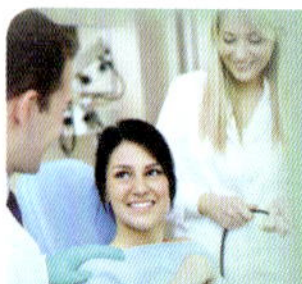

Follow-up Questions

"What type of thyroid problem do you have? How well controlled is your condition? Have you ever had a problem during dental treatment?"

Acute dental infection or stressful dental procedures have precipitated thyroid storm in individuals with uncontrolled hyperthyroidism.[3]

APPLICATION TO PRACTICE

Because both hyperthyroidism and hypothyroidism are associated with an increased incidence of cardiovascular disease, vital signs should be measured at each appointment.[2]

Monitor not only the blood pressure but also the pulse and the functional capacity to determine whether the thyroid condition is controlled. The client with thyroid disease should be able to meet a 4 metabolic equivalent functional capacity (discussed in Chapter 1).[2] The clinical examination should include examination for facial edema or intraoral edema. The midline of the base of the tongue should be examined for presence of a thyroid nodule. The anterior neck region should be examined for surgical scars or the presence of an enlarged thyroid. The area superior and lateral to the thyroid cartilage should be palpated for the presence of enlargement and coordinated with having the client swallow while the fingers remain on the soft tissue area of the neck. Nodules due to hyperplasia may feel rubbery and soft, whereas enlargement from autoimmune disease is usually firm.[3]

The symptomatic client should be referred for medical evaluation, and a physician consultation should be made to assure disease control before oral procedures are scheduled. Elective treatment should be delayed until control has been achieved. Clients with hypothyroidism have a low risk for medical emergencies during oral health care, but side effects of a common medication to treat the condition (e.g., Synthroid®) may induce a hyperthyroid state. Poorly controlled hypothyroid clients may be unable to tolerate CNS depressant drugs. Epinephrine should not be used in the uncontrolled hyperthyroid client. If signs of hyperthyroidism are noted in the client taking thyroid hormone, refer the client to the physician to have the thyroid levels checked. Signs of thyroid disease are listed in Box 14-4.

POTENTIAL EMERGENCIES

Although unlikely to occur during oral health care because of its slow onset, myxedemic coma is the medical emergency associated with uncontrolled hypothyroidism. It is most likely to occur in the undiagnosed client. Myxedemic coma is characterized by severe hypotension, hypothermia, swelling or edema, and hypoventilation.[3] Stressful situations such as cold, surgery, infection, and trauma can precipitate myxedemic coma.

Thyroid storm is the most likely medical emergency in uncontrolled *hyperthyroidism*. It has a rapid onset and results when the client is unable to respond to physiologic stress. Elevation of blood pressure (≥180/110) or a pulse rate over 100 bpm may indicate thyroid storm. Symptoms include restlessness, fever, tachycardia, pulmonary edema, tremors, stupor, coma, and, finally, death if treatment is not provided.[3] Precipitating factors can involve trauma, surgery, and acute oral infection.

Prevention

The physical examination with vital sign measurement should be able to identify signs of uncontrolled thyroid disease so that the client can be referred for medical evaluation. Oral health care should not be provided in the client who shows signs of uncontrolled thyroid disease. Vital signs are a significant tool to identify poorly controlled thyroid conditions. Extraoral examination for the presence of a goiter and swelling of head and neck tissues may indicate a need for medical evaluation before treatment. For individuals taking thyroid hormone, the use of epinephrine or other vasoconstrictors should be limited, even in euthyroid clients. If acute oral infection occurs, consultation with the client's physician is recommended before dental management.[3]

Management

Because thyroid storm (also called thyrotoxic crisis) has a rapid onset and is the most likely emergency situation during oral health care, the discussion will be limited to management of this condition. The clinician should recognize the signs of the condition onset, activate the 911 emergency system as the client will need hospital care, place cold towels on the client to bring down the body temperature, monitor and record vital signs, and provide basic life support (airway, breathing, and circulation).[3] If cardiac arrest occurs, cardiopulmonary resuscitation should be provided until the emergency medical personnel arrive. If the equipment and drugs are available in the dental office, 100 to 300 mg of hydrocortisone can be administered by the dentist and an IV infusion of hypertonic glucose initiated.[3]

Self-Study Review

9. Maintenance of body temperature, growth, and regulation of body functions is controlled by which gland?
   a. Adrenal
   b. Thyroid
   c. Parathyroid
   d. Pituitary
10. Myxedema represents:
    a. Hypothyroidism in children.
    b. Hypothyroidism in adults.
    c. Hyperthyroidism in children.
    d. Hyperthyroidism in adults.
11. The two most common forms of hyperthyroidism are:
    a. graves disease and Hashimoto thyroiditis.
    b. toxic goiter and Graves disease.
    c. toxic goiter and Hashimoto thyroiditis.
    d. hashimoto thyroiditis and TSH syndrome.
12. The medical emergency most likely to occur in hypothyroidism is:
    a. thyroid storm.
    b. bradycardia.
    c. thyrotoxic crisis.
    d. myxedema coma.
13. Hashimoto thyroiditis leads to hyperthyroidism, while Graves disease leads to hypothyroidism. Both conditions cause enlargement of the thyroid gland.
    a. Both statements are true.
    b. Both statements are false.
    c. The first statement is true, and the second statement is false.
    d. The first statement is false, and the second statement is true.

CHAPTER SUMMARY

This chapter highlighted significant information concerning glaucoma, kidney disease, and thyroid disease. Potential emergencies and management strategies have been included to allow the clinician to feel prepared to address these situations appropriately during the health history review. Follow-up questions are included to guide clinical practice. The next chapter will include a discussion of reporting summary information about the health history, preparation of healthcare personnel for emergency management, and federal regulations regarding privacy of healthcare information.

Review

1. Define the following terms: euthyroid, glaucoma, and hemodialysis.
2. List the symptoms of open-angle glaucoma and narrow-angle glaucoma.
3. Describe the treatment needed for a client who experiences an acute narrow-angle glaucoma attack.

Case Study

Case A

John Rizzo presents with a history of glomerulonephritis and ESRD. He has been treated with hemodialysis and is awaiting a kidney transplant. Vital signs include pulse, 80 bpm; respiration, 18 breaths/min; blood pressure, 180/110 mm Hg, right arm, sitting.

1. What oral complications are associated with hemodialysis?
2. If the client has his dialysis treatment on Mondays, Wednesdays, and Fridays, when during the week can his maintenance appointment be scheduled? Why?
3. If the client has a shunt in his right arm, which arm should be used for taking blood pressure? Why?
4. What management strategies should be used for this client?
5. What is the leading cause of death in cases of ESRD?
6. If this client does have a kidney transplant, when is it safe for him to return for dental hygiene care?

Case B

Ann Myerson presents with a history of hypothyroidism after treatment for hyperthyroidism. Vital signs include pulse, 66 bpm; respiration, 14 breaths/min; blood pressure, 116/62 mm Hg, right arm, sitting.

1. List the signs of hyperthyroidism.
2. List the signs of hypothyroidism.
3. If the client reports taking Synthroid and demonstrates evidence of a hyperthyroid state, what medical emergency might occur? How would you treat this emergency?
4. Describe the medical emergency associated with hypothyroidism and give two examples of situations that can cause this emergency.

Chapter Fifteen

Analysis of Information with Clinical Applications

Objectives

After completing the self-study chapter the reader will be able to:

- Identify appropriate clinical recording information and describe the rationale for analyzing clinical data.
- Describe the advantages of documenting the analysis of the health history.
- Identify regulations to assure client information is kept private.
- Describe reasons for establishing emergency management protocols and staff practice sessions for those protocols.

MEDICAL CONDITION

INTRODUCTION

This final section provides verification that the information provided in the health history and the indicated follow-up information has been considered by the practitioner. It contains a summary of critical thinking analysis used to determine professional judgments made by the oral healthcare provider (HCP).

"Has a physician or previous dentist recommended that you take antibiotics prior to your dental treatment? Name of physician or dentist making recommendation and phone number."

This question is an additional area on the health history questionnaire to get information regarding previous instructions to the client regarding antibiotic prophylaxis. It helps the practitioner to contact other healthcare practitioners to discuss the indication for antibiotic prophylaxis for the client's health history. The intention would be to resolve practitioner recommendations and assist the client in understanding recommendations. It may result in the previous medical recommendation to be rescinded, based on the current guidelines.

"Do you have any disease, condition, or problem not listed above that you think I should know about? Please explain."

This question provides the opportunity for the client to address any condition not included on the health history form. Whatever information is reported would require analysis of the impact on planned procedures or the effects of medications used to manage symptoms of the newly reported condition.

CLIENT SIGNATURE OR LEGAL GUARDIAN, DATE OF HEALTH HISTORY

This section is prefaced by a NOTE statement regarding the importance of discussing all relevant patient health issues prior to treatment. The client is asked to sign a statement that the information given on the form is accurate and that the client understands the importance of providing truthful information. This is followed by an oath that the dentist or any member of the dental staff will not be held responsible for errors made due to errors or omissions within the health history. The health history is a legal record and must contain the signature of the client to verify that the information was provided by the client or the legal guardian of the client. In most states, the client is a minor when under the age of 18, and the parent or legal guardian must sign the document to verify the accuracy. The date identifies when the information was provided. Health history information should be updated periodically, usually at recall or maintenance appointments in the private dental office. It is recommended to update the health history information on each appointment as the information can change on a day-to-day basis.

"FOR COMPLETION BY DENTIST" SECTION

This section provides space for analysis of health history information. It should include clinical decisions regarding analysis of information obtained from responses provided on the history. Management decisions based on the information gained from the health examination would be recorded. Recording significant information as it pertains to (1) the verification of information reported by the client, (2) medical consultations completed, (3) consideration of pertinent laboratory data, and (4) the relationship of the information to planned oral healthcare procedures is essential to legally document that information was evaluated.

This section provides a medicolegal purpose, in case the client's record is requested by an attorney. In a discussion regarding steps to take to avoid medical lawsuits, one author states, "Taking time to consider how dentists can avoid being sued and what they can do to win when they are sued is invaluable. One important step requires that the dentist ask patients to fill out medical history questionnaires. Each dentist then should keep the forms and continually update them."[1] Well-documented records demonstrate good client care and discourage an attorney from accepting a lawsuit case.

Unlike past editions of the American Dental Association (ADA) Health History, the 2008 revision contains no specific area to verify that the health history was updated, when the update occurred, or to describe changes reported during an update. This omission may not meet the legal obligations of the oral HCP, and a section should be added in order to verify the client's "permission to treat" acceptance.

PRIVACY OF HEALTH INFORMATION AND HIPAA REGULATIONS

The Health Insurance Portability and Accountability Act (HIPAA) was established in 1996 to make it easier and more affordable for Americans to obtain health insurance. Group health insurance providers were prohibited from using a person's past health information as a reason to deny coverage or increase coverage cost.[2] Insurance portability was protected for workers who had lost job-covered insurance. A provision for supplying medical claims electronically was included in the 1996 law. It became evident that circulating health information electronically posed a risk for keeping information private. The U.S. Department of Health and Human Services enacted the current regulations to assure privacy when electronic data were transmitted. These regulations took effect with an April 14, 2003, effective date for implementation by healthcare facilities. The act protects personal health information from being provided to others without the written approval of those involved, except in the case of a medical emergency.[3] Health providers may disclose client information only to the degree necessary to accomplish a given purpose.[2] Information must be kept where it can be seen only by those who have a legitimate reason to see it. For example, written appointment schedules of client names should not be posted in public view. Clients are allowed access to their health information and can request that errors be corrected. HCP must provide written office policies to clients outlining procedures to protect client information, secure their signatures to verify receipt of the office policy, and keep records documenting compliance with the law. In addition to privacy safeguards, the office policy must also include descriptions of security safeguards for administrative, physical, and technical situations. For example, these descriptions should include how information is kept private by staff, how room design provides protection of information from being seen by office visitors or the public, and how computerized information is kept secure. The law also requires that when health information is shared with other business associates, agencies, or companies, such as a client name and information on an order to a dental laboratory, and that the company sign an agreement assuring protection of private information. Healthcare offices must establish separate policies for privacy and for security. A privacy policy notice must be posted in a conspicuous area detailing how the information will be kept from unauthorized use. The client's written consent is required before personal health information can be used for marketing purposes, such as information provided to another HCP not associated with the primary office.

Allowed Privacy Behaviors

Dental office personnel are allowed to call out client names when it is time to be seated for treatment. Clients can sign on a sheet when presenting for treatment. Reasonable precautions must be taken to ensure privacy when discussing client treatment needs in the office. When dental charts are secured before treatment, the chart must be stored away from public view, such as in a drawer within the operatory area. Chart markers related to safety issues are allowed to be placed within the chart to alert the treating professional to allergies or premedication requirements.

HIPAA Checklist (from ADA Material)

The dental office must:

- Learn HIPAA requirements, appoint a compliance officer to enforce requirements and receive complaints, and establish office security and privacy mechanisms.
- Develop office policies on security and privacy protocols and provide written policies to clients. Secure client signature to verify receipt of policies.
- Develop training sessions for employees on policies and have an employee discipline protocol for violations of policy.
- Prepare agreements for business associates that may receive client information, requiring privacy of information.
- Establish a written document for policies and procedures, staff training, and technical electronic safeguards and physical safeguards for maintaining privacy and security of client data.
- Establish office policies to ensure client privacy during verbal communication within the office.
- Post written notice of privacy assurance in public area of office with person to contact if privacy issues develop.

- Make reasonable efforts to keep client information private and communicated only to those who are intended to get the information.
- Provide to clients the right to access personal health information, identify errors, and request changes. Costs associated with securing the information must be disclosed.
- Develop a self-audit procedure to monitor compliance.
- Document training sessions, specify personnel trained, client acknowledgments of receiving policies, and all issues relative to compliance.

These policies are still in the process of review and may be modified as healthcare facilities establish compliance. Some HIPAA privacy Web sites are:

http://www.ada.org/goto/hipaa
http://www.hhs.gov/ocr/hipaa

Compliance standards for HIPAA regulations can be found at:

http://www.hhs.gov/hipaafaq/about/190.html

OFFICE PREPARATION FOR EMERGENCY MANAGEMENT

All members of the dental team should be prepared to handle emergency situations and have completed basic life support (BLS) and cardiopulmonary resuscitation (CPR) training on a regular basis.[4] A written emergency plan for management of emergency situations should be prepared, and office protocol should be practiced on a regular basis, such as every 6 months. All dental offices should maintain the basic recommended emergency equipment and drugs. The ADA Council on Scientific Affairs recommends the following drugs as a minimum: epinephrine 1:1,000, histamine-blocking injectable agents (both adult and child dosage forms), oxygen with positive-pressure administration capability, nitroglycerin (sublingual tablet or spray), bronchodilator inhaler, sugar, and aspirin.[4] In situations in which emergency medical system (EMS) personnel cannot arrive within a reasonable time frame, an automated external defibrillator may be used. Training to use this device is included in current CPR courses. In essence, the content and design of the office kit should be based on each practitioner's training and knowledge. The emergency management protocol should include responsibilities of each member of the staff, for example, dentist gives injectable drug, receptionist calls 911, assistant gets oxygen and emergency kit, hygienist monitors vitals and records information, and so forth. A suggested emergency management protocol might include:

- All office staff must have current BLS certification and be familiar with didactic information on emergency medicine.
- Periodic office emergency drills should be conducted, telephone numbers of EMS or appropriate trained HCPs should be posted at telephones, and all staff must be aware of the protocol established.
- Recognize emergency situation, position client to open airway, assess carotid pulse; manage emergency based on most likely cause.
- Notify dentist or nearby staff member, being careful not to alert other clients in the office.
- Observe client behavior, identify signs of an emergency situation, respond first to immediate life-threatening situations.
- Unconsciousness? Place in supine position, retrieve oxygen for possible use. Cardiac arrest? Call 911, monitor airway, breathing, and circulation, provide CPR if no pulse found. Conscious? Place in upright position, monitor, and respond to signs of emergency.
- Secure emergency equipment (oxygen, medical kit), place blood pressure cuff, monitor vital signs every 5 minutes, and record data; dentist and staff must have knowledge to properly use all items in emergency kit.
- Provide oxygen by face mask at 10 L/minute unless contraindicated.
- Document events of emergency in client treatment record, include vital sign information; describe management and resolution of emergency.
- Inform family and get information relevant to current situation.

The best way to manage medical emergency situations is to prevent the emergency from occurring. Never treat a stranger! Know the information provided on the health history form and question the client to gain appropriate information related to identifying when risks of treatment are increased. Gain information through medical consultation when conditions require it. Use information gained in this self-study to guide preparatory procedures associated with oral health care.

MEDICAL CONSULTATION FORM

There are a variety of medical consultation forms available. Some are open-ended and allow the practitioner to identify the specific medical condition that requires additional information and physician recommendations for oral care, while others are more detailed. Several examples of medical consultation forms are available on "the Point" Web site that accompanies this text. When forms are faxed to the dental office, the original form with the original physician signature should be requested and placed within the client record. This meets the requirement for legal verification that the information was provided by the physician who received the medical consultation document.

CHAPTER SUMMARY

This chapter describes the necessity for and components of the analysis of the health history. It allows the clinician to use critical thinking skills to determine what services can be provided in a safe and effective manner.

Review

1. Identify the four components that comprise the analysis of health history information section.
2. Explain why the client signature and date of history should be included in the health history form.
3. Describe the significance of asking the client if he or she has any other disease or problem not listed on the medical history form.
4. Describe the purpose of documenting the analysis of the health history.

Case Study

Case A: Refer to Figure 15.1.

Mr. Joseph Antonio Lopez presents for a routine dental hygiene appointment. He is a 79-year-old man with a history of coronary artery disease treated with coronary artery bypass graft surgery in 2000 and has recovered well.

Recently, this client developed bradycardia and a pacemaker was placed in December 2012. Within 2 weeks, the client had a mild myocardial infarction (MI) and was rehospitalized. During the course of hospitalization, he developed significant arrhythmia wherein his heart would stop beating on a regular basis. The client was treated with laser surgery that corrected the problem. Also, during the course of hospitalization, the client developed facial cellulitis. An infectious disease specialist was consulted, and intravenous (IV) antibiotics were administered. Upon being discharged from the hospital after 10 days of care, the client was placed on oral antibiotics. Since the client was not complaining of dental pain and the cause of the facial swelling was unknown, he was advised to defer any dental treatment or dental hygiene care for 1 month.

Mr. Lopez notes that his health has improved significantly since his hospitalization and treatment, but he still fatigues easily and has mild chest pain upon exertion. He can walk upstairs to his bedroom without shortness of breath, but tires easily with grocery shopping and attending follow-up medical appointments. He has lost 20 pounds. In addition, he continues to have mild facial swelling, but is no longer taking antibiotics. He states that he was told he would not require antibiotic premedication for dental care.

Mr. Lopez reports that he takes several medications for his heart condition as noted on his medical history form (Fig. 15.1). Vital signs include pulse, 72 bpm; respiration, 17 breaths/min; blood pressure, 130/84 mm Hg, right arm, sitting.

1. What findings, if any, from the medical history would you consider significant? Record your notations as if you were completing the section of the medical history entitled "significant findings from the questionnaire or oral interview."
2. Mr. Lopez reports taking the following medications for his coronary artery disease: Plavix, felodipine, and metoprolol (Toprol-XL®). Look up each medication in a drug reference manual and note any dental management considerations appropriate for dental hygiene care, as if you were completing the "dental management considerations" section of the medical history form.
3. What follow-up questions and dental considerations are appropriate for the history of facial swelling?
4. What potential medical emergency should you be prepared to address during this appointment?
5. What strategies should you use to avoid this emergency?

Case B: Refer to Figure 15.2

Victoria Davis presents for caries restoration of tooth number 30. She is a 27-year-old woman who feels she is in good health although she recently has experienced "heartburn" and right upper quadrant pain for which she was recently diagnosed with gastritis and sludge in the gallbladder. She is currently on a low-fat diet and taking omeprazole daily. She is an occupational therapist who maintains excellent oral hygiene, and this is her first caries experience. She typically has 6-month continuing care dental hygiene appointments. She has a history of mitral valve prolapse with minor regurgitation, and hypothyroidism for which she takes a T3 supplement. Her vital signs include pulse, 68 bpm; respiration, 14 breaths/min; blood pressure, 116/60 mm Hg, right arm, sitting. Review the client's medical history (see attached) and answer the following items.

1. Given the client's gastrointestinal history, what oral changes would you look for during the oral examination?
2. Given the client's medical history, what notations would you make in the section entitled "significant findings from questionnaire or oral interview"?
3. Given the client's medical history, what notations would you make in the section entitled "dental management considerations?"
4. Give an example of using professional judgment for treatment recommendations, given the client's health history.
5. Is this client at risk for medical emergency during this appointment? Is so, what prevention strategies would you use?

Health History Form

ADA. American Dental Association www.ada.org

E-mail: VictoRia davis @ gmail.com Today's Date: 2/15/13

As required by law, our office adheres to written policies and procedures to protect the privacy of information about you that we create, receive or maintain. Your answers are for our records only and will be kept confidential subject to applicable laws. Please note that you will be asked some questions about your responses to this questionnaire and there may be additional questions concerning your health. This information is vital to allow us to provide appropriate care for you. This office does not use this information to discriminate.

Name: Last DAVIS First Victoria Middle M
Home Phone: *Include area code* (856) 767-2275
Business/Cell Phone: *Include area code* (856) 429-1467

Address: Mailing address 439 Blackwood Circle
City: Clementon State: NJ Zip: 08021

Occupation: Occupational Therapist
Height: 5'5" Weight: 135 lbs. Date of birth: 6/19/86 Sex: M (F)

SS# or Patient ID: 43297 Emergency Contact: Jordan Davis Relationship: brother Home Phone: (856) 767-2275 Cell Phone: (856) 767-6847 *Include area codes*

If you are completing this form for another person, what is your relationship to that person?

Your Name Relationship

Do you have any of the following diseases or problems: ***(Check DK if you Don't Know the answer to the question)***

	Yes	No	DK
Active Tuberculosis	☐	☑	☐
Persistent cough greater than a 3 week duration	☐	☑	☐
Cough that produces blood	☐	☑	☐
Been exposed to anyone with tuberculosis	☐	☑	☐

If you answer yes to any of the 4 items above, please stop and return this form to the receptionist.

Dental Information

For the following questions, please mark (X) your responses to the following questions.

	Yes	No	DK
Do your gums bleed when you brush or floss?	☐	☑	☐
Are your teeth sensitive to cold, hot, sweets or pressure?	☐	☑	☐
Does food or floss catch between your teeth?	☐	☑	☐
Is your mouth dry?	☐	☑	☐
Have you had any periodontal (gum) treatments?	☐	☑	☐
Have you ever had orthodontic (braces) treatment?	☐	☑	☐
Have you had any problems associated with previous dental treatment?	☐	☑	☐
Is your home water supply fluoridated?	☐	☐	☑
Do you drink bottled or filtered water?	☑	☐	☐
If yes, how often? Circle one: DAILY / WEEKLY / (OCCASIONALLY)			
Are you currently experiencing dental pain or discomfort?	☑	☐	☐

What is the reason for your dental visit today? Fix molar that has a cavity

How do you feel about your smile? good

	Yes	No	DK
Do you have earaches or neck pains?	☐	☑	☐
Do you have any clicking, popping or discomfort in the jaw?	☐	☑	☐
Do you brux or grind your teeth?	☐	☑	☐
Do you have sores or ulcers in your mouth?	☐	☑	☐
Do you wear dentures or partials?	☐	☑	☐
Do you participate in active recreational activities?	☑	☐	☐
Have you ever had a serious injury to your head or mouth?	☐	☑	☐

Date of your last dental exam: 8/12

What was done at that time? Cleaning + dental exam

Date of last dental x-rays: 8/12

Medical Information

Please mark (X) your response to indicate if you have or have not had any of the following diseases or problems.

	Yes	No	DK
Are you now under the care of a physician?	☐	☑	☐

Physician Name: Michael Mancinello Phone: *Include area code* (856) 767-6955

Address/City/State/Zip: 1437 White Horse Ave, Berlin, NJ, 08009

	Yes	No	DK
Are you in good health?	☑	☐	☐
Has there been any change in your general health within the past year?	☐	☑	☐

If yes, what condition is being treated?

Date of last physical exam: 7/12

	Yes	No	DK
Have you had a serious illness, operation or been hospitalized in the past 5 years?	☐	☑	☐

If yes, what was the illness or problem?

	Yes	No	DK
Are you taking or have you recently taken any prescription or over the counter medicine(s)?	☑	☐	☐

If so, please list all, including vitamins, natural or herbal preparations and/or diet supplements:

Omeprazole
T3 supplement

Form S500

Figure 15.1 ■ Medical history for Case Study A.

Medical Information

Please mark (X) your response to indicate if you have or have not had any of the following diseases or problems.

(Check DK if you Don't Know the answer to the question)	Yes	No	DK
Do you wear contact lenses?	☐	☑	☐
Are you taking, or have you taken, any diet drugs such as Pondimin (fenfluramine), Redux (dexphenfluramine) or phen-fen (fenfluramine-phentermine combination)?	☐	☑	☐
Are you taking or scheduled to begin taking either of the medications, alendronate (Fosamax®) or risedronate (Actonel®) for osteoporosis or Paget's disease?	☐	☑	☐
Since 2001, were you treated or are you presently scheduled to begin treatment with the intravenous bisphosphonates (Aredia® or Zometa®) for bone pain, hypercalcemia or skeletal complications resulting from Paget's disease, multiple myeloma or metastatic cancer?	☐	☑	☐

Date Treatment began: ________

	Yes	No	DK
Do you use controlled substances (drugs)?	☐	☑	☐
Do you use tobacco (smoking, snuff, chew, bidis)? If so, how interested are you in stopping? (Circle one) VERY / SOMEWHAT / NOT INTERESTED	☐	☑	☐
Do you drink alcoholic beverages? If yes, how much alcohol did you drink in the last 24 hours? ____ If yes, how much do you typically drink In a week? ____	☐	☑	☐

WOMEN ONLY Are you:
Pregnant? NO
Number of weeks: —
Taking birth control pills or hormonal replacement? NO
Nursing? NO

	Yes	No	DK
Joint Replacement. Have you had an orthopedic total joint (hip, knee, elbow, finger) replacement? Date: ____ If yes, have you had any complications?	☐	☑	☐

Allergies - Are you allergic to or have you had a reaction to:
To all **yes** responses, specify type of reaction.

	Yes	No	DK
Local anesthetics	☐	☑	☐
Aspirin	☐	☑	☐
Penicillin or other antibiotics	☐	☑	☐
Barbiturates, sedatives, or sleeping pills	☐	☑	☐
Sulfa drugs never used	☐	☐	☑
Codeine or other narcotics never used	☐	☐	☑
Metals	☐	☑	☐
Latex (rubber)	☐	☑	☐
Iodine	☐	☑	☐
Hay fever/seasonal to pollen + oak trees	☑	☐	☐
Animals	☐	☑	☐
Food	☐	☑	☐
Other	☐	☑	☐

Please mark (X) your response to indicate if you have or have not had any of the following diseases or problems.

	Yes	No	DK
Heart murmur	☑	■	☐
Mitral valve prolapse	☐	☑	☐
Artificial heart valves	☐	☑	☐
Rheumatic fever	☐	☑	☐
Cardiovascular disease	☐	☑	☐
Angina	☐	☑	☐
Arteriosclerosis	☐	☑	☐
Congestive heart failure	☐	☑	☐
Coronary artery disease	☐	☑	☐
Damaged heart valves	☐	☑	☐
Heart attack	☐	☑	☐
Low blood pressure	☐	☑	☐
High blood pressure	☐	☑	☐
Congenital heart defects	☐	☑	☐
Pacemaker	☐	☑	☐
Rheumatic heart disease	☐	☑	☐
Abnormal bleeding	☐	☑	☐
Anemia	☐	☑	☐
Blood transfusion If yes, date:	☐	☑	☐
Hemophilia	☐	☑	☐
AIDS or HIV infection	☐	☑	☐
Arthritis	☐	☑	☐
Autoimmune disease	☐	☑	☐
Rheumatoid arthritis	☐	☑	☐
Systemic lupus erythematosus	☐	☑	☐
Asthma	☐	☑	☐
Bronchitis	☐	☑	☐
Emphysema	☐	☑	☐
Sinus trouble	☐	☑	☐
Tuberculosis	☐	☑	☐
Cancer/Chemotherapy/ Radiation Treatment	☐	☑	☐
Chest pain upon exertion	☐	☑	☐
Chronic pain	☐	☑	☐
Diabetes Type I or II	☐	☑	☐
Eating disorder	☐	☑	☐
Malnutrition	☐	☑	☐
Gastrointestinal disease	☑	☐	☐
G.E. Reflux/persistent heartburn	☑	☐	☐
Ulcers	☐	☑	☐
Thyroid problems	☑	☐	☐
Stroke	☐	☑	☐
Glaucoma	☐	☑	☐
Hepatitis, jaundice or liver disease	☐	☑	☐
Epilepsy	☐	☑	☐
Fainting spells or seizures	☐	☑	☐
Neurological disorders If yes, Specify:	☐	☑	☐
Sleep disorder	☐	☑	☐
Mental health disorders Specify:	☐	☑	☐
Recurrent Infections Type of infection:	☐	☑	☐
Kidney problems	☐	☑	☐
Night sweats	☐	☑	☐
Osteoporosis	☐	☑	☐
Persistent swollen glands in neck	☐	☑	☐
Severe headaches/ migraines	☐	☑	☐
Severe or rapid weight loss	☐	☑	☐
Sexually transmitted disease	☐	☑	☐
Excessive urination	☐	☑	☐

	Yes	No	DK
Has a physician or previous dentist recommended that you take antibiotics prior to your dental treatment?	☐	☑	☐

Name of physician or dentist making recommendation: Phone:

	Yes	No	DK
Do you have any disease, condition, or problem not listed above that you think I should know about? Please explain:	☐	☑	☐

NOTE: Both Doctor and patient are encouraged to discuss any and all relevant patient health issues prior to treatment.
I certify that I have read and understand the above and that the information given on this form is accurate. I understand the importance of a truthful health history and that my dentist and his/her staff will rely on this information for treating me. I acknowledge that my questions, if any, about inquiries set forth above have been answered to my satisfaction. I will not hold my dentist, or any other member of his/her staff, responsible for any action they take or do not take because of errors or omissions that I may have made in the completion of this form.

Signature of Patient/Legal Guardian: Victoria Davis Date: 2/15/13

FOR COMPLETION BY DENTIST

Comments: ________

Figure 15.1 ■ continued

Health History Form

ADA. American Dental Association www.ada.org

E-mail: jala gmail.com Today's Date: 3.05.13

As required by law, our office adheres to written policies and procedures to protect the privacy of information about you that we create, receive or maintain. Your answers are for our records only and will be kept confidential subject to applicable laws. Please note that you will be asked some questions about your responses to this questionnaire and there may be additional questions concerning your health. This information is vital to allow us to provide appropriate care for you. This office does not use this information to discriminate.

Name: Last Lopez First Joseph Middle A

Home Phone: *Include area code* (609) 567.2369

Business/Cell Phone: *Include area code* (—)

Address: Mailing address 625 Plum Street City: Hammonton State: NJ Zip: 08037

Occupation: Retired Height: 5'10" Weight: 195 Date of birth: 7.29.34 Sex: (M) F

SS# or (Patient ID:) 43578 Emergency Contact: Luisa Lopez Relationship: Daughter Home Phone: (609) 567.2369 Cell Phone: (609) 567-4131 *include area codes*

If you are completing this form for another person, what is your relationship to that person?

Your Name Relationship

Do you have any of the following diseases or problems: ***(Check DK if you Don't Know the answer to the question)***

	Yes	No	DK
Active Tuberculosis		X	
Persistent cough greater than a 3 week duration		X	
Cough that produces blood		X	
Been exposed to anyone with tuberculosis		X	

If you answer yes to any of the 4 items above, please stop and return this form to the receptionist.

Dental Information *For the following questions, please mark (X) your responses to the following questions.*

	Yes	No	DK
Do your gums bleed when you brush or floss?		X	
Are your teeth sensitive to cold, hot, sweets or pressure?		X	
Does food or floss catch between your teeth?		X	
Is your mouth dry?	X		
Have you had any periodontal (gum) treatments?		X	
Have you ever had orthodontic (braces) treatment?		X	
Have you had any problems associated with previous dental treatment?		X	
Is your home water supply fluoridated?			X
Do you drink bottled or filtered water?		X	
If yes, how often? Circle one: DAILY / WEEKLY / OCCASIONALLY			
Are you currently experiencing dental pain or discomfort?	X		

What is the reason for your dental visit today? Facial Swelling

How do you feel about your smile? Ok

	Yes	No	DK
Do you have earaches or neck pains?		X	
Do you have any clicking, popping or discomfort in the jaw?		X	
Do you brux or grind your teeth?			X
Do you have sores or ulcers in your mouth?		X	
Do you wear dentures or partials?		X	
Do you participate in active recreational activities?		X	
Have you ever had a serious injury to your head or mouth?		X	

Date of your last dental exam: 3/12

What was done at that time? Dental Checkup

Date of last dental x-rays: Don't Know

Medical Information *Please mark (X) your response to indicate if you have or have not had any of the following diseases or problems.*

	Yes	No	DK
Are you now under the care of a physician?	X		

Physician Name: Kevin Carpenter Phone: *include area code* (609) 561.2506

Address/City/State/Zip: 1355 Flemington Pike, Hammonton, NJ

	Yes	No	DK
Are you in good health?		X	
Has there been any change in your general health within the past year?	X		

If yes, what condition is being treated? Heart Attack

Date of last physical exam: 1/13

	Yes	No	DK
Have you had a serious illness, operation or been hospitalized in the past 5 years?	X		

If yes, what was the illness or problem? Heart Attack and Heart Problems

	Yes	No	DK
Are you taking or have you recently taken any prescription or over the counter medicine(s)?	X		

If so, please list all, including vitamins, natural or herbal preparations and/or diet supplements:

Plavix
Toprol
Felodipine

Figure 15.2 ■ Medical history for Case Study B.

Medical Information

Please mark (X) your response to indicate if you have or have not had any of the following diseases or problems.

(Check DK if you Don't Know the answer to the question)	Yes	No	DK
Do you wear contact lenses?		X	
Are you taking, or have you taken, any diet drugs such as Pondimin (fenfluramine), Redux (dexphenfluramine) or phen-fen (fenfluramine-phentermine combination)?		X	
Are you taking or scheduled to begin taking either of the medications, alendronate (Fosamax®) or risedronate (Actonel®) for osteoporosis or Paget's disease?		X	
Since 2001, were you treated or are you presently scheduled to begin treatment with the intravenous bisphosphonates (Aredia® or Zometa®) for bone pain, hypercalcemia or skeletal complications resulting from Paget's disease, multiple myeloma or metastatic cancer?		X	

Date Treatment began: ______

	Yes	No	DK
Do you use controlled substances (drugs)?		X	
Do you use tobacco (smoking, snuff, chew, bidis)?		X	

If so, how interested are you in stopping?
(Circle one) VERY / SOMEWHAT / NOT INTERESTED

	Yes	No	DK
Do you drink alcoholic beverages?		X	

If yes, how much alcohol did you drink in the last 24 hours? ______
If yes, how much do you typically drink In a week? ______

WOMEN ONLY Are you:
Pregnant?
Number of weeks: ______
Taking birth control pills or hormonal replacement?
Nursing?

	Yes	No	DK
Joint Replacement. Have you had an orthopedic total joint (hip, knee, elbow, finger) replacement?		X	

Date: ______ If yes, have you had any complications?

Allergies - Are you allergic to or have you had a reaction to:
To all **yes** responses, specify type of reaction.

	Yes	No	DK
Local anesthetics		X	
Aspirin		X	
Penicillin or other antibiotics tetracyclene	X		
Barbiturates, sedatives, or sleeping pills		X	
Sulfa drugs		X	
Codeine or other narcotics		X	
Metals		X	
Latex (rubber)		X	
Iodine		X	
Hay fever/seasonal		X	
Animals		X	
Food		X	
Other		X	

Please mark (X) your response to indicate if you have or have not had any of the following diseases or problems.

	Yes	No	DK
Heart murmur		X	
Mitral valve prolapse		X	
Artificial heart valves		X	
Rheumatic fever		X	
Cardiovascular disease	X		
Angina	X		
Arteriosclerosis	X		
Congestive heart failure		X	
Coronary artery disease	X		
Damaged heart valves		X	
Heart attack	X		
Low blood pressure		X	
High blood pressure		X	
Congenital heart defects		X	
Pacemaker	X		
Rheumatic heart disease		X	
Abnormal bleeding		X	

	Yes	No	DK
Anemia		X	
Blood transfusion		X	
If yes, date: ______			
Hemophilia		X	
AIDS or HIV infection		X	
Arthritis	X		
Autoimmune disease		X	
Rheumatoid arthritis		X	
Systemic lupus erythematosus		X	
Asthma		X	
Bronchitis		X	
Emphysema		X	
Sinus trouble		X	
Tuberculosis		X	
Cancer/Chemotherapy/ Radiation Treatment		X	
Chest pain upon exertion	X		

	Yes	No	DK
Chronic pain		X	
Diabetes Type I or II		X	
Eating disorder		X	
Malnutrition		X	
Gastrointestinal disease		X	
G.E. Reflux/persistent heartburn		X	
Ulcers		X	
Thyroid problems		X	
Stroke		X	
Glaucoma		X	
Hepatitis, jaundice or liver disease		X	
Epilepsy		X	
Fainting spells or seizures		X	
Neurological disorders		X	
If yes, Specify: ______			

	Yes	No	DK
Sleep disorder		X	
Mental health disorders		X	
Specify: ______			
Recurrent Infections	X		
Type of infection: Cellulitis			
Kidney problems		X	
Night sweats		X	
Osteoporosis		X	
Persistent swollen glands in neck		X	
Severe headaches/ migraines		X	
Severe or rapid weight loss	X		
Sexually transmitted disease		X	
Excessive urination		X	

	Yes	No	DK
Has a physician or previous dentist recommended that you take antibiotics prior to your dental treatment?		X	

Name of physician or dentist making recommendation: ______ Phone: ______

	Yes	No	DK
Do you have any disease, condition, or problem not listed above that you think I should know about?		X	

Please explain:

NOTE: Both Doctor and patient are encouraged to discuss any and all relevant patient health issues prior to treatment.
I certify that I have read and understand the above and that the information given on this form is accurate. I understand the importance of a truthful health history and that my dentist and his/her staff will rely on this information for treating me. I acknowledge that my questions, if any, about inquiries set forth above have been answered to my satisfaction. I will not hold my dentist, or any other member of his/her staff, responsible for any action they take or do not take because of errors or omissions that I may have made in the completion of this form.

Signature of Patient/Legal Guardian: Joseph Lopez Date: 3/05/13

FOR COMPLETION BY DENTIST

Comments: ______

Figure 15.2 ■ continued

References

Chapter One

1. Fleisher LA, Beckman JA, Brown KA, et al. ACC/AHA 2007 guidelines on perioperative cardiovascular evaluation and care for noncardiac surgery: executive summary: a report of the American College of Cardiology/American Heart Association Task Force on Practice Guidelines (Writing Committee to Revise the 2002 Guidelines on Perioperative Cardiovascular Evaluation for Noncardiac Surgery). Circulation 2007;116(17):1971–1996.
2. American Society of Anesthesiologists: New Classification of Physical Status. Anesthesiology 1963;24:111.
3. Little JW, Falace DA, Miller CS, Rhodus NL. Dental Management of the Medically Compromised Patient. 8th Ed. St. Louis: Mosby Elsevier, 2013:15, DM5, DM53, 12(54):6–7.
4. James PA, Oparil S, Carter BL, et al. 2014 Evidence-Based Guideline for the Management of High Blood Pressure in Adults. Report From the Panel Members Appointed to the Eighth Joint National Committee (JNC 8). JAMA. 2014;311(5):507–520. doi:10.1001/jama.2013.284427.
5. Rosendorff C, Black HR, Cannon CP, et al. Treatment of hypertension in the prevention and management of ischemic heart disease: a scientific statement from the American Heart Association Council for High Blood Pressure Research and the Councils on Clinical Cardiology and Epidemiology and Prevention. Circulation 2007;115(21):2761 2788.
6. American Dental Association Council on Dental Health and Health Planning and Bureau of Health Education and Audiovisual Services. Breaking the silence on hypertension: a dental perspective. J Am Dent Assoc 1985;10:781–789.
7. The Fourth Report on the Diagnosis, Evaluation, and Treatment of High Blood Pressure in Children and Adolescents. National High Blood Pressure Evaluation Program Working Group on High Blood Pressure in Children and Adolescents. Pediatrics 2004;114(2):555–576.
8. Bennett JD, Rosenberg MB. Medical Emergencies in Dentistry. Philadelphia: WB Saunders, 2002:147.
9. Tyler MT, Lozada-Nur F, Glick M. Ed. Clinician's Guide to Treatment of Medically Complex Dental Patients. 2nd Ed. Seattle: The American Academy of Oral Medicine 2001:12, 13.
10. Stapleton ER, et al. Fundamentals of BLS for Healthcare Providers. American Heart Association 2001:1.
11. Wilkins E. Clinical Practice of the Dental Hygienist. 11th Ed. Philadelphia: Lippincott Williams & Wilkins, 2013:131.

Chapter Two

1. Centers for Disease Control and Prevention. Tuberculosis Data and Statistics—2011. Available at http://www.cdc.gov/tb/publications/factsheets/statistics/TBTrends.htm. Accessed February 5, 2013.
2. Jensen PA, Lambert LA, Iademarco MF, Ridzoa R. Guidelines for preventing the transmission of *Mycobacterium tuberculosis* in healthcare settings, 2005. Centers for Disease Control and Prevention. MMWR 2005;54(RR-17): 1–121.
3. Cleveland JL, Kent J, Gooch BF, et al. Multidrug-resistant *Mycobacterium tuberculosis* in an HIV dental clinic. Infect Control Hosp Epidemiol 1995;16:7–11.
4. CDC. Guidelines for infection control in dental healthcare settings, 2003. Available at http://www.cdc.gov/OralHealth/infectioncontrol/guidelines/. Accessed February 2, 2013.
5. CDC. Core Curriculum on Tuberculosis. What the Clinician Should Know. 6th Ed. Atlanta: Centers for Disease Control and Prevention, National Center for HIV, STD, and TB Prevention, Division of Tuberculosis Elimination, 2013. Available at to http://www.cdc.gov/tb/education/corecurr/pdf/corecurr_all.pdf. Accessed April 2, 2014.
6. Steingart KR, Sohn H, Schiller I, Kloda LA, Boehme CC, Pai M, Dendukuri N. Xpert® MTB/RIF assay for pulmonary tuberculosis and rifampicin resistance in adults. Cochrane Database Syst Rev 2013;(1): CD009593. DOI:10.1002/14651858. Available at http://onlinelibrary.wiley.com/doi/10.1002/14651858.CD009593.pub2/full. Accessed February 3, 2013.

Chapter Three

1. Rethman MP, Beltran-Aguilar ED, Billings RJ, et al. Nonfluoride caries-preventive agents. Executive summary of evidence-based clinical recommendations. JADA 2011;142(9):1065–1071. Available at http://jada.ada.org/content/142/9/1065.full.pdf+html. Accessed January 29, 2013.
2. Ly KA, Milgrom P, Roberts M et al. Linear response of mutans streptococci to increasing frequency of xylitol chewing gum use: a randomized controlled trial. BMC Oral Health 2006;6:6. Accessed at www. biomedcentral.com/1472-6831/6/6 on May 8, 2008.
3. Bollen AM, Cunha-Cruz J, Huang GJ, Hujoel PP. The effects of orthodontic therapy on periodontal health. A systematic review of controlled evidence. J Am Dent Assoc 2008;139(4):413–422.

4. American Dental Association Council on Scientific Affairs. Professionally applied topical fluoride. Evidence-based clinical recommendations. J Am Dent Assoc 2006;137(8):1151–1159.
5. Elter JR, Strauss RP, Beck JD. Assessing dental anxiety, dental care use and oral status in older adults. J Am Dent Assoc 1997;128(5):591–597.
6. Lahmann C. Schoen R, Henningsen P et al. Brief relaxation versus music distraction in the treatment of dental anxiety. J Am Dent Assoc 2008;139(3):317–324.
7. Malamed SF. Medical Emergencies in the Dental Office. 6th Ed. St. Louis, MO: Mosby, 2007:124–125, 129, 138–139.
8. Blakey G. Syncope. In: Bennett J, Rosenberg M, eds. Medical Emergencies in Dentistry. Philadelphia, PA: WB Saunders, 2002:184.
9. Little JW, Falace DA, Miller CS, Rhodus NL. Dental Management of the Medically Compromised Patient. 8th Ed. St. Louis, MO: Mosby, 2013:553.
10. Ward BB, Feinberg SE. Hyperventilation. In: Bennett JD, Rosenberg MB, eds. Medical Emergencies in Dentistry. Philadelphia, PA: WB Saunders, 2002:105–109.
11. American Dental Association Council on Scientific Affairs. Professionally applied topical fluoride: evidence-based clinical recommendations. JADA 2006;137(8):1151–1159. Available at http://ebd.ada.org/contentdocs/clinical_recommendations_non_fluoride_caries_preventive_agents_full_report.pdf. Accessed January 29, 2013.
12. Council on Scientific Affairs. American Dental Association. Fluoride Supplementation Guidelines. Available at jada.ada.org/content/141/12/1480.full. Accessed January 29, 2013.
13. ADA Council on Scientific Affairs. U.S. Department of Health and Human Services (FDA). Dental Radiographic Examinations: Recommendation for Patient Selection and Limiting Radiation Exposure. Available at http://www.ada.org/sections/professionalResources/pdfs/Dental_Radiographic_Examinations_2012.pdf. Accessed 2013.
14. Krasse B. The Vipeholm dental caries study: recollections and reflections 50 years later. J Dent Res 2001;80(9): 1785–1788. Available at http://jdr.sagepub.com/content/80/9/1785.full.pdf. Accessed January 29, 2013.

Chapter Four

1. American Academy of Orthopaedic Surgeons. American Dental Association. Prevention of orthopaedic implant infection in patients undergoing dental procedures. Evidence-based guideline and evidence report. V0.22.2.2012. Available at http://www.aaos.org/research/guidelines/PUDP/PUDP_guideline.pdf. Accessed January 29, 2013.
2. Little JW, Falace DA, Miller CS, Rhodus NL. Dental Management of the Medically Compromised Patient. 8th Ed. St. Louis, MO: Mosby, 2013:DM-5, DM-53, 546, 548.
3. Moore TJ, Cohen MR, Furberg CD. Serious adverse drug events reported to the Food and Drug Administration, 1998–2005. Arch Intern Med 2007;167:1752–1759.
4. Alexander RE. Unregulated herbal products: potential interactions and side effects in dental patients. Texas Dent J 2007;124:365–385.
5. Malamed SF. Medical Emergencies in the Dental Office. 6th Ed. St. Louis, MO: Mosby, 2007:121, 151.
6. Pickett F, Terezhalmy G. Management of Medical Emergencies in the Oral Health Care. In: Pickett F, Terezhalmy G, eds. Dental Drug Reference with Clinical Implications. 2nd Ed. Baltimore, MD: Lippincott Williams & Wilkins, 2010:145.
7. Ardekian L, Gaspar R, Peled M, Brener B, Laufer D. Does low-dose aspirin therapy complicate oral surgical procedures? J Am Dent Assoc 2000;131:331–335.
8. Grines CL, Bonow RO, Gardner TJ, et al. AHA/ACC/SCAI/ACS/ADA Science Advisory. Prevention of premature discontinuation of dual antiplatelet therapy in patients with coronary artery stents. Circulation 2007;115:813–818.
9. Glick M. The new blood pressure guidelines: a digest. J Am Dent Assoc 2004;135:585–586.

Chapter Five

1. American Academy of Orthopaedic Surgeons. American Dental Association. Prevention of orthopaedic implant infection in patients undergoing dental procedures. Evidence-based guideline and evidence report. V0.22.2.2012. Available at http://www.aaos.org/Research/guidelines/PUDP/PUDP_guideline.pdf. Decision Making Tool at http://www.ada.org/sections/professionalResources/pdfs/DentalSDMTool.pdf. Accessed January 29, 2013.
2. Jevsevar DS, Abt E. Editorial: The new AAOS/ADA clinical practice guidelines on prevention or orthopaedic implant infection in patients undergoing dental procedures. Available at http://www.aaos.org/Research/guidelines/PUDP/dentaleditorial.pdf. Accessed January 29, 2013.
3. Roberts GJ. Dentists are innocent! "Everyday" bacteremia is the real culprit: a review and assessment of the evidence that dental surgical procedures are a principal cause of bacterial endocarditis in children. Pediatric Cardiol 1999;20:317–325.
4. Forner L, Larsen T, Kilian M, Holmstrup P. Incidence of bacteremia after chewing, toothbrushing and scaling in individuals with periodontal inflammation. J Clin Periodontol 2006;33:401–407.
5. Brennan MI, Kent ML, Fox PC, et al. The impact of oral disease and nonsurgical treatment in bacteremia in children. J Am Dent Assoc 2007;138(1):80–85.
6. Pallasch TJ. Perspectives on the 2007 AHA endocarditis prevention guidelines. CDA J 2007;35(7):507–513.
7. Lockhart PB, Loven B, Brennan MT, et al. The evidence base for the efficacy of antibiotic prophylaxis in dental practice. J Am Dent Assoc 2007;138(4):458–474.
8. Lockhart PB, Brennan MT, Sasser HC, et al. Bacteremia associated with toothbrushing and dental extraction. Circulation 2008;117(24):3118–25.
9. Pickett FA. Bisphosphonate-associated osteonecrosis of the jaw: a literature review and clinical practice guidelines. J Dent Hyg 2006;80(3):1–12.
10. Hellstein JW, Adler RA, Edwards B, et al. American Dental Association. Managing the care of patients receiving antiresorptive therapy for prevention and treatment of osteoporosis. November 2011. Available at http://www.ada.org/2594.aspx?currentTab=2. Accessed January 29, 2013.
11. Ruggiero SL, Mehrotra B, Rosenberg TJ, et al. Osteonecrosis of the jaws associated with the use of bisphosphonates: a review of 63 cases. J Oral Maxillofac Surg 2004;62:527–534.

12. Marx R, Sawatari Y, Fortin M, Broumand V. Bisphosphonate-induced bone (osteonecrosis/osteopetrosis) of the jaws: risk factors, recognition prevention, and treatment. J Oral Maxillofac Surg 2005;63:1567–1575.
13. Yip JK, Borrell LN, Cho S-C, Francisco H, Tarnow DP. Association between oral bisphosphonate use and dental implant failure among middle-aged women. J Clin Periodontol 2012; 39: 408–414.
14. Ficarra G, et al. Osteonecrosis of the jaws in periodontal patients with a history of bisphosphonate treatment. J Clin Periodontol 2005;32(11):1123–1128.
15. American Association of Oral and Maxillo-facial Surgeons. American Association of Oral and Maxillofacial Surgeons Position Paper on bisphosphonate-related osteonecrosis of the jaws. J Oral Maxillofac Surg 2007;65:369–376.
16. Grbic JT, Landesberg R, Lin SQ, et al. Incidence of osteonecrosis of the jaw in women with postmenopausal osteoporosis in the Health Outcomes and Reduced Incidence with Zoledronic Acid Once Yearly Pivotal Fracture Trial. J Am Dent Assoc 2008;139(1):32–40.
17. Freiberger JJ, Padilla-Burgos R, Chhoeu AH, et al. Hyperbaric oxygen treatment and bisphosphonate-induced osteonecrosis of the jaw: a case series. J Oral Maxillofac Surg 2007;65(7):1321–1327.

Web Resources

American Association of Endodontists. Position statement on endodontic implications of bisphosphonate-associated osteonecrosis of the jaws. http://www.aae.org/uploadedFiles/Publications_and_Research/Endodontics_Colleagues_for_Excellence_Newsletter/fall2012ecfe.pdf. Accessed February 5, 2012.

Executive Summary of ADA/AAOS 2012 guideline for antibiotic prophylaxis and patient with prosthetic joint. Rethman M, Watters W, Abt E, et al. Prevention of Orthopaedic Implant Infection in Patients Undergoing Dental Procedures Executive Summary on the AAOS/ADA Clinical Practice Guideline. Available at http://ebd.ada.org/contentdocs/dentalexecsumm.pdf. Accessed February 4, 2013.

Chapter Six

1. Malamed S. Medical Emergencies in the Dental Office. 6th Ed. St. Louis, MO: Mosby, 2007:399, 410, 419.
2. Pickett F, Terezhalmy G. Basic Pharmacology with Dental Hygiene Applications. Baltimore, MD: Lippincott Williams & Wilkins, 2009:48–56.
3. Boorin MR. Drug allergy and anaphylaxis. In: Bennett JD, Rosenberg MB, eds. Medical Emergencies in Dentistry. Philadelphia, PA: WB Saunders, 2001:163, 169, 176.
4. Center for Drug Evaluation and Research. FDA panel wants more restrictions on hydrocodone. Meeting of the Drug Safety and Risk Management Advisory Committee. January 24–25, 2013. Available at http://www.medicinenet.com/script/main/art.asp?articlekey=167382. Accessed February 4, 2013.
5. Hamann CP, Turjanmaa K, Rietschel R, et al. Natural rubber latex hypersensitivity: incidence and prevalence of type 1 allergy in the dental professional. J Am Dent Assoc 1998;129:43–54.
6. Dillard SF, MacCollum MA. Reports to FDA: allergic reactions to latex containing medical devices. In: Program and Proceedings, International Latex Conference: Sensitivity to Latex in Medical Devices. November 5–7, 1992;23.
7. American Heart Association. 2012 Hands Only CPR. American Heart Association Fact Sheet. Available at http://www.heart.org/idc/groups/heart-public/@wcm/@ecc/documents/downloadable/ucm_441302.pdf. Accessed February 4, 2013.

Chapter Seven

1. Rees T. Oral effects of drug abuse. Crit Rev Oral Biol Med 1992;3:163–184.
2. Thomson WM, et al. Cannabis smoking and periodontal disease among young adults. JAMA 2008;200(5): 525–531.
3. Klasser GD, Epstein J. Methamphetamine and its impact on dental care. J Can Dent Assoc 2005;71(10): 759–762.
4. Wentworth RB. Ethical moment. J Am Dent Assoc 2008;139(5):623–624.
5. Pallasch TJ, McCarthy FM, Jastak, JT. Cocaine and sudden cardiac death. J Oral Maxillofac Surg 1989;47: 1188–1191.
6. McCord J, et al. Management of cocaine-associated chest pain and myocardial infarction. Circulation 2008;117:1897–1907.
7. Mukamal KJ, et al. An exploratory prospective study of marijuana use and mortality following acute myocardial infarction. Am Hear J 2008;155(3):465–470.
8. Horowitz L, Nersasian R. A review of marijuana in relation to stress-response mechanisms in the dental patient. J Am Dent Assoc 1978;96:983–986.
9. National Institute on Drug Abuse. Research Report Series. Methamphetamine abuse and addiction. Available at http://www.drugabuse.gov/drugs-abuse/methamphetamine. Accessed February 4, 2013.
10. Abel PW, Bockman CS. Drugs of abuse. In: Yagiela JA, Neidle EA, Dowd FJ, eds. Pharmacology and Therapeutics for Dentistry. 4th Ed. St. Louis, MO: Mosby, 1998:660.
11. Yukna RA. Cocaine periodontitis. Int J Periodontics Restor Dent 1991;11(1):73–79.
12. Hill EE, Herijgers P. Infective endocarditis: changing epidemiology and predictors of 6-month mortality. A prospective cohort study. European Heart J 2007;28:196–203.
13. Bullock K. Dental care of patients with substance abuse. Dent Clin North Am 1999;43(3):513–526.
14. Centers for Disease Control and Prevention. Current Tobacco use, among middle and high school students—United States, 2012. Morbidity and Mortality Weekly Report [serial online]. 2012;61(31):581–585. Available at http://www.cdc.gov/mmwr/preview/mmwrhtml/mm6131a1.htm. Accessed February 4, 2013.
15. Rahman M, Sakamoto J, Fukui T. Bidi smoking and oral cancer: a meta-analysis. Int J Cancer 2003;106:600–604.
16. Rahman M, Fukui T. Bidi smoking and health. Public Health 2000;114:123–127.
17. Sankaranarayanan R, Duffy SW, Padmakumary G, Nair Sm, Day NE, Padmanabhan TK. Risk factors for cancer of the oesophagus in Kerala, India. Int J Cancer 1991;49:485–489.
18. Pais P, et al. Risk factors for acute myocardial infarction in Indians: a case-control study. Lancet 1996;348:358–363.

19. American Dental Hygienists' Association. Tobacco Cessation Protocols for the Dental Practice. Available at http://www.askadviserefer.org/continueEducation.asp. Accessed February 10, 2013.
20. Friedlander AH, Norman DC. Geriatric alcoholism: pathophysiology and dental implications. J Am Dent Assoc 2006;137:330–338.
21. Glick M. Medical considerations for dental care of patients with alcohol-related liver disease. J Am Dent Assoc 1997;128:61–69.
22. Kuffner EK, Dart RC, Bogdan GM, Hill RE, Casper E, Darton L. Effect of maximal daily doses of acetaminophen on the liver of alcoholic patients: a randomized, double-blind, placebo controlled trial. Arch Intern Med 2001;161:2247–2252.
23. Leyes BJL, et al. Efficacy of chlorhexidine mouthrinses with and without alcohol: a clinical study. J Periodontol 2002;73:317–321.
24. Dickey KW. Ethical moment. J Am Dent Assoc 2007;138(2):245–246.

Chapter Eight

1. Wilkins E. Clinical Practice of the Dental Hygienist. 11th Ed. Baltimore, MD: Lippincott Williams & Wilkins, 2013:774, 776, 828.
2. Little JW, et al. Dental Management of the Medically Compromised Patient. 8th Ed. St. Louis, MO: Mosby, 2013:270, 273, 275.
3. Donaldson M, Goodchild JH. Pregnancy, breast-feeding and drugs used in dentistry. JADA 2012;143(8):858–871.
4. Frommer HH. Radiology for Dental Auxiliaries. 7th Ed. St. Louis, MO: Mosby, 2001:76, 271.
5. Mauriello SM, Overman VP, Platin E. Radiographic Imaging for the Dental Team. Philadelphia, PA: Lippincott, 1995:256.
6. Assail LA. The pregnant patient. In: Bennett JD, Rosenberg MB, eds. Medical Emergencies in Dentistry. Philadelphia, PA: WB Saunders, 2002:494–500.
7. Steer PJ, et al. Maternal blood pressure in pregnancy, birth weight, and perinatal mortality in first birth: prospective study. BMJ 2004;329:1312–1314.
8. ADA Council on Scientific Affairs. Antibiotic interference with oral contraceptives. J Am Dent Assoc 2002;133:880.
9. Hersh EV. Adverse drug reactions in dental practice: interactions involving antibiotics. J Am Dent Assoc 1999;130:236–251.
10. Cerel-Suhl SL, Yeager BF. Update on oral contraceptive pills. Am Fam Physician 1999;60:2073–2084.
11. Kuo LC, Polson AM, Kang T. Associations between periodontal diseases and systemic diseases: a review of the inter-relationships and interactions with diabetes, respiratory diseases, cardiovascular diseases and osteoporosis. Public Health 2007; doi:10.1016/j.puhe.2007.07.004.
12. Phipps KR, et al. Longitudinal study of bone density and periodontal disease in men. J Dent Res 2007;86(11):1110–1114.
13. Pilgram TK, et al. Relationships between clinical attachment level and spine and hip bone mineral density: data from healthy postmenopausal women. J Periodontol 2002;73:298–301.
14. Edwards BJ, Migliorati CA. Osteoporosis and its implications for dental patients. J Am Dent Assoc 2008;139(5):545–552.
15. Wilson W, Taubert KA, Gewitz M, et al. AHA Guideline: prevention of infective endocarditis. Circulation 2007;116:1736–1754.
16. Pallasch TJ. Antibiotic prophylaxis: problems in paradise. Dental Clin N Am 2003;47:665–679.
17. Pallasch TJ. Perspectives on the 2007 AHA endocarditis prevention guidelines. J Calif Dent Assoc 2007;35(7):507–513.
18. Lockhart PB, Loven B, Brennan MT, Fox PC. The evidence base for the efficacy of antibiotic prophylaxis in dental practice. J Am Dent Assoc 2007;138(4):458–474.
19. Pasquali SK, He X, Mohamad Z, et al. Trends in Endocarditis Hospitalizations at US Children's Hospitals. Am Heart J 2012;163(5):894–899.

Chapter Nine

1. Tyler MT, Rhodus NL, Miller CS. Clinician's Guide to Treatment of Medically Complex Dental Patients. 4th Ed. Seattle, WA: American Academy of Oral Medicine, 2011.
2. Little JW, Falace DA, Miller CS, Rhodus NL. Dental Management of the Medically Compromised Patient. 8th Ed. St. Louis, MO: Mosby, 2013:145–162.
3. The National Heart, Lung, and Blood Institute. Guidelines for diagnosis and management of von Willebrand's disease. Haemophilia 2008;14:171–232.
4. Royzman D, et al. The effect of aspirin intake on bleeding on probing in patients with gingivitis. J Periodontol 2004;75:679–684.
5. Ardekian L, Gaspar R, Peled M, Brener B, Laufer D. Does low-dose aspirin therapy complicate oral surgical procedures? J Am Dent Assoc 2000;131:331–335.
6. Brennan MT, Wynn RL, Miller CS. Aspirin and bleeding in dentistry: an update and recommendations. Oral Surg Oral Med Oral Pathol Oral Radiol Endod 2007;104:316–323.
7. Grines CL, Bonow RO, Casey DE Jr., et al. Prevention of premature discontinuation of dual antiplatelet therapy in patients with coronary artery stents. Circulation 2007;115:813–818.
8. Oake N, Jennings A, Forster AJ, et al. Anticoagulant intensity and outcomes among patients prescribed oral anticoagulant therapy: a systematic review and meta-analysis. CMAJ 2008;179:235–244.
9. Buller H. A higher international normalized ratio may be better for your patient. CMAJ 2008;179(3):217.
10. Wahl MJ. Myths of dental surgery in patients receiving anticoagulant therapy. J Am Dent Assoc 2000;131:77–81.
11. Souto JC, Oliver A, Zuazu-Jausoro I, Vives A, Fontcuberta J. Oral surgery in anticoagulated patients without reducing the dose of oral anticoagulant: a prospective randomized study. J Oral Maxillofac Surg 1996;54:27–32.
12. DePaola LG. Managing the care of patients infected with bloodborne diseases. J Am Dent Assoc 2003;134:350–358.
13. Perry JL, Pearson RD, Jagger J. Infected healthcare workers and patient safety: a double standard. Am J Infect Control 2006;34:313–319.
14. Redd JT, Baumbach J, Kohn W, et al. Patient-to-patient transmission of hepatitis B virus associated with oral surgery. J Infect Dis 2007;195:1311–1314.
15. Wilkins E. Clinical Practice of the Dental Hygienist. 11th Ed. Baltimore: Lippincott, Williams & Wilkins, 2013:32, 34–37, 43–50.

16. Hall HI, et al. Estimation of HIV incidence in the United States. JAMA 2008;300(5):520–529.
17. Reznik DA, Bednarsh H. HIV and the dental team. Dimen Den Hyg 2006;4(6):14–16.
18. Campo J, et al. Oral complication risks after invasive and non-invasive dental procedures in HIV-positive patients. Oral Dis 2007;13:110–116.
19. Kuhar DT, Henderson DK, Struble KA, et al. Updated U.S. Public Health Service Guidelines for the Management of Occupational Exposures to Human Immunodefiiency Virus and Recommendations for Postexposure Prophylaxis. Infect Control Hosp Epidemiol 2013;34(9): 875–892.
20. Perdue B, Wolderufael D, Mellors J, et al. HIV-1 transmission by a needlestick injury despite rapid initiation of four-drug postexposure prophylaxis [Abstract 210]. In: Program and Abstracts of the 6th Conference on Retroviruses and Opportunistic Infections. Chicago: Foundation for Retrovirology and Human Health in scientific collaboration with the National Institute of Allergy and Infectious Diseases and CDC, 1999:107.
21. Patton LL, Shugars DA, Bonito AJ. A systematic review of complication risks for HIV-positive patients undergoing invasive dental procedures. J Am Dent Assoc 2002;133:195–202.
22. Updated U.S. Public Health Service guidelines for the management of occupational exposures to HBV, HCV, and HIV and recommendations for postexposure prophylaxis. MMWR Recomm Rep, June 29, 2001;50 (RR-11):1–12, appendix B 45–46.
23. Weinstock H, Berman S, Cates W. Sexually transmitted disease among American youth: incidence and prevalence estimates, 2000. Perspect Sex Reprod Health 2004;36(1):6–10.
24. Kent ME, Romanelli F. Reexamining syphilis: an update on epidemiology, clinical manifestations, and management. Ann Pharmacother 2008;42(2):226–236.
25. Centers for Disease Control and Prevention. Sexually Transmitted Disease, Surveillance 2004 Supplement: Syphilis Surveillance Report. Atlanta, GA: Department of Health and Human Services, Centers for Disease Control and Prevention, 2005.
26. Tramont EC. *Treponema pallidum* (syphilis). In: Mandell GL, Bennett JE, Dolin R, eds. Principles and Practice of Infectious Diseases. 6th Ed. Orlando, FL: Churchill Livingstone, 2005:2768–2784.
27. Center for Disease Control and Prevention. 2010 Sexually transmitted diseases treatment guidelines, 2010. MMWR Recomm Rep 2010;59(RR-12):1–96. Available at http://www.cdc.gov/std/treatment/2010/default.htm. Accessed February 9, 2013.
28. Bennett J, Rosenberg MG. Medical Emergencies in Dentistry. Philadelphia, PA: WB Saunders, 2002:393.

Chapter Ten

1. Little JW, Falace DA, Miller CS, Rhodus NL. Dental Management of the Medically Compromised Patient. 8th Ed. St. Louis, MO: Mosby, 2013:23, 250–256, 480.
2. Friedlander AH, Sung EC, Child JS. Radiation-induced heart disease after Hodgkin's disease and breast cancer treatment: dental implications. J Am Dent Assoc 2003;134:1615–1620.
3. Peterson DE, Öhrn K, Bowen J, et al. Systematic review of oral cryotherapy for management of oral mucositis caused by cancer therapy. Support Care Cancer 2013;21: 327–332. DOI 10.1007/s00520-012-1562-0.
4. Migliorati C, Hewson I, Lalla RV, et al. Systematic review of laser and other light therapy for the management of oral mucositis in cancer patients. Support Care Cancer 2013;21:333–341. DOI 10.1007/s00520-012-1605-6.
5. Oral Care Provider's Reference Guide for Oncology Patients. NIDCR pamphlet, US patent number 5,063,637.
6. Cole P, Rodu B, Mathisen A. Alcohol-containing mouthwash and oropharyngeal cancer. J Am Dent Assoc 2003;134(8):1079–1087.
7. Harris DJ, Eilers J, Harriman A, Cashavelly BJ, Maxwell C. Putting evidence into practice: evidence-based interventions for the management of oral mucositis. Clin J Oncol Nurs 2008;12(1):141–152. Available at http://guideline.gov/content.aspx?id=15700&search=management+of+oral+mucositis+and+chemotherapy. Accessed January 31, 2013.
8. Oral Complications of Cancer Treatment: What the Oncology Team Can Do. NIDCR pamphlet, publication #99-4360:2–4.
9. Dental Oncology Education Program. Oral Health in Cancer Therapy. 3rd Ed. February 2008. Available at http://www.doep.org/images/OHCT_III_FINAL.pdf. Accessed February 5, 2013.
10. What the Oral Health Team Can Do. NIDCR pamphlet, publication #99-4372:4.
11. Pallasch TJ, Slots J. Antibiotic prophylaxis and the medically compromised patient. Periodontol 2000 1996;10:107–138.
12. Centers for Disease Control and Prevention. 2011 National Diabetes Fact Sheet: General Information and National Estimates on Diabetes in the United States, 2010. Atlanta, GA: U.S. Department of Health and Human Services, Centers for Disease Control and Prevention, 2011. Available at http://www.cdc.gov/diabetes/pubs/pdf/ndfs_2011.pdf. Accessed February 2, 2013.
13. American Diabetes Association. 2013 Clinical Practice Recommendations. Diabetes Care 2013; 36:S3; DOI:10.2337/dc13-S003. Published online at http://professional.diabetes.org/ResourcesForProfessionals.aspx?cid=84160. Accessed February 3, 2013.
14. Vernillo AT. Dental considerations for the treatment of patients with diabetes mellitus. J Am Dent Assoc 2003;133(suppl):24S–33S.
15. Malamed S. Medical Emergencies in the Dental Office. 6th Ed. St. Louis, MO: Mosby, 2007:145–158, 276–279.
16. DeRossi S, Glick M. Lupus erythematosus: considerations for dentistry. J Am Dent Assoc 1998;129:330–339.
17. Khalaf MW, Khader R, Cobetto G, et al. Risk of adrenal crisis in dental patients. JADA 2013;144(2):152–160.
18. Bennett JD, Rosenberg MB. Medical Emergencies in Dentistry. Philadelphia, PA: WB Saunders, 2002:353.
19. Tornwall RD, Chow AK. The association between periodontal disease and the systemic inflammatory conditions of obesity arthritis, Alzheimer's and renal disease. Can J Dent Hyg 2012;46(2):115–123.
20. Treister N, Glick M. Rheumatoid arthritis: a review and suggested dental care considerations. J Am Dent Assoc 1999;130(5):689–698.
21. NIDCR. Dental Management of the Organ Transplant Patient. Publication. NIH publication 11-6270. Available at http://www.nidcr.nih.gov/OralHealth/Topics/OrganTransplantationOralHealth/OrganTransplantProf.htm. Accessed February 10, 2013.

Chapter Eleven

1. Fang J, et al. Disparities in adult awareness of heart attack warning signs and symptoms—14 states. MMWR 2008;57(7):175–179. Available at http://www.cdc.gov/mmwr/preview/mmwrhtml/mm5707a3.htm?s_cid mm5707a3_e.
2. Kreiner M, et al. Craniofacial pain as the sole symptom of cardiac ischemia. J Am Dent Assoc 2007;138(1):74–79.
3. Pickett F. American College of Cardiology/American Heart Association updated guidelines for perioperative care cardiovascular evaluation prior to noncardiac surgery: implications for dental hygiene treatment in post-myocardial infarction. Access 2008;22(7):36–40.
4. Tyler MT, Lozada-Nur F, Glick M, eds. Clinician's Guide to Treatment of Medically Complex Dental Patients. 2nd Ed. Baltimore: American Academy of Oral Medicine, 2001:6–19.
5. Little JW, Falace DA, Miller CS, Rhodus NL. Dental Management of the Medically Compromised Patient. 8th Ed. St. Louis, MO: Mosby, 2013:DM5, 22–24, 78, 87–88, 423, 471–474.
6. Baddour LM, et al. A summary of the update on cardiovascular implantable electronic device infections and their management. A scientific statement from the American Heart Association. JADA 2011;142(2):159–165.
7. Pallasch TJ. Antibiotic prophylaxis: problems in paradise. Dent Clin N Am 2003;47:665–679.
8. Hunt SA, et al. ACC/AHA 2005 Guideline update for the diagnosis and management of chronic heart failure in the adult—summary article. Circulation 2005;112: 1825–1852.
9. Field JM, Hazinski MF, Sayre MR, et al. Part 1: executive summary: 2010 American Heart Association Guidelines for Cardiopulmonary Resuscitation and Emergency Cardiovascular Care. Circulation 2010;122(suppl 3): S640–S656.
10. Glick M. Screening for traditional risk factors for cardiovascular disease. J Am Dent Assoc 2002;133:291–300.
11. Mudawi TO, Kaye GC. Implantable cardiac devices—past, present and future. Br J Cardiol 2008;15(1):23–28.
12. Maisel W, et al. Pacemaker and ICD generator malfunctions: analysis of Food and Drug Administration annual reports. JAMA 2006;295:1901–1906.
13. Boston Scientific. Cardiac Myths and Facts. www.bostonscientific.com; Medtronic. Frequently asked questions. www.medtronic.com; St. Jude. What electrical equipment is safe to use? www.sjm.com.
14. Conlin K. Treating patients with implanted heart devices. Dimen Den Hyg 2008;6:14–17.
15. Brand HS, et al. Interference of electrical dental equipment with implantable cardio-defibrillators. Br Dent J 2007;203(10):577–579.
16. Gurenlian JR, Kleiman C. Cerebrovascular accident. Access 2002;6:40–47.
17. Verdelho A, Ferro JM, Melo T, et al. Headache in acute stroke. A prospective study in the first 8 days. Cephalalgia 2008;28:346–354.
18. Ovbiagele B, et al. Early stroke risk after transient ischemic attack among individuals with symptomatic intracranial artery stenosis. Arch Neurol 2008;65(6):733–737.
19. Jauch ED, Saver JL, Adams HP, et al. Guidelines for the Early Management of Patients with Acute Ischemic Stroke : A Guideline for Healthcare Professionals from the American Heart Association/American Stroke Association. *Stroke.* Published online January 31, 2013. Available at http://stroke.ahajournals.org/content/early/2013/01/31/STR.0b013e318284056a.full.pdf+html. Accessed February 1, 2013.
20. Pickett F. State of evidence: Chronic periodontal disease and Stroke. Can J Dent Hyg 2012;46(2):124–128.
21. Lockhart P, Bolger AF, Papapanou PN, et al. Periodontal disease and atherosclerotic vascular disease: does the evidence support an independent association?: a scientific statement from the American Heart Association. Circulation 2012;125:2520–2544.

Chapter Twelve

1. Ragalis K. The patient with a seizure disorder. In: Wilkins E, ed. Clinical Practice of the Dental Hygienist. 10th Ed. Baltimore: Lippincott Williams & Wilkins, 2009: 957–968.
2. Jacobsen PL, Eden O. Epilepsy and the dental management of the epileptic patient. J Contemp Dent Pract 2008;9(1):1–9.
3. Rados C. Epilepsy and seizures can occur at any age. FDA Consum 2005;39:31–35.
4. Tuxhorn I, Kotagal P. Classification. Semin Neurol 2008;28(3):277–288.
5. Berg AT, Schaeffer IE. New concepts in classification of the epilepsies. Entering the 21st Century. Epilepsia 2011;52(6):1058–1062. Available at http://www.ilae.org/Visitors/Centre/ctf/documents/NewConcepts-Classification_2011_000.pdf. Accessed February 4, 2013.
6. Mehmet Y, Senem O, Sulun T, et al. Management of epileptic patients in dentistry. Surg Sci 2012;3:47–52. Available at www.scirp.org/journal/PaperDownload.aspx?paperID=17010. Accessed February 6, 2013.
7. Modi AC, Morita DA, Glauser TA. Adherence to antiepileptic drug therapy in newly diagnosed pediatric patients. Pediatrics 2008;121:e961–e966.
8. Zhang W, Moskowitz RW, Nuki G, et al. OARSI recommendations for the management of hip and knee osteoarthritis, Part II: OARSI evidence-based, expert consensus guidelines. Osteoarthritis Cartilage 2008;16:137–162.
9. Friedlander AH, Marder SR. The psychopathology, medical management and dental implications of schizophrenia. J Am Dent Assoc 2002;133:603–610.
10. Clark DB. Dental care for the patient with bipolar disorder. J Can Dent Assoc 2003;69(1): 20–24.
11. Little JW, Falace DA, Miller CS, Rhodus NL. Dental Management of the Medically Compromised Patient. 8th Ed. St. Louis: Mosby Elsevier, 2013:474–481.
12. Friedlander AH, Norman DC, Mahler ME, et al. Alzheimer's disease. Psychopathology, medical management and dental implications. J Am Dent Assoc 2006;137(9):1240–1251.
13. Grover S, Rhodus N. Dental Implications of Parkinson's Disease. Northwest Dent J. 2011;11:357. Available at http://www.mndental.org/features/2011/11/01/357/dental_implications_of_parkinsons_disease. Accessed February 10, 2013.
14. Prajer R, Kacerik M. Treating patients with Alzheimer's Disease. Dimen Den Hyg 2006;4:24–26.
15. Southern Association of Institutional Dentists, Special Care Advocates in Dentistry Modules. Available at http://saiddent.org/modules.php

16. Hernandez P, Ikkanda Z. Applied behavior analysis: behavior management of children with autism spectrum disorders in dental environments. J Am Dent Assoc 2011;142(3):281–287.
17. Barros de Carvalho R, Mendes RF, Prado RR, Neto JMM. Oral Health and oral motor function in children with cerebral palsy. Spec Care Dentist 2011;31(2):58–62.

Chapter Thirteen

1. Carlaio RG, Grassi RF, Losacco T, et al. Gastroesophageal reflux disease and dental erosion. A case report and review of the literature. Clin Ter 2007;158:349–353.
2. Guyton AC, Hall JE. Textbook of Medical Physiology. 10th Ed. Philadelphia, PA: WB Saunders, 2000:766.
3. Ali DA, Brown RS, Rodriguez LO, et al. Dental erosion caused by silent gastroesophageal reflux disease. J Am Dent Assoc 2002;133:734–737.
4. Wilkins EM. Clinical Practice of the Dental Hygienist. 10th Ed. Baltimore, MD: Lippincott Williams & Wilkins, 2009:990–993, 1017–1031.
5. Christensen GJ. Oral care for patients with bulimia. J Am Dent Assoc 2002;133:1689–1691.
6. Pickett F, Terezhalmy G. Basic Pharmacology with Dental Hygiene Applications. Baltimore, MD: Lippincott Wilkins & Williams, 2009:200–210.
7. Alexander RE, Grogan DM. Management of dental patients with obstructive lung diseases. Tex Dent J 2008;125:228–240.
8. Little JW, Falace DA, Miller CS, Rhodus NL. Dental Management of the Medically Compromised Patient. 8th Ed. St. Louis: Mosby, 2013:95–97.
9. Steinbacher DM, Glick M. The dental patient with asthma. An update and oral health considerations. J Am Dent Assoc 2001;132:1229–1239.
10. Narang A. Oral health and related factors in cystic fibrosis and other chronic respiratory disorders. Arch Dis Child 2003;88:702–707.
11. Bennett JD, Rosenberg MB. Medical Emergencies in Dentistry. Philadelphia, PA: WB Saunders, 2002:22–29, 63, 103.
12. Handbook of Emergency Cardiovascular Care for Healthcare Providers. Dallas, TX: American Heart Association, 2012.

Chapter Fourteen

1. Guyton AC, Hall JE. Textbook of Medical Physiology. 10th Ed. Philadelphia, PA: WB Saunders, 2000:577.
2. Pickett F, Terezhalmy G. Basic Pharmacology with Dental Hygiene Applications. Baltimore, MD: Lippincott Wilkins & Williams, 2009:43–44, 173–189, 304.
3. Little JW, Falace DA, Miller CS, Rhodus NL. Dental Management of the Medically Compromised Patient. 8th Ed. St. Louis, MO: Mosby, 2013.
4. Werner CW, Saad TF. Prophylactic antibiotic therapy prior to dental treatment for patients with end-stage renal disease. Spec Care Dentist 1999;19:106–111.
5. Lockhart PB, Loven B, Brennan MT, et al. The evidence base for the efficacy of antibiotic prophylaxis in dental practice J Am Dent Assoc 2007;138: 458–474.
6. Baddour LM, Bettmann MA, Bolger AF, et al. Nonvalvular cardiovascular device-related infection. Circulation 2003;108:2015–2031.
7. DeRossi S, Glick M, Bettmann MA, Bolger AF, et al. Dental considerations for the patient with renal disease receiving hemodialysis. J Am Dent Assoc 1996;127:211–219.
8. Shultis WA, Weil J, Looker HC, et al. Effect of periodontitis on overt nephropathy and end-stage renal disease in type 2 diabetes. Diabetes Care 2007;30:306–311.
9. Jover-Cerveró A, Bagán JV, Jiménez-Soriano Y, Poveda-Roda R. Dental management in renal failure: patients on dialysis. Med Oral Patol Oral Cir Bucal. 2008;13(7):E419–E426.

Chapter Fifteen

1. Robbins KS. Medicolegal considerations. In: Malamed S, ed. Medical Emergencies in the Dental Office. 5th Ed. St. Louis, MO: Mosby, 2000:94.
2. Ring T. HIPAA and its implications for dental hygiene. Chicago, IL: ADA Publishing, April 2003:21–28.
3. American Dental Association's HIPAA Privacy Kit for Dentists. Chicago, IL: ADA Publishing, 2002:1–137.
4. ADA Council on Scientific Affairs. Office emergencies and emergency kits. J Am Dent Assoc 2002;133: 364–365.

Review and Case Study Answers

Chapter 1: Self-Study, Review and Case Study Answers

Self-Study Answers and Page Numbers

1. e *page 2*
2. a *pages 2–3*
3. c *page 2*
4. b *page 3*
5. c *page 4*
6. c *page 5*
7. c *page 11*
8. b *pages 9–10*
9. a, c *page 12*
10. b *page 12*
11. a *page 12*
12. c *pages 12–13*
13. b *page 13*
14. b *page 13*
15. d *pages 13–14*
16. b *page 14*
17. c *page 15*
18. c *page 15*

If you answered any items incorrectly, refer to the page number and review that information before proceeding to the next chapter.

Review Answers

1. Blood pressure (BP)—the pressure in the arteries when the heart beats and the pressure when the heart rests
   Systolic BP—the pressure in the arteries when the heart beats
   Diastolic BP—the pressure in arteries when the heart rests or between beats
   Pulse—the heart rate or a reflection of the heartbeat
   Respiration—the inhalation and exhalation of air
   Functional capacity—the ability to complete various physical activities; a measure of cardiac risk assessment
   Metabolic equivalents (METs)—a measure of the ability to perform common daily tasks
2. All questions on the medical history form should be answered to help predict potential medical emergencies.
3. Recheck BP after 5 minutes when client has rested; if still elevated, inform client of readings; refer for medical evaluation if dental procedure is stressful or if anesthesia is required; provide routine treatment; consider using a stress-reduction protocol during oral health treatment; and keep appointments short.
4. Failure to adhere to antihypertensive therapy and lifestyle changes are factors that contribute to insufficient BP control.
5. BP should be measured routinely after age 3.
6. Palpate the carotid artery found in the middle of the neck along the sternocleidomastoid muscle.
7. Presence of sounds or noises, and depth of respirations.
8. Disease or infection transmission.

Case A

1. Prehypertension
2. Lifestyle modifications including weight management and BP control
3. Routine dental treatment can be provided; remeasure BP at continuing care appointments as a screening strategy for hypertension
4. Mr. Farnsworth presents with stage 1 hypertension
5. Mr. Farnsworth presents with ASA classification IV.
6. Postpone elective treatment, such as a dental hygiene appointment, until his condition has improved and medical consultation verifies that he has moved to the ASA III category.

Chapter 2: Review and Case Study Answers

Self-Study Answers and Page Numbers

1. b *page 18*
2. d *page 20*
3. c *page 19*
4. a *page 20*
5. a *pages 20–21*
6. d *page 22*
7. a *pages 21–22*
8. d *page 23*
9. a *page 23*

If you answered any items incorrectly, refer to the page number and review that information before proceeding to the next chapter.

Review Answers

1. TB is an infectious, inflammatory disease caused by *M. tuberculosis* that primarily affects the pulmonary system. TB infection refers to a person who has inhaled the TB bacillus and whose immune system has developed antibodies to the bacillus, but has not developed active disease. Active TB disease refers to a person who presents with symptoms of the disease.
2. The screening questions for active TB are as follows: Have you had any of the following diseases or problems? Active TB, persistent cough for more than 3 weeks, cough that produces blood? Other signs include night sweats, recent unexplained weight loss, and close association with someone who has active TB.
3. Etiologies of a persistent cough may include cigarette smoking, chronic bronchitis, asthma, and respiratory infection.
4. Criteria for determining noninfectious status in clients with active TB include effective anti-TB drugs have been taken for three or more weeks, three consecutive negative sputum smears are documented, and the client is not in a coughing stage.

Case A

1. Have you seen a physician about this condition? How long has the cough lasted? Do you have night sweats, elevated temperature, unexplained weight loss? Do you smoke cigarettes? Do you have any other chronic respiratory conditions such as bronchitis or asthma? Are you taking any medications for this condition? Is there anyone else that you work with or a resident who has the same type of cough?
2. Elective dental care is contraindicated in clients with active TB. If you suspect active TB, refer the client for a medical evaluation.
3. Utilize the criteria of the CDC: not in the coughing stage, three consecutive negative sputum smears, and has taken effective anti-TB medications for at least 3 weeks. You can also request the results of a culture-negative sputum smear after 3 weeks of drug treatment to ensure that the disease is not resistant to the medications used.
4. No contraindication to treatment, but monitor history for signs of active disease in the future.

Case B

1. Even if active TB disease is ruled out, the physician may prescribe a single anti-TB drug to prevent disease from developing.
2. The employee would likely be directed to take INH for 6 months.
3. If the staff member has no symptoms of active disease, she can continue working. She is not contagious and cannot transmit the disease.

Chapter 3: Review and Case Study Answers

Self-Study Answers and Page Numbers

1. a, d, e, f *page 26*
2. d *page 27*
3. a *page 27*
4. e *page 29*
5. a, b, c, d, f, g *pages 27–36*
6. d *page 30*
7. c *page 34*
8. b *page 32*
9. d *page 32*
10. b *page 33*
11. a *page 35*
12. b *page 37*

If you answered any items incorrectly, refer to the page number and review that information before proceeding to the next chapter.

Review Answers

1. Hyperventilation: excessive intake of oxygen and exhalation of carbon dioxide. Vasodepressor syncope: fainting.
2. During hyperventilation the client is inspiring excessive oxygen, and providing additional oxygen would compromise the situation further.
3. The client's chief complaint reflects the client's primary reason for seeking oral health care and their oral health concerns, which may be different from the concerns of the clinician.
4. Strategies for reducing stress include discussing topics to occupy the client's mind, ensuring adequate pain control, considering the use of nitrous oxide conscious sedation, and prescribing an antianxiety medication.
5. Signs and symptoms of pre-syncope include facial paleness, perspiration or feelings of warmth, nausea, and increased pulse rate. Signs of syncope include yawning, dilated pupils, feeling cold, dizziness, and hypotension. Post-syncope signs include facial pallor, nausea, weakness, and disorientation.
6. A clinical examination should precede the decision to take dental X-rays.
   - Exposures should be limited to the fewest number needed for diagnosis.
   - Factors to consider: age, dental developmental stage (primary dentition, transitional dentition, adolescent with permanent dentition, dentate adult, partially edentulous adult, or edentulous adult)
   - Clinical circumstances (symptomatic or asymptomatic)
   - New patient or continuing care (recall) patient
   - Risk factors for caries or dental disease

Case A

1. Hyperventilation
2. Syncope
3. Cup hands over mouth, or have client breathe into a paper bag.
4. Record the incident, vital signs, treatment sequence and response, how long before normal breathing was restored, and client's decision to continue or postpone treatment.

Case B

1. Vasodepressor syncope
2. Anxiety: fear of injection
3. Lack of blood flow to the brain or cerebral ischemia as a result of hypotension
4. Place the client in the supine position with the feet elevated, monitor vital signs, record incident in dental chart, determine with client whether treatment should continue or be postponed after recovery, and observe client for signs of recurrent syncope should treatment continue.
5. The Trendelenburg position has been shown to restrict respiration and diminish the effects of breathing. It is more appropriately used to manage airway obstruction.

Chapter 4: Review and Case Study Answers

Self-Study Answers and Page Numbers

1. d *page 41*
2. b *page 42*
3. a *page 42*
4. d *page 43*
5. a *page 43*
6. c, d *page 43*
7. a *page 44*
8. a *page 45*
9. c *page 45*
10. a *page 46*
11. c *page 46*
12. d *page 49*
13. a *page 49*

If you answered any of the items incorrectly, refer to the page number and review that information before proceeding to the next chapter.

Review Answers

1. If a client is under the care of a physician, consider whether there is a risk for medical problems arising during treatment, whether there might be drug side effects relevant to a medical emergency from those medications being taken, and the potential for cross-contamination from the medical condition being treated. A recent history of hospitalization must be investigated for the same reasons.
2. Thrombocytopenia: a decrease in the number of platelets in circulating blood

   Leukopenia: a reduction in the number of leukocytes in the blood with the count being 5,000 or less

   Agranulocytosis: a dramatic decrease in the production of granulocytes

Neutropenia: a diminished number of neutrophils in the blood

3. The major side effects that can represent a risk for medical emergency include postural hypotension, bleeding, hypertension/tachycardia/arrhythmia, nausea/vomiting/gastrointestinal (GI) reflux, and leukopenia/blood dyscrasias.
4. Adverse effects can occur from herbal or dietary supplements. Niacin can cause postural hypotension; kava, valerian, and St. John's wort can cause interference with sedative drugs; ephedrine can cause hypertension and tachycardia; and ginkgo, ginseng, and garlic supplements have been known to cause increased bleeding.
5. Criteria used to investigate medications include the action of the drug, the dose, side effects relevant to oral changes or to treatment modification, interactions between the client's drug and drugs used during treatment, and dental treatment considerations for both the medical condition or disease the drug is being used for and the relevant side effects of the drug.
6. Vital signs can identify hypotensive and hypertensive states and abnormal values of pulse rhythm that may predispose the client to a medical emergency during oral health care.

Case A

1. Elective oral health care should be postponed for 1 month after the myocardial infarction and the functional capacity determined to meet the 4 MET level, before elective care is provided. A medical clearance with a cardiologist is advised.
2. The clinician should request the most recent prothrombin time or international normalized ratio data prior to providing oral health care.
3. The combination of Plavix, aspirin, and ginseng may result in increased bleeding. Antihypertensive medications frequently have postural hypotension as a potential side effect.
4. Allowing an upright, seated position for a few minutes before dismissing the client provides time for vasoconstriction of blood vessels and prevents postural hypotension from occurring.

Case B

1. Given that the client sleeps with the bed elevated, she would most likely be comfortable in a semiupright or semisupine position.
2. Nausea, GI discomfort, and gas are the most common GI side effects. Dry mouth is the most common oral side effect.
3. The client may be presenting with leukopenia or neutropenia, both rare side effects, but which occurred in some patients in clinical trials. These side effects can result in increased infection.

Chapter 5: Review and Case Study Answers

Self-Study Answers and Page Numbers

1. c *page 55*
2. b *page 54*
3. a *page 54*
4. b *page 55*
5. a *page 57*
6. d *page 56*
7. c *page 57*
8. e *page 57*
9. b *page 57*
10. b *page 57*
11. c *page 57*
12. c *page 57*

If you answered any of the items incorrectly, refer to the page number and review that information before proceeding to the next chapter.

Review Answers

1. Bacteremia: the presence of bacteria in the circulation, which can be transferred to distant sites within the body

   Immunosuppression: a reduced immune response resulting in reduced healing and increased risk of infection

   Innocuous: harmless
2. Safety glasses are used to protect the eyes from aerosols and spatter during oral procedures.
3. According to the ADA and AAOS guidelines, there is no scientific evidence to support the routine use of antibiotic premedication in patients with prosthetic knee implants. Therefore, prophylactic antibiotics are not recommended for this patient.
4. The characteristics to be diagnosed with ARONJ include: the client is currently receiving or has received BIS in the past; exposed bone that has persisted for more than 8 weeks is present; and there is no history of radiation therapy to the jaws.

Case A

1. The client is not considered to be at risk for infection. According to the ADA/AAOS, there is no scientific evidence that indicates this patient is at an increased risk of PJI.
2. Prophylactic antibiotic therapy is NOT recommended for this client.
3. Consult with orthopedic surgeon and share new guidelines; discuss benefits and risks of prophylactic antibiotics; record recommendation of the orthopedic surgeon in the client's chart; discuss with client recommendation and inform client of scientific evidence; reach final decision and note it in client's chart.

Case B

1. A history of corticosteroid therapy, chemotherapy, diabetes mellitus, smoking, alcohol, and poor oral hygiene are other risk factors that may be associated with ONJ.
2. There is no evidence that delaying therapy will reduce the risk of ARONJ.
3. Recommend the client to maintain meticulous oral health and have regular oral examinations to identify any disease early. The goal is to avoid the need for surgery.
4. Eliminate pain, control infection of soft and hard tissues, minimize progression of necrosis, and removal of necrotic bone or infected teeth in the area of necrotic bone.

Chapter 6: Review and Case Study Answers

Self-Study Answers and Page Numbers

1. b *page 64*
2. c *page 67*
3. c *page 65*
4. a, b, d, e, f *page 67*
5. a *page 65*
6. d *page 65*
7. c *page 65*
8. c, f *page 66*
9. b *page 67*
10. d *page 67*
11. c *page 68*
12. c *page 69*
13. b *page 71*
14. b *page 72*

If you answered any items incorrectly, refer to the page number and review that information before proceeding to the next chapter.

Review Answers

1. Anaphylactic shock: a severe and sometimes fatal allergic reaction characterized by respiratory distress and cardiovascular collapse.
   Hypersensitivity reaction: an abnormal condition characterized by an excessive reaction to a particular stimulus such as allergy.
   Sensitization: an acquired reaction in which specific antibodies develop in response to an antigen.
2. Signs of a mild allergy include skin rash, erythema, hives, and urticaria. Signs of a severe allergic reaction include bronchiolar constriction, asphyxiation, reduction of blood pressure, and cardiovascular collapse.
3. Follow-up questions should include "Which LA caused your reaction? What were your symptoms?"
4. Items in the dental office that can cause a latex allergy include rubber tubing, stethoscope, blood pressure cuff, gloves, latex barriers, elastic on face masks, rubber polishing cups, and rubber dam material.

Case A

1. The child appears to be allergic to lidocaine.
2. This allergic reaction represents a type I reaction.
3. The dentist should inject epinephrine sublingually while the dental assistant activates 911 office emergency protocol.
4. Record the event in the clinical record, place information regarding possible lidocaine allergy on the front of the health history, and avoid using lidocaine at future appointments. As there is no cross-sensitivity among the amide group of LA, the child should be sent for immunologic evaluation to determine whether one of the other LA in the amide group can be used.
5. Nausea is typically NOT a sign of an allergic reaction. It is usually a side effect of medication. In this case, it may also be related to anxiety.

Case B

1. The name of this condition is contact stomatitis.
2. The most likely cause of this contact stomatitis is use of the new toothpaste.
3. Discontinue the use of the new toothpaste product and record findings in the dental record for future reference.

Chapter 7: Review and Case Study Answers

Self-Study Answers and Page Numbers

1. b *page 76*
2. d *page 75*
3. a *page 79*
4. a *page 77*
5. b *page 77*
6. a, c *page 79*
7. c *page 80*
8. c, d, e, g, h *pages 80–81*
9. c *pages 79–80*
10. a *page 85*
11. a *page 83*
12. c *page 84*
13. c *page 83*
14. b *page 82*
15. c *page 84*
16. b *page 84*

If you answered any of the items incorrectly, refer to the page number and review that information before proceeding to the next chapter.

Review Answers

1. Aspects that must be considered when treating an individual who abuses recreational drugs include medical consultation, client instruction regarding refraining from use of drugs before dental or dental hygiene appointments, use of non-narcotic pain medications for postoperative pain management, monitoring of bleeding time during treatment, and management of increased dental caries.
2. A smoking cessation protocol should include three steps: Ask, Advise, and Refer. Recommending use of a tobacco quitline and providing follow-up support is helpful for achieving success.
3. Issues related to treating individuals with a history of alcohol abuse vary and may include any of the following: nutritional deficiency, increased oral disease, liver dysfunction, increased bleeding and liver disease, behavior management, oral manifestations of alcohol abuse, oral care product selection, and tobacco and alcohol use.

Case A

1. With a history of infective endocarditis (IE), the client should take amoxicillin as a preventive agent. The client should have taken 2 g of amoxicillin 1 hour before the appointment.
2. During a crown preparation, gingivae in the area are likely to bleed. The dentist may need to use a gingival retraction cord with epinephrine to stop the bleeding and improve the impression for the crown. For clients who recently used marijuana, there is the risk that the epinephrine in the retraction cord may enhance tachycardia and cause increased blood pressure.
3. It is recommended that treatment be postponed for at least 1 week for this client because he used marijuana the evening before the appointment. An alternative suggestion is for the dentist to use products that do not contain epinephrine or other vasoconstrictors.
4. Advise the client to refrain from using any recreational drugs before the dental appointment because epinephrine will need to be used as part of treatment and can cause significant cardiovascular effects. Also, because the client took amoxicillin for the scheduled appointment, the dentist should prescribe a different antibiotic for the next appointment.

Case B

1. Clinical findings may include periodontal disease, increased dental caries, increased bleeding, candidiasis, xerostomia, and evidence of squamous cell carcinoma.
2. Recommend treatment be postponed until the client is sober.
3. Non-narcotic analgesics such as acetaminophen are preferred. Aspirin or nonsteroidal anti-inflammatory drugs may be recommended depending on whether or not the client has any GI bleeding or ulcers. Narcotic medications are contraindicated.
4. Acetaminophen, 4 g/day.

Chapter 8: Review and Case Study Answers

Self-Study Answers and Page Numbers

1. b *page 89*
2. a *pages 89–90*
3. c *page 91*
4. a *page 92*
5. d *page 90*
6. b *page 94*
7. c *pages 94–95*
8. c *page 97*
9. d *page 95*
10. b *page 97*
11. c *pages 95–96*
12. a, b, d *page 97*

If you answered any items incorrectly, refer to the page number and review that information before proceeding to the next chapter.

Review Answers

1. Parturition is the act of giving birth to a child. Teratogen refers to any drug capable of causing a birth defect in the fetus. Valvulopathy is a disorder of valve function causing a variety of cardiac disorders.
2. Side effects of birth control and hormone replacement therapy relevant for oral health care include increased blood pressure, nausea, increased bleeding, and increased incidence of dry socket.
3. To prevent syncope in the pregnant woman, place a pillow under the client's right hip to displace the weight of the fetus to the left and away from the vena cava vein.
4. Antibiotic prophylaxis is no longer indicated in the following conditions: cardiac-native heart valve disease; prosthetic heart valve and pacemakers; hip, knee, and shoulder prosthetic joints; renal dialysis shunts; cerebrospinal fluid shunts; vascular grafts; immunosuppression secondary to cancer and cancer chemotherapy; systemic lupus erythematosus; and type 1 diabetes mellitus.

Case A

1. Lidocaine is considered safe for use with pregnant clients.
2. NSAIDs delay parturition.
3. Radiographs can be performed for this client, but only if deemed necessary (to determine the extent of the decay); a protective lead apron is used, and only the minimum number of radiographs should be taken.
4. Recommend that the client take antibiotics as prescribed until completed and that the client use a backup nonhormonal contraceptive method while taking the antibiotics and for 1 week after antibiotic therapy is completed.

Case B

1. According to the 2007 AHA guideline for prevention of IE, prophylactic antibiotic coverage is not recommended, given this client's medical history.
2. In most cases, osteoporosis is asymptomatic for years. Low back pain and fractures develop later in the course of the disease.

Chapter 9: Review and Case Study Answers

Self-Study Answers and Page Numbers

1. a *pages 104–105*
2. b *page 103*
3. a *page 102*
4. c *page 102*
5. c, d, e *page 102*
6. a *page 103*
7. b *page 103*
8. a, e *page 107*
9. b *page 109*
10. a *page 108*
11. c *page 108*
12. b *page 108*
13. a, b, c *page 112*
14. a, d *page 111*
15. b *page 110*
16. a *page 111*
17. c *page 112*
18. c *page 115*
19. b *page 116*
20. a *page 116*
21. d *page 117*

If you answered any items incorrectly, refer to the page number and review that information before proceeding to the next chapter.

Review Answers

1. Idiopathic: the cause for the condition is unknown.
   Petechiae: small collections of blood under the skin or mucous membrane. Ecchymosis: discoloration of the skin caused by blood within the local tissue. Seroconvert: the development of antibodies in response to vaccination.
2. Four major causes of abnormal bleeding include blood dyscrasias, bleeding disorders, liver dysfunction, and drug-induced clotting abnormalities.
3. The major components of an occupation exposure report are summarized in Box 9.4.
4. Follow-up questions for a client with a history of blood transfusion include "Why did you need to have a blood transfusion? Have you had any complications as a result of the transfusion? Have you been tested for bloodborne disease as a result of the transfusion?"

Case A

1. Coumadin inhibits the formation of vitamin K–related coagulation factors; it reduces the formation of blood clots within blood vessels.
2. Myocardial infarction, stroke, artificial heart valves, and total joint replacement are other conditions for which Coumadin might be prescribed.
3. Blood tests used to measure anticoagulation in clients taking Coumadin include PT and INR.
4. Preventive measures include consulting with the client's physician or hematologist, PT/INR laboratory testing before treatment, and continued use of therapeutic levels of Coumadin or change of therapy as recommended by physician.
5. Management strategies include rinsing with tranexamic acid or using another antifibrinolytic medication, local application of an absorbable gelatin sponge or other hemostatic agent, application of digital pressure, dismiss client once bleeding is stopped or controlled, offer postoperative instructions such as mild rinsing with cold water or applying a moistened tea bag to the affected site.

Case B

1. What treatment is being used for the sickle cell anemia? How long have you been in control? What problems do you have with healing? Are you having any symptoms now?
2. Symptoms of uncontrolled sickle cell anemia would include facial pallor, fatigue, muscle weakness, shortness of breath, and sore, painful tongue, bald tongue, or loss of taste sensation.
3. Management of any client with anemia includes frequent, short appointments, stressing plaque control, use of low epinephrine local anesthetics, prophylactic antibiotics if oral surgery is planned, use of acetaminophen or opioid/APAP for oral pain, and use of diazepam or nitrous oxide with oxygen levels greater than 50% if sedation is needed.

Chapter 10: Review and Case Study Answers

Self-Study Answers and Page Numbers

1. a *page 123*
2. c *page 124*
3. a, b, c *page 124*
4. d *page 125*
5. d *page 125*
6. b *page 125*
7. a, b, c, e, f *pages 129*
8. b *page 130*
9. a *page 131*
10. a *pages 131–133*
11. b *page 135*
12. c *page 135*
13. a *page 136*
14. c *pages 137–138*
15. a, b, c, d, e, f, g *page 141*

If you answered any items incorrectly, refer to the page number and review that information before proceeding to the next chapter.

Review Answers

1. Hyperglycemia: greater amounts of glucose in the blood.
   Hypoglycemia: abnormally low levels of glucose in the blood usually caused by taking too much insulin.
   Osteoradionecrosis: the destruction and death of bone tissue from radiation.
2. Signs of undiagnosed diabetes include frequent urination, frequent thirst, healing slowly, and frequent infections, although the client may be asymptomatic.
3. Type 1 DM occurs in approximately 5% to 10% of individuals and usually during adolescence. Causes include heredity, idiopathic, and autoimmune destruction of pancreatic beta cells. Type 2 DM occurs in 90% to 95% of cases usually in

individuals older than 45 years. Causes include hereditary predisposition, obesity, and sedentary lifestyle. High-risk ethnic groups for type 2 diabetes include African-Americans, Hispanics, and Native Americans.

4. Conditions that involve swollen glands or unexpected weight loss may include metastatic malignancy, metabolic disorders, and diseases of lymphatic tissues.

Case A

1. Identify and treat existing infections, problem teeth, and tissue injury or trauma; stabilize or eliminate potential sites of infection; extract teeth that may pose a future problem; and instruct client on oral hygiene, use of fluoride gel, nutrition, and the need to avoid tobacco and alcohol.
2. Reduces the risk and severity of oral complications; improves the likelihood that the individual will tolerate optimal doses of treatment; prevents oral infection that could lead to potentially fatal systemic infections; prevents or minimizes complications that can compromise nutrition; prevents, eliminates, or controls pain; prevents or reduces the incidence of bone necrosis in radiation clients; preserves or improves oral health; and improves quality of life.
3. Encourage frequent sips of water, suggest using liquids to soften or thin foods, recommend using sugarless gum or sugar-free hard candies to help stimulate saliva, suggest using a commercial oral lubricant, consider prescribing a saliva stimulant drug, and daily fluoride therapy.
4. What is the client's complete blood count, including absolute neutrophil and platelet counts? If an invasive oral health procedure needs to be done, are there adequate clotting factors? Does the individual have a central venous catheter? What is the scheduled sequence of treatments so that safe oral health treatment can be planned?
5. Postpone treatment as client is at risk of hemorrhage and infection.
6. Research does not support the use of chlorhexidine for prevention or treatment of oral mucositis as it is not effective.

Case B

1. What have your recent blood sugar levels been? How often do you test for control of diabetes? Have you experienced hypoglycemia recently? Have you had any problems during dental treatment? When was your last appointment with your physician?
2. Hypoglycemia
3. Provide a sugar source such as candy, juice, or glucose tablet. If the client is uncooperative or loses consciousness, dial 911 and provide basic life support. Either 50% dextrose intravenously or intramuscular glucagon can be administered.
4. The best way to prevent hypoglycemia is to ensure that the client has eaten a meal after taking antidiabetic medication and observe for signs of hypoglycemia, avoid scheduling appointments around the peak effect of taking diabetes medications, and avoid lengthy appointments that extend into the client's snack or meal time.

Chapter 11: Review and Case Study Answers

Self-Study Answers and Page Numbers

1. a *page 146*
2. c *page 146*
3. d *page 147*
4. c *page 148*
5. d *page 145*
6. c *page 148*
7. c *pages 147–148*
8. a, b *page 151*
9. a *page 151*
10. d *page 152*
11. b *page 153*
12. a, b *page 153*
13. a *page 154*
14. c *page 157*
15. a, b, c, d, f *page 156*
16. b *page 159*

If you answered any items incorrectly, refer to the page number and review that information before proceeding to the next chapter.

Review Answers

1. Dyspnea: shortness of breath.
   Ischemia: lack of oxygen to a tissue.
   Orthopnea: an abnormal condition in which the person must sit or stand to breathe deeply or comfortably.
2. Directing the overhead dental light into the client's eyes may precipitate a migraine headache.
3. Cardiac conditions that do not require antibiotic prophylaxis are isolated secundum atrial septal defect, surgical repair of septal defects, previous

coronary artery bypass graft, mitral valve prolapse without regurgitation, physiologic murmurs, previous Kawasaki disease or rheumatic fever without valvular dysfunction, and cardiac pacemakers and implanted defibrillators.

4. Oral health procedures requiring antibiotic prophylaxis include procedures in which significant bleeding is anticipated, extractions, periodontal surgery, scaling and debridement, oral prophylaxis, subgingival placement of antibiotic fibers or strips, implant placement, tooth implantation, placement of orthodontic bands, endodontic surgery or instrumentation beyond apex of tooth, and intraligamentary injections.

Case A

1. MI and angina pectoris
2. Reassure client, measure and record vital signs, place nitroglycerin sublingually if systolic pressure is >100 mm Hg, provide 100% oxygen, readminister nitroglycerin up to three tablets in 10 minutes, if pain is not relieved summon 911 EMS, and record events in dental record.
3. Activate EMS and perform CPR until EMS arrives.
4. How long has it been since your heart attack? How is your health now? Can you walk up a flight of stairs without having to stop and rest? What medications are you taking?
5. Antibiotic prophylaxis is not recommended for coronary grafts. This is considered a low risk for endocarditis.

Case B

1. CVA.
2. Anticoagulant medications.
3. Visual abnormalities, confusion, inability to speak, loss of feeling on one side of the body, and unequal pupil size are all signs of a stroke.
4. If the client experiences signs of a stroke, stop the procedure, place the client in a supine position with the head elevated, activate EMS, provide basic life support, administer 100% oxygen if respiratory distress occurs, monitor vital signs, and record the emergency in the dental record.
5. Aspirin can now be part of emergency care; however, this client already took that medication. A physician consult is needed to determine if additional aspirin therapy can be provided.

Chapter 12: Review and Case Study Answers

Self-Study Answers and Page Numbers

1. b *page 164*
2. a *page 164*
3. b *page 165*
4. d *page 165*
5. d *page 167*
6. a *page 166*
7. b *page 165*
8. a *page 169*
9. b *page 169*
10. c *page 169*
11. c *page 169*
12. c *page 170*
13. a *page 172*
14. d *page 173*
15. b *page 172*
16. a *page 174*
17. c *page* 174
18. *a page 175*

If you answered any item incorrectly, refer to the page number and review that information before proceeding to the next chapter.

Review Answers

1. Seizure: a hyperexcitation of neurons in the brain leading to convulsions or abnormal behaviors.
   Absence seizures: a type of generalized seizure with a variety of symptoms in which the person is unaware of the seizure, but does not fall to the floor.
   Tonic-clonic seizure: a prolonged contraction of muscles followed by rhythmic contraction and relaxation of muscle groups.
2. The two major etiologic categories of epilepsy are idiopathic and acquired.
3. Oral healthcare practices or procedures that can precipitate a seizure include directing the overhead dental light into the client's eyes and use of the ultrasonic scaler or drill.

4. Insomnia refers to the inability to sleep during normal sleeping hours and ranges from restlessness to complete sleeplessness. Narcolepsy refers to an irresistible urge to sleep, usually at inappropriate times.

Case A

1. Generalized convulsive seizure.
2. An aura may include headache, drowsiness, yawning, and tingling sensations.
3. Prevent the client from being injured by moving the client to the floor or by moving materials out of the way; allow the client to have the seizure; place a pillow under the client's head; place the client in a position such that vomitus cannot be inhaled; and move the client to a recovery room to sleep while calling someone to transport the client home.
4. Activate 911 system and administer Valium intravenously or intramuscularly.
5. Seizures that continue for more than 5 minutes without regaining consciousness between attacks (status epilepticus); breathing difficulties after a seizure; persistent confusion or unconsciousness for more than 5 minutes; injuries sustained during a seizure; a first seizure and no history of prior seizure; and seizure during pregnancy or in a person with diabetes all require contacting EMS/911.

Case B

1. Alzheimer disease
2. If the client becomes significantly stressed, she is at risk for syncope or a cardiovascular event.
3. Use patience, understanding, and a calm approach; provide reassurance and reduce fear; call a family member or caregiver for assistance; monitor client's vital signs if concern that this stress could cause a medical emergency.

Chapter 13: Review and Case Study Answers

Self-Study Answers and Page Numbers

1. b *page 181*
2. c *page 181*
3. a, b, d, f *page 181*
4. a *page 181*
5. d *page 183*
6. d *page 183*
7. c *page 184*
8. c *page 186*
9. d *page 185*
10. b *page 186*
11. d *page 187*
12. c *page 188*

If you answered any item incorrectly, refer to the page number and review that information before proceeding to the next chapter.

Review Answers

1. GI reflux: backflow of stomach contents into the esophagus.
   Perimylolysis: erosion of enamel and dentin as a result of chemical effects.
2. Follow-up questions include "Has your medication controlled the symptoms of your condition? Can you tolerate being placed in a supine position?"
3. Oral changes associated with GI disease include erosion of teeth and increased risk of caries.
4. Oral changes associated with bulimia nervosa include perimylolysis, increased caries, restorations that appear raised or floating, xerostomia, tooth sensitivity, impaired taste sensation, and enlargement of the parotid salivary glands.
5. Wheezing can be heard as the client attempts to breathe during partial airway obstruction. In total obstruction, the airway is characterized by complete absence of sound.

Case A

1. GERD is caused by stomach contents flowing backward into the esophagus because of reduced function of the lower esophageal sphincter.
2. Symptoms of GERD include pain in the middle of the chest, burping, cramps, flatulence, and a feeling of fullness in the stomach.
3. Choking is the medical emergency most likely to occur.
4. To avoid choking during oral health care, place the client in a semiupright position for treatment, schedule the appointment at least 3 hours after a meal, and inform the client to indicate if short breaks are needed.
5. If the client experiences reflux during treatment, stop the procedure and raise the head so the client is less likely to choke, provide some water to clear the throat area, and let the client decide whether treatment should continue or be rescheduled.

Case B

1. Use of a local anesthetic with vasoconstrictor that contains a sulfite is the most likely cause of the asthma episode.

2. Seat the client in an upright position, allow her to use her bronchodilator as prescribed, and provide supplemental oxygen as needed. If treatment is successful, reappoint or reschedule the client.
3. Activate 911 and transport the client to the hospital.
4. Note that the emergency occurred, the cause if known, list of medications used by the healthcare provider, list of procedures used during the emergency, and the outcomes.
5. Determine if the client has an allergy to sulfites and use a local anesthetic without a vasoconstrictor.

Chapter 14: Review and Case Study Answers

Self-Study Answers and Page Numbers

1. a *page* 192
2. b *page 192*
3. a *page 192*
4. c *page 193*
5. a *page 196*
6. a, d, e, f, g *page 194*
7. c *page 194*
8. c *page 195*
9. b *page 199*
10. b *page 199*
11. b *page 199*
12. d *page 200*
13. d *pages* 198–199

If you answered any item incorrectly, refer to the page number and review that information before proceeding to the next chapter.

Review Answers

1. Euthyroid: normal thyroid gland function
   Glaucoma: a condition of the eye characterized by increased pressure in the eyeball.
   Hemodialysis: the removal of wastes and other undesirable substances from the blood by means of a medical device.
2. Symptoms of open-angle glaucoma are progressive loss of peripheral vision, blurred vision, difficulty adjusting to brightness and darkness, a halo surrounding a light, and mild pain. Symptoms of narrow-angle glaucoma include sudden, severe pain, and abrupt, blurred vision.
3. Activate 911 emergency medical system to transport the client to a facility where ophthalmic surgery can be performed.

Case A

1. Oral complications associated with this client may include mucosal ecchymosis, oral malodor, xerostomia, taste changes, and tongue and mucosal pain.
2. Maintenance appointments can be scheduled on alternate days (Tuesday, Thursday, Saturday) when the effects of heparin are no longer present and blood waste products have been removed.
3. The left arm should be used for taking blood pressure to avoid collapsing the arteriovenous shunt.
4. Medical consultation regarding antibiotic prophylaxis, encouragement of excellent oral hygiene habits, laboratory testing to determine the risk of hemorrhage, frequent continuing care appointments, avoidance of nephrotoxic drugs, monitoring of blood pressure, and avoidance of air-polishing devices.
5. Cardiovascular disease is the leading cause of death in ESRD.
6. Six months is the time frame from transplant to resuming dental hygiene care during which time antirejection medications are adjusted and the client is monitored for evidence of organ rejection.

Case B

1. Signs of hyperthyroidism are bulging eyes, increased body temperature, sweating, weight loss, increased basal metabolic rate, tachycardia, hyperactivity, nervousness, tremors, emotional instability, and hypertension.
2. Signs of hypothyroidism include reduced growth patterns in children; anemia; bradycardia; sluggishness; fatigue; edema in the tongue, face, neck, and hands; depression; weight gain; dry skin and hair; recurrent infections; and intolerance to cold temperature.
3. Thyroid storm could occur. Activate 911 emergency medical system, place cold towels on the client, monitor and record vital signs, and provide basic life support or cardiopulmonary resuscitation as needed.
4. Myxedema coma is the emergency associated with hypothyroidism and is characterized by bradycardia, severe hypotension, and swelling. Stressful situations such as cold, surgery, infection, and trauma are associated with this emergency.

Chapter 15: Review and Case Study Answers

Review Answers

1. The four components are comments on patient interview concerning health history; significant findings from questionnaire or oral interview; dental management considerations; and health history update, information, and signature of patient and dentist or HCP.
2. The client signature is used to verify that the client or legal guardian provided the information. The date is noted as a means to measure current reporting of information.
3. This question allows an opportunity for the client to discuss any other information that was not addressed on the health history form. The oral health clinician must then determine the significance of that information in relation to providing oral health care.
4. The analysis of health history information demonstrates that all medical conditions have been considered in a thorough manner so that comprehensive care can be provided to the client.

Case A

1. Client reports history of coronary artery disease treatment with coronary artery bypass graft surgery in 2000, recent history of MI, pacemaker placed and laser surgery to correct arrhythmia; client is post 1-month recovery period; client reports onset of concomitant facial cellulitis of undetermined etiology; treated with IV and oral antibiotics, mild swelling persists, takes multiple medications; vital signs within normal limits.
2. Plavix: avoid prescribing aspirin, caution in use with nonsteroidal anti-inflammatory drugs, monitor bleeding during treatment; consider local hemostasis measure to prevent excessive bleeding; medical consultation on bleeding time; caution to prevent trauma when using oral hygiene aids, advise client to report any unusual or prolonged bleeding episodes after dental treatment.

   Felodipine: take vital signs at each appointment because of cardiovascular disease and cardiovascular drug side effects (MI, pulmonary edema, dysrhythmia, congestive heart failure, hypotension); use stress reduction protocol to prevent stress-induced angina during appointment; have client sit more than 2 minutes to avoid orthostatic hypotension after supine positioning; place on continuing care appointment to monitor gingival overgrowth; if using local anesthesia, use vasoconstrictors in low doses and with careful aspiration; assess salivary flow and if dry mouth, use same protocol as with Norvasc.

   Metoprolol: same as felodipine; also, in clients with symptoms of blood dyscrasias, request a medical clearance for blood studies and postpone treatment until normal values are established.
3. Onset of symptoms; other oral symptoms present; other treatment provided beside antibiotic therapy; current symptoms and any other evaluations/treatment rendered for this condition.
4. Given the client's significant cardiac history, an MI is the most likely medical emergency that could occur during this appointment.
5. Prevention strategies include monitoring vital signs throughout appointment, stress reduction protocol, request medical clearance to assess for adequate functional capacity, review medications taken for drug actions and adverse effects, and observe client for signs of MI or other cardiac problems during treatment.

Case B

1. If the client has heartburn and frequent burping as a result of gastrointestinal reflux disease and gallbladder disease, evaluate her teeth for signs of enamel erosion.
2. If taking medications for seasonal allergies, the client may have xerostomia; gastrointestinal disease and gall bladder disease may predispose to enamel erosion.
3. Client may require semisupine or upright positioning depending on extent of reflux symptoms; evaluate for signs of enamel erosion related to gastrointestinal disease.
4. The client with healthy gingival tissue in whom significant bleeding is not expected would not be a candidate for antibiotic prophylaxis.
5. Given the client's vital signs, she does not appear to be at risk for myxedema coma. Continued monitoring of vital signs during the appointment and limited use of local anesthetic with epinephrine should be considered.

Index

Note: Page numbers followed by b indicate material in boxes; page numbers followed by f indicate figures; and page numbers followed by t indicate tables

B

C